I0055113

Nutrition in Critical Care–Where Are We Now?

Editors

PAUL E. WISCHMEYER
EMMA J. RIDLEY

CRITICAL CARE CLINICS

www.criticalcare.theclinics.com

Consulting Editor
GREGORY S. MARTIN

April 2025 • Volume 41 • Number 2

ELSEVIER

1600 John F. Kennedy Boulevard ● Suite 1800 ● Philadelphia, Pennsylvania, 19103-2899

http://www.theclinics.com

CRITICAL CARE CLINICS Volume 41, Number 2
April 2025 ISSN 0749-0704, ISBN-13: 978-0-443-31690-6

Editor: Joanna Gascoine
Developmental Editor: Anirban Mukherjee

© **2025 Elsevier Inc. All rights are reserved, including those for text and data mining, AI training, and similar technologies.**

This periodical and the individual contributions contained in it are protected under copyright by Elsevier, and the following terms and conditions apply to their use:

Photocopying
Single photocopies of single articles may be made for personal use as allowed by national copyright laws. Permission of the Publisher and payment of a fee is required for all other photocopying, including multiple or systematic copying, copying for advertising or promotional purposes, resale, and all forms of document delivery. Special rates are available for educational institutions that wish to make photocopies for non-profit educational classroom use. For information on how to seek permission visit www.elsevier.com/permissions or call: (+44) 1865 843830 (UK)/(+1) 215 239 3804 (USA).

Derivative Works
Subscribers may reproduce tables of contents or prepare lists of articles including abstracts for internal circulation within their institutions. Permission of the Publisher is required for resale or distribution outside the institution. Permission of the Publisher is required for all other derivative works, including compilations and translations (please consult www.elsevier.com/permissions).

Electronic Storage or Usage
Permission of the Publisher is required to store or use electronically any material contained in this periodical, including any article or part of an article (please consult www.elsevier.com/permissions). Except as outlined above, no part of this publication may be reproduced, stored in a retrieval system or transmitted in any form or by any means, electronic, mechanical, photocopying, recording or otherwise, without prior written permission of the Publisher.

Notice
No responsibility is assumed by the Publisher for any injury and/or damage to persons or property as a matter of products liability, negligence or otherwise, or from any use or operation of any methods, products, instructions or ideas contained in the material herein. Because of rapid advances in the medical sciences, in particular, independent verification of diagnoses and drug dosages should be made.

Although all advertising material is expected to conform to ethical (medical) standards, inclusion in this publication does not constitute a guarantee or endorsement of the quality or value of such product or of the claims made of it by its manufacturer.

Critical Care Clinics (ISSN: 0749-0704) is published quarterly by Elsevier Inc., 360 Park Avenue South, New York, NY 10010-1710. Months of issue are January, April, July, and October. Business and Editorial Offices: 1600 John F. Kennedy Blvd., Suite 1800, Philadelphia, PA 19103-2899. Customer Service Office: 6277 Sea Harbor Drive, Orlando, FL 32887-4800. Periodicals postage paid at New York, NY and additional mailing offices. Subscription prices are $285.00 per year for US individuals, $100.00 per year for US students and residents, $323.00 per year for Canadian individuals, $369.00 per year for international individuals, $100.00 per year for Canadian students/residents, and $150.00 per year for foreign students/residents. For institutional access pricing please contact Customer Service via the contact information below. To receive student/resident rate, orders must be accompanied by name of affiliated institution, date of term, and the signature of program/residency coordinator on institution letterhead. Orders will be billed at individual rate until proof of status is received. Foreign air speed delivery is included in all *Clinics* subscription prices. All prices are subject to change without notice. Orders, claims, and journal inquiries: Please visit our Support Hub page https://service.elsevier.com for assistance.

Reprints. For copies of 100 or more of articles in this publication, please contact the Commercial Reprints Department, Elsevier Inc., 360 Park Avenue South, New York, NY 10010-1710. Tel.: 212-633-3874; Fax: 212-633-3820; E-mail: reprints@elsevier.com.

Critical Care Clinics is also published in Spanish by Editorial Inter-Medica, Junin 917, 1er A, 1113, Buenos Aires, Argentina.

Critical Care Clinics is covered in *MEDLINE/PubMed (Index Medicus), EMBASE/Excerpta Medica, Current Concepts/Clinical Medicine, ISI/BIOMED,* and *Chemical Abstracts.*

Contributors

CONSULTING EDITOR

GREGORY S. MARTIN, MD, MSc
Professor, Division of Pulmonary, Allergy, Critical Care and Sleep Medicine, Research Director, Emory Critical Care Center, Director, Emory/Georgia Tech Predictive Health Institute, Co-Director, Atlanta Center for Microsystems Engineered Point-of-Care Technologies, President, Society of Critical Care Medicine, Atlanta, Georgia, USA

EDITORS

PAUL E. WISCHMEYER, MD, EDIC, FASPEN, FCCM
Professor with Tenure of Anesthesiology and Surgery, Division of Critical Care Medicine, Department of Anesthesiology and Surgery, Duke University School of Medicine, Durham, North Carolina, USA

EMMA J. RIDLEY, BNutriDietet, APD, MPH, PhD
Associate Professor, Faculty of Medicine, Nursing and Health Sciences, Australian and New Zealand Intensive Care Research Centre, Monash University, Melbourne, Australia

AUTHORS

ASHLEY L. ARTESE, PhD
Assistant Professor, Department of Exercise Science and Health Promotion, Florida Atlantic University, Boca Raton, Florida, USA

DANIELLE E. BEAR, PhD, MRes, BHealthSci (Nutr&Diet)
Consultant Dietitian – Critical Care, Department of Nutrition and Dietetics, St Thomas' Hospital, London, United Kingdom

METTE M. BERGER, MD, PhD
Honorary Professor, Faculty of Biology and Medicine, Lausanne University Hospital, Lausanne, Switzerland

MEGAN BEYER, MS, RD, LDN
Clinical Research Coordinator, Department of Anesthesiology, Duke University School of Medicine, Durham, North Carolina, USA

Dr GEORGIA BROWN, MBBS, MD
Cardiac ICU Consultant - Paediatric Intensive Care Unit, The Royal Children's Hospital, Melbourne; Honorary Research Fellow, Murdoch Children's Research Institute; Clinical Lecturer, Department of Critical Care, The University of Melbourne, Melbourne, VIC, Australia

ANNIKA REINTAM BLASER, MD, PhD
Associate Professor, Department of Anaesthesiology and Intensive Care, University of Tartu, Tartu, Estonia; Department of Intensive Care Medicine, Lucerne Cantonal Hospital, Lucerne, Switzerland

MARTIN B. BRODSKY, PhD, ScM
Speech-Language Pathologist, Department of Otolaryngology–Head and Neck Surgery, Cleveland Clinic, Cleveland, Ohio, USA; Department of Medicine and Rehabilitation, Pulmonary and Critical Care, Johns Hopkins University, Baltimore, Maryland, USA

NICOLA A. CLAYTON, BAppSc (Speech Pathology), MScMed, PhD
Speech-Language Pathologist, Department of Speech Pathology, Concord Repatriation General Hospital, Concord, New South Wales, Australia; Faculty of Medicine and Health, University of Sydney, Sydney, New South Wales, Australia; School of Health and Rehabilitation Sciences, University of Queensland, Brisbane, Queensland, Australia

AMY FREEMAN-SANDERSON, BAppSc (Speech Pathology), PhD
Senior Lecturer, Graduate School of Health, Faculty of Health, University of Technology Sydney, Sydney, Australia; Speech Pathology and Intensive Care Service, Royal Prince Alfred Hospital, Sydney, Australia; Division of Critical Care, The George Institute for Global Health, Faculty of Medicine, UNSW Sydney, Sydney, Australia; Australian and New Zealand Intensive Care Research Centre (ANZIC-RC), School of Public Health and Preventive Medicine, Monash University, Melbourne, Australia

DASHIELL GANTNER, MBBS, PhD
Adjunct Senior Lecturer, Australian and New Zealand Intensive Care Research Centre, School of Public Health and Preventive Medicine, Monash University; Senior Staff Specialist, Intensive Care Unit, Alfred Health, Melbourne, Australia

MARIA CRISTINA GONZALEZ, PhD, MD
Professor, Postgraduate Program in Nutrition and Food, Federal University of Pelotas, Pelotas, Rio Grande do Sul, Brazil

KRISTA L. HAINES, DO
Assistant Professor, Division of Trauma, Critical Care, and Acute Care Surgery, Department of Surgery, Duke University Medical Center, Durham, North Carolina, USA

STEPHEN A. McCLAVE, MD
Professor, Division of Gastroenterology, Hepatology, and Nutrition, Department of Medicine, University of Louisville School of Medicine, Louisville, Kentucky, USA

GEORGIA HARDY, BSc, MNutrDiet
PhD Candidate, Australian and New Zealand Intensive Care Research Centre, School of Public Health and Preventive Medicine, Monash University, Senior ICU Dietitian, Department of Nutrition and Dietetics, Alfred Health, Melbourne, Australia

RYAN T. HURT, MD, PhD
Professor, Division of General Internal Medicine, Department of Medicine, University of Louisville, Louisville, Kentucky, USA

KATE J. LAMBELL, MNutrDiet, BHSc, PhD
ICU Clinical Lead Dietitian, Department of Nutrition and Dietetics, Alfred Health, Affiliate Research Fellow, Australian and New Zealand Intensive Care Research Centre, Monash University, Melbourne, Australia

SEOHO LEE, BA
Fourth Year Medical Student, Department of Anesthesiology, Johns Hopkins University School of Medicine, Baltimore, Maryland, USA

MATTHEW J. LEES, PhD
Postdoctoral Fellow, Exercise Metabolism Research Group, Department of Kinesiology, McMaster University, Hamilton, Ontario, Canada

ANDREA P. MARSHALL, RN, PhD
Professor of Intensive Care Nursing, Intensive Care Unit, Gold Coast Health, Gold Coast University Hospital, School of Nursing and Midwifery, Griffith University, Gold Coast, Queensland, Australia

ROBERT G. MARTINDALE, MD, PhD
Professor, Department of Surgery, Oregon Health and Sciences University, Portland, Oregon, USA

CYRUS D. MINTZ, MD, PhD
Associate Professor, Department of Anesthesiology and Critical Care, Johns Hopkins University School of Medicine, Baltimore, Maryland, USA

JEROEN MOLINGER, MSc, PhDc
Senior Research Lab Analyst, Human Pharmacology and Physiology Lab, Department of Anesthesiology, Duke University Medical Center, Durham, North Carolina, USA

MANPREET MUNDI, MD
Professor, Division of Endocrinology, Diabetes, Metabolism, and Nutrition, Department of Medicine, Mayo Clinic, Rochester, Minnesota, USA

SAIRA NAZEER, Physiotherapy BSC(Hons)
Research Therapist, Critical Care and PeriOperative Medicine Research Group, The William Harvey Research Institute, Barts and the London School of Medicine and Dentistry, Queen Mary University of London, London, United Kingdom

MICHAEL T. PARIS, PhD
Assistant Professor, Faculty of Health, School of Kinesiology and Health Science, York University, Toronto, Canada

AMY M. PASTVA, PhD
Professor, Department of Orthopaedic Surgery, Director of Research, Division of Physical Therapy, Duke University School of Medicine, Senior Fellow, Center for the Study of Aging and Human Development, Duke University Medical Center, Durham, North Carolina, USA

MICHELLE CARMEN PAULUS, MD
Medical Doctor, Department of Intensive Care Medicine and Research, Gelderse Vallei Hospital, Ede, The Netherlands; PhD Candidate, Division of Human Nutrition and Health, Nutritional Biology, Wageningen University and Research, Wageningen, The Netherlands

STUART M. PHILLIPS, PhD
Professor, Exercise Metabolism Research Group, Department of Kinesiology, McMaster University, Hamilton, Ontario, Canada

CARLA M. PRADO, PhD, RD
Distinguished University Professor, Division of Human Nutrition, Department of Agricultural, Food and Nutritional Science, University of Alberta, Edmonton, Canada

ZUDIN PUTHUCHEARY, MBBS, BMedSci, DUHM, PGCME, EDICM, FRCP, FHEA, FFICM, PhD
Clinical Senior Lecturer, The William Harvey Research Institute, Barts and The London School of Medicine and Dentistry, Queen Mary University of London, Consultant in Intensive Care, Royal London Hospital, Barts Health NHS Trust, London, United Kingdom

ORIT RAPHAELI, PhD
Lecturer, Department of Industrial Engineering and Management, Ariel University, Ariel, Israel

EMMA J. RIDLEY, BNutriDietet, APD, MPH, PhD
Associate Professor, Faculty of Medicine, Nursing and Health Sciences, Australian and New Zealand Intensive Care Research Centre, Monash University, Melbourne, Australia

MARA A. SERBANESCU, MD
Assistant Professor in Anesthesiology, Critical Care Division, Duke University School of Medicine, Durham, North Carolina, USA

PIERRE SINGER, MD
Emeritus Full Professor, Department of Anesthesia and Intensive Care, Faculty for Medical and Health Sciences, Tel Aviv University, Herzlia Medical Center, General Intensive Care Department, Beilinson Hospital, Rabin Medical Center, Petah Tikva, Israel

CHRISTIAN STOPPE, MD, PhD
Professor, Department of Anaesthesiology, Intensive Care, Emergency and Pain Medicine, University Hospital, Würzburg, Würzburg, Germany; Department of Cardiac Anesthesiology and Intensive Care Medicine, Charité Berlin, Berlin, Germany

ANNA-LIISA SUTT, BA, MA, PhD
Speech-Language Pathologist, Critical Care Research Group, The Prince Charles Hospital, Institute of Molecular Bioscience, University of Queensland, Brisbane, Australia; Department of Speech and Language Therapy, The Royal London Hospital, London, United Kingdom

ANDREW A. UDY, BHB, MB ChB, PGCert(AME), FCICM, PhD
Professor, Deputy Director (Research), Department of Intensive Care and Hyperbaric Medicine, The Alfred, Professor and Deputy Director, Australian and New Zealand Intensive Care Research Centre, Monash University, Melbourne, Victoria, Australia

ARTHUR RAYMOND HUBERT VAN ZANTEN, MD, PhD
Chair, Department of Intensive Care Medicine and Research, Gelderse Vallei Hospital, Ede, The Netherlands; Division of Human Nutrition and Health, Chair Group Nutritional Biology, Wageningen University and Research, Wageningen, The Netherlands

Dr NAOMI WATSON, BMBCH, MA, PGDIP, MRCP
Academic Clinical Fellow in Anaesthesia, The William Harvey Research Institute, Barts and the London School of Medicine and Dentistry, Queen Mary University of London, London, United Kingdom

Ms JACINTA WINDERLICH, BNutDietet, MCLinRes
PhD candidate, Australian and New Zealand Intensive Care Research Centre, Monash University; Paediatric Clinical Specialist Dietitian, Nutrition and Dietetics, and Paediatric Intensive Care Unit, Monash Children's Hospital, Melbourne, VIC, Australia

HILARY M. WINTHROP, MS, RD, LDN, CNSC
Registered Dietitian, Duke Office of Clinical Research, Duke University School of
Medicine, Durham, North Carolina, USA

PAUL E. WISCHMEYER, MD, EDIC, FASPEN, FCCM
Professor with Tenure of Anesthesiology and Surgery, Division of Critical Care Medicine,
Department of Anesthesiology and Surgery, Duke University School of Medicine, Durham,
North Carolina, USA

CHARISSA J. ZAGA, BSpPath, MPH, PhD
Speech-Language Pathologist, Department of Speech Pathology, Austin Health,
Heidelberg, Victoria, Australia; Implementation Science Unit, Institute for Breathing and
Sleep, Austin Health, Department of Critical Care, University of Melbourne, Department of
Audiology and Speech Pathology, University of Melbourne, Victoria, Australia

Contents

to mitigate muscle loss are early mobilization and adequate nutrient supply, especially protein, using an individualized approach to support skeletal muscle maintenance and recovery.

During critical illness and while recovering, patients may experience varied nutrition interventions, nutrition-impacting symptoms, and challenges relating to the systems of hospital food services. All of these factors can directly impact their experiences and nutrition intake. External factors that may indirectly influence the patient experience of nutrition include family involvement, clinician knowledge and communication, and the hospital environment. The experience of patients during hospitalization may affect behavior and ability to comply with nutrition-related recommendations. However, understanding and including these experiences may help to improve clinical practice, hospital food service systems, and research design.

During the past decade, there has been an increased research focus on the prevalence, nature, and impact of newly acquired critical illness dysphagia. Disordered function can impact the safety and efficiency across all stages of the swallow mechanism, with detrimental impacts on patients' body systems, function, and participation. Accurate assessment of swallow function is key to informed diagnosis and enhances intervention planning. We discuss the current evidence base around dysphagia pathophysiology with a detailed discussion considering the modes of ventilation commonly received in intensive care units. Assessment and management across critical illness are evaluated and future research efforts are presented.

In this review, we outline key practical components of the nutritional management of critically-ill children in the context of the current peer reviewed literature and identify vital knowledge gaps for further investigation. Emerging areas of research are discussed, including skeletal muscle ultrasonography for measurement of skeletal muscle, and the potential future role of pre- and probiotics.

Selecting appropriate outcome measures is a critical component of clinical trial design. Core outcome sets, which utilize stakeholder input to define the most important outcomes for a particular research question, are

CRITICAL CARE CLINICS

SERIES OF RELATED INTEREST

Emergency Medicine Clinics
https://www.emed.theclinics.com/
Clinics in Chest Medicine
https://www.chestmed.theclinics.com/

THE CLINICS ARE AVAILABLE ONLINE!
Access your subscription at:
www.theclinics.com

Preface

Nutrition in Critical Care—Where Are We Now?

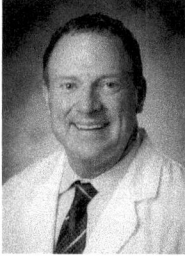

Paul E. Wischmeyer, MD, EDIC, FASPEN, FCCM   Emma J. Ridley, BNutriDietet, APD, MPH, PhD

Editors

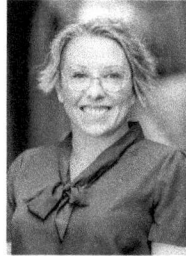

It has been 14 years since an issue of *Critical Care Clinics* has focused on nutrition in critical care. Since then, an explosion of research in the field has informed the field with high-quality data, which has significantly advanced critical care nutrition practice. However, it has also led to controversies and confusion for clinicians at the bedside who are trying to apply this evidence and ensure they provide the best patient care. In this issue, we provide you with an update of "where are we now" for critical care nutrition internationally. Importantly, it covers the most controversial topics currently, providing a guide to clinicians with the hard bedside decisions we are faced with every day. Furthermore, the issue is multidisciplinary, including experts in medicine, dietetics, speech pathology, and nursing.

This issue focuses on a wide breadth of contemporary topics related to nutrition and includes both adult and pediatric critical illness. The issue begins with an overview of how clinical nutrition has changed over the past 75 years by eminent Professors McClave and Martindale, who have shaped the field of critical care nutrition over many years with their knowledge, research, and guidance of new clinicians. Following this, challenging topics with a wealth of recent data, including optimizing early feeding, protein dose and timing in the ICU, and why a "one-size-fits-all" approach will not work for ICU nutrition are covered in detail. Timely pieces cover the latest evidence for personalizing ICU rehabilitation and its interaction with nutrition, body composition measurement, and the role of skeletal muscle in ICU recovery. Two unique articles cover the patient experience of nutrition during and after ICU and the impact of dysphagia. Finally, key topics, such as pediatric critical care nutrition, and which outcomes are best for ICU nutrition trial, are addressed, as are novel concepts such as the role of the microbiome in critical illness.

Crit Care Clin 41 (2025) xv–xvii
https://doi.org/10.1016/j.ccc.2024.11.004
0749-0704/25/© 2024 Published by Elsevier Inc.

criticalcare.theclinics.com

While it is impossible to predict the future, the next decade will be one of much research and activity in critical care nutrition. While advances have been made, there remain more questions than answers, with aspects of care we once felt as beneficial needing to be adapted to reflect the latest data (such as new recommendations to "ramp-up" calories and protein vs early full provision of energy and protein); these aspects and the timing of nutrition to be of greatest benefit are key questions for continued investigation. Applying nutrition in a personalized manner (ie, via use of indirect calorimetry and CPET testing for guiding rehabilitation exercise), not in a one-size-fits-all approach, is also paramount to our understanding. Although these new advances are often not easy to implement in practice, this should now be the goal for best care in ICUs worldwide, as we hope the lower cost of these technologies makes them more accessible. Further research is also urgently needed to find optimal methods to incorporate nutrition, rehabilitation, and potentially anabolic nutrients/anabolic agents to best combat the epidemic of post-ICU syndrome–related physical and cognitive disability. Finally, understanding the ideal, patient-preferred outcomes for research and the patient experience of nutrition during and following critical care is also key.

It is an exciting time for the field, and we hope you enjoy reading this specially curated list of topics, written by global experts in critical illness nutrition therapy.

DISCLOSURES

Dr E.J. Ridley has received honorarium from Baxter Healthcare (United States and "Australia), and Nestle and Nutricia" (Australia) and is supported by a National Health and Medical Research Council (NHMRC) Emerging Leadership Fellowship. Dr P.E. Wischmeyer reports receiving investigator-initiated grant funding from National Institutes of Health, Department of Defense, Abbott Nutrition, Baxter, and Fresenius, has served as a consultant to Abbott Nutrition, Fresenius, Baxter, Mend Inc, and Nutricia, has received unrestricted gift donations for nutrition research from Musclesound and

DSM, and has received honoraria or travel expenses for CME lectures from Abbott Nutrition, Baxter, Danone-Nutricia, Mend, and Nestlé.

Paul E. Wischmeyer, MD, EDIC, FASPEN, FCCM
Department of Anesthesiology
Duke University Hospital
Duke Clinical Nutrition Fellowship
Duke University School of Medicine
DUMC, Box 3094 Mail # 41
2301 Erwin Road, 5692 HAFS
Durham, NC 27710, USA

Emma J. Ridley, BNutriDietet, APD, MPH, PhD
Australian and New Zealand
Intensive Care Society Research Centre
School of Public Health and Preventive Medicine
Monash University

Department of Dietetics and Nutrition
Alfred Health
Level 3, 553 St Kilda Road
Melbourne, Victoria 3004, Australia

E-mail addresses:
Paul.Wischmeyer@Duke.edu (P.E. Wischmeyer)
emma.ridley@monash.edu (E.J. Ridley)

The History of Critical Care Nutrition

Seventy-Five Years of Evolution

Robert G. Martindale, MD, PhD[a],*, Ryan T. Hurt, MD, PhD[b],
Manpreet Mundi, MD[c], Stephen A. McClave, MD[d]

KEYWORDS

- Critical care • Nutritional therapy • Enteral nutrition • Parenteral nutrition
- Nutritional risk

KEY POINTS

- Early critical care nutrition tried a one-size-fits-all approach and overfeeding was common.
- Parenteral nutrition (PN) early in its use was the mainstay of intensive care unit (ICU) nutrition. Now PN is used for focused need in specific populations, reporting much more consistent benefits.
- Macronutrients remain the mainstay of critical care nutrition, with evidence now to support appropriate levels of protein, carbohydrates, and lipids.
- The concepts of disease-specific or organ-specific nutrient solutions in the ICU have come and mostly gone, with only immunonutrition in the surgical population showing consistent favorable studies to support use.
- The most recent critical care nutrition "evolution" has been the wide-spread use of societal guidelines and protocols globally.

INTRODUCTION

Beginning in the period following World War II, the specialty of critical care medicine began to emerge as greater understanding of the complexity of critical illness necessitated designation of specialized units within the hospital system staffed by highly trained health care professionals. As innovations evolved in areas such as ventilatory support, renal dialysis, wound management, and sepsis control, the need for more

[a] Department of Surgery, Oregon Health and Sciences University, Portland, OR, USA; [b] Division of General Internal Medicine, Department of Medicine, University of Louisville, KY, USA; [c] Division of Endocrinology, Diabetes, Metabolism, and Nutrition, Department of Medicine, Mayo Clinic, Rochester, MN, USA; [d] Division of Gastroenterology, Hepatology, and Nutrition, Department of Medicine, University of Louisville School of Medicine, Louisville, KY, USA
* Corresponding author. Department of Surgery, Oregon Health Sciences University, Portland, OR.
E-mail address: martindr@ohsu.edu

Crit Care Clin 41 (2025) 199–211
https://doi.org/10.1016/j.ccc.2024.09.001
0749-0704/25/© 2024 Elsevier Inc. All rights reserved, including those for text and data mining, AI training, and similar technologies.
criticalcare.theclinics.com

comprehensive nutritional therapy became apparent. Over the decades that followed, advances in enteral and parenteral access devices, formulations, and strategies to provide early aggressive nutritional therapy developed to meet that need. The adoption of evidence-based medicine and the publication of prospective randomized controlled trials helped fine-tune issues of management involving the timing, content, route, safety, and tolerance of the nutrition regimens, leading to the modern era of critical care nutrition. This study reviews these advances over the past several decades, showing how a greater understanding of the pathophysiology of critical illness, the stress response, and fuel utilization led to more effective nutritional therapy, documenting its role in improving outcomes in the intensive care unit (ICU).

EMERGENCE OF THE SPECIALTY OF CRITICAL CARE AND STRATEGIES TO PROVIDE NUTRITIONAL THERAPY

The concept of specialized ICUs began to take shape in the early 1950s in Copenhagen, Denmark, during one of the last polio epidemics, where patients with failing pulmonary function were placed in specific sections of the hospital allowing for more focused care.[1] Following this conceptional introduction from the Copenhagen reports, the practice of concentrating care for the severely ill was adopted by a Los Angeles, California group led by Max Harry Weil. Under his leadership, the group formed specialized units with positive pressure ventilation and provided a multidisciplinary team consisting of physicians, nurses, dieticians, pharmacists, respiratory therapists, occupational therapists, and physical therapists. With these specialized ICU teams, the mortality of the patients treated in the ICU plummeted from 80% to 40% over 2 decades.[1]

Early efforts to provide enteral nutrition (EN), although reported by Osler in 1874, involved feeding patients with rubber tubes. The concept of specialized nutrition therapy via feeding tubes into the gastrointestinal (GI) tract was rudimentary, and the early tubes used were rigid and uncomfortable for the patients. The 1960s saw improvements in the design and use of more patient-friendly, flexible, and softer feeding tubes. In addition, refinements in blenderized commercial formulae became more available. The 1960s also brought an increased focus on the safety and efficacy of enteral feeding with the growing contribution from commercial formulae and delivery pump system technology.

Simultaneous with the refinements in enteral feeding came the ability to access the central circulation for high-volume resuscitation. These techniques were developed in the Korean War and were brought back to the University of Pennsylvania by Jonathan Rhoads. This application allowed Stanley Dudrick, a surgical resident training under Dr Rhoads, to apply this technique to deliver hyperosmolar intravenous (IV) nutritional formulations.[2] The development of long-term total parenteral nutrition (TPN) delivered by a central venous catheter, published by Dudrick in 1968, is credited with launching the modern era of clinical nutrition and specialized ICU nutrition support.[3] Parenteral nutrition (PN) now allowed for lifesaving nutrient delivery for various patients who would have otherwise died from GI failure, triggering the rapid growth of nutrition support teams and the widespread use of TPN in hospitalized patients by the early and mid-1970s.[2] By the late 1960s, the first comprehensive TPN solutions including amino acids, glucose, vitamins, lipids, and minerals were developed and rapidly adopted for use in well-established ICUs.

These initial PN formulations started with a protein source derived from protein hydroxylates, with crystalline amino acids not becoming available until the 1970s. Although protein hydrozylates were sufficiently tolerated, a significant number of contaminates were often included in the solution. Conversion to crystalline amino acids reduced contamination significantly, however, resulted in micronutrient deficiencies as demonstrated by a variety of reported cases of copper, zinc, selenium, and other trace mineral deficiencies. These micronutrient and trace mineral deficiencies were not observed with protein hydrozylates a finding that led to the need for trace mineral PN supplementation.

Lipid emulsions utilizing cottonseed oil as the lipid source were initially approved by the Federal Drug Administration in the mid-1950s but then rapidly removed from the market after significant pulmonary complications were reported, raising concern for fat emboli.[4] The development of a soy-based formula by Arvid Wretlind, which became available outside of the United States in 1961, enabled the delivery of safe intravenous lipid emulsions (IVLEs) that subsequently proved to be consistently effective for patient use.[5] In addition to innovation in macronutrients and micronutrients, the next 2 decades from the 1960s to 1980s also saw a series of innovations and developments in IV access catheter made based on landmark work by Scribner, Broviac, Hickman, and Groshong. These innovations have led to the majority of catheters used today.[6,7]

ERA OF HYPERALIMENTATION

Once parenteral access and delivery of IV calories became feasible, the concept of "hyperalimentation" emerged as the leading strategy for critical care nutrition.[8] A common belief at this time was that "if more calories can be delivered, the hyperdynamic response to critical illness could be reversed." The 1970s were marked by the widespread adoption of the hyperalimentation concept into clinical practice. Consequently, the early days of feeding in the ICU were associated with significant overfeeding and related complications such as hyperglycemia and the development of PN-associated liver disease.[9] By the end of the 1970s, guidelines and protocols for the administration of PN were developed, focusing on the prevention of complications such as infection and metabolic disturbances.[10]

CONCEPT OF EARLY ENTERAL FEEDING

The 1980s brought a paradigm shift driven by the change from parenteral-based ICU nutrition to enteral based. The concept of "early enteral feeding" for patients in ICU began to gain traction in the late 1970s and early 1980s. Pioneering work by Eugene and Frederick Moore led to the publication of several prospective randomized trials reporting fewer ICU infections and complications with EN when compared to PN.[11,12] Initially, increased rate of infections was blamed on the need for central line access required when providing PN leading many clinicians to not push enteral feeding. This changed with clinical trial by Ken Kudsk in patients with trauma, again comparing EN with PN. In addition to the reduction in infection risk, Kudsk's study showed EN had benefits in maintaining gut integrity, modulating immune responses, and reducing inflammatory responses.[13] The impact of this study in changing practice was attributed to the fact that all patients enrolled had both central lines and feeding jejunostomies, conclusively sealing the concept that enteral was superior to parenteral feeding in reducing ICU infections.[13] These studies were key for emphasizing the importance of initiating nutritional support soon after ICU admission. Early meta-analyses demonstrated EN to be superior to PN in improving clinical outcomes.[14] The practice of initiating EN within the first 24 to 48 hours of ICU admission was shown to be associated with reduced infection rates, shorter hospital stays, and decreased mortality.[15] This approach, although somewhat modified by changes in quantity and timing over the past 3 decades, remains a cornerstone of critical care nutrition today.

The 1990s emphasized evidence-based practices in ICU nutritional support. A key concept explored during this period was the timing of delivery of nutrients into the GI tract. Numerous protocols and trials reported benefits of receiving nutrition into the GI tract within 24 hours of admission to the ICU.[15] McDonald reported that immediate enteral feeding in patients with burn, defined as being delivered within 6 hours of injury, was safe and effective.[16] This study involved patients with burns over greater than 20% of total body surface area and showed no increase in problems of intolerance to the prescribed regimen. The study was interpreted to suggest that very early feeding was important for supporting patient tolerance and improving clinical outcomes.[16]

ADVANCES IN ENTERAL ACCESS AND DEVELOPMENT OF SPECIALIZED FORMULATIONS

Another paradigm shift in nutrition support occurred with the introduction of percutaneous endoscopic gastrostomy tubes by Dr Michael WL Gauderer and Dr Jeffery Ponsky, which provided a less invasive method for long-term enteral feeding, although these were not commonly placed early on following admission to the ICU.[17] Although relatively short-lived, another innovation in enteral access occurred in the late 1970s with the introduction of the needle catheter jejunostomy, 5 and 7 FR tubes primarily placed at the time of surgery for use with an elemental formula of very low viscosity.[18] The "Vivonex" formula containing crystalline amino acids, simple carbohydrates, and a small amount of lipid was originally developed for the space program but was felt by many clinicians to be the ideal formula for an patient in ICU presumed to have reduced absorptive and digestive capabilities.[15] When well-controlled trials could not show benefit of this formula over standard formulations, widespread use of elemental formulations began to wane.[15] Similarly the needle catheter jejunostomy went out of favor due to problems with clogging and the fact that elemental formulas were no longer being utilized.[15]

Commercially prepared enteral feeding formulas soon became widely available, providing balanced and nutrient-rich options tailored to specific patient needs. The concept of disease-specific formulas began with the introduction of a specialized formula for patients with renal failure. The rationale for such a formula was derived from the presumption that reducing the total content of protein and increasing the percentage amount of essential amino acids (or just the alpha-keto amino acid backbone of essential amino acids) would help minimize the buildup of nitrogenous waste products, by recycling nitrogen through transamination to make nonessential amino acids.[15] In actuality, less than 1% of the nitrogen could be recycled through these pathways, a finding that coupled with the advent of dialysis being readily available rendered these formulas to have limited value. The renal formulae today are used primarily for their electrolyte profile, with reduced potassium and phosphorus concentrations.[15,19]

Also in this relative time frame, hepatic formulas were introduced, available in both enteral and parenteral options, designed for the patients with decompensated cirrhosis. These formulas were initially low in protein and were fortified with branch chain amino acids, designed to compete with aromatic amino acids crossing the blood–brain barrier, as a strategy to manage portosystemic encephalopathy (PSE).[20] Again in actual practice, use of these formulas had little impact on symptoms in the hospitalized patient with cirrhosis (shown only in randomized trials to reduce readmission rates for outpatients with cirrhosis and mild PSE).[19,20] Ironically, both groups of patients (renal and hepatic failure) tended to require normal amounts of protein, with renal patients on dialysis requiring even greater doses, contradicting the original design of these formulas.[20]

The period of the 1980s also saw the introduction of specifically designed pulmonary formulas for respiratory failure, which was immediately extrapolated to the ICU for use in patients on ventilators to minimize CO_2 production.[21] These formulas were made with a higher lipid/lower carbohydrate content, based on the knowledge that the oxidative metabolism of fatty acids yields a respiratory quotient (ratio of CO_2 produced/O_2 consumed) of 0.7, while that for carbohydrate was 1.0 (indicating less CO_2 production from the metabolism of fat).[21] Subsequently, numerous studies showed that the ratio of fat/carbohydrate in a formula only influenced CO_2 production when patients were overfed by an amount of calories exceeding requirements. The irony of their design that the excess fat (which was nearly double the normal content in other formulas) was comprised pro-inflammatory potentially immunosuppressive omega-6 fatty acids eventually led to their waning use in the ICU. Similar to these organ failure formulations, diabetic formulas designed with alternative carbohydrate sources were found to have limited or no benefit for the population in ICU.[15]

The potential for metabolic and immune modulation with specific enteral formulations leads to the derivation of the concept of immunonutrition. Introduced in 1989, these immune-enhancing formulas were conclusively shown to benefit the surgical population by showing favorable modulation of the inflammatory response to surgery, traumatic injury, and infection, thereby improving clinical outcomes.[22,23] The nutritional components of these formulations that showed the most consistent data included arginine, omega-3 fatty acids (eicosapentanoic acid [EPA] and docosahexaenoic acid [DHA]), and nucleotides.[22,23] Glutamine was another frequently utilized amino acid given as a pharmaconutrient for the population in ICU in this decade, as it was shown to support the mucosal barrier function by being the primary fuel for enterocytes in addition to numerous other metabolic benefits.[24] Glutamine remained as a supplemental mainstay in the surgical ICU until 2013, when a major prospective randomized trial reported increased mortality from use of glutamine in patients with organ failure, primarily hepatic, and renal.[25] After that trial, glutamine found little use in the ICU. Inconsistent results in medical ICU clinical trials suggest that the mechanisms by which immune-modulating formulations activate immune function and accelerate wound healing processes are somewhat selective and depend on several factors including metabolic state, genetics, dose of specific nutrient and/or timing of delivery.[19,26] Although use of immunonutrition in medical patients in ICU is now more limited, robust data demonstrate benefits including reduced infections and shorter length of ICU stay for wide variety of surgical patients undergoing major surgery who require admission to a surgical ICU.[26]

ESTABLISHING MONITORS FOR TOLERANCE OF THE NUTRITION REGIMEN

Tolerance became a major issue in ICU enteral support and a significant amount of literature was directed at reducing risk of aspiration and subsequent pneumonia. Factors shown to significantly reduce risk of aspiration included post-pyloric feeding, the use of prokinetic agents, and elevation of the head of bed.[27] A poorly documented concept that appeared early in the nursing literature involved measurement of gastric residual volumes (GRVs) to monitor tolerance, gastric emptying, and risk of aspiration, its interpretation leading to the practice that GRVs greater than 150 cc should direct cessation of gastric feeding.[28] Subsequent studies showed that GRVs correlated poorly with gastric emptying, actual aspiration, and pneumonia.[29] In international trials, Montejo showed that raising the GRV to 500 cc (vs 200 cc) had similar outcomes but nearly doubled the volume of EN infused, while Reignier showed that avoiding use of GRVs altogether (vs continued practice) again had similar outcomes with a much greater volume of feeding delivered.[30] The hypothesis that bolus feeding might be better tolerated then continuous infusion and possibly offer a metabolic advantage in protein dynamics was tested in several RCTs without firm consistent data supporting the benefit of one over the either.[31,32]

IMPROVEMENTS IN THE PROVISION OF PARENTERAL NUTRITION

Innovations in PN during this time included the development of multichamber bags, allowing for convenient mixing without the need for a compounding pharmacy. Most hospital pharmacies at major medical centers still do compounding, due to the versatility of PN needed for their more complex patients. Smaller hospitals and other regions globally are more likely to utilize the convenient ready-mix to use, all-in-one commercial PN bags for their more routine, less complex patients.[33] The multichamber bags were initially marketed with the belief that they reduce the risk of contamination and waste, but such concepts could not be confirmed in large trials.[34,35] The 1990s also saw the PN research focused on optimizing the composition of PN solutions to better meet the metabolic demands of critically ill patients. Combining data from indirect calorimetry and PN to specifically manage metabolic needs have not caught on globally and appear to offer little benefit in outcome data.[19]

Advances in PN during this decade primarily revolved around technology, which included the use of computerized systems to individualize and optimize nutrient delivery. The continued focus on reducing catheter-related bloodstream infections led to the implementation of stricter aseptic techniques and the use of antimicrobial-impregnated catheters.[36]

PUBLICATION OF GUIDELINES AND PROTOCOLS FOR DELIVERY

In the decade beginning in the year 2000, clinicians began integrating ICU nutrition protocols into practice, derived from national and international critical care nutrition guidelines. As EN became recognized as the preferred, more optimal route of delivery of nutrients in the ICU, protocols were published with the emphasis on getting to goal feeding (meeting 100% of protein/calorie requirements) within 24 hours.[37] The concept of reducing the caloric deficit (determined daily by subtracting calories infused from calories expended) in the early days of the ICU stay became a primary focus, as retrospective studies showed that large caloric deficits greater than 4000 to 10,000 kcal were associated with worsened outcomes.[38] Protocols such as PEP-UP and volume-based feeding were developed for those periods where enteral feeding was held; directing nurses once feeding was resumed to accelerate the rate of infusion to make up for lost nutrient delivery.[39,40] While such protocols were primarily popular in North America, Europe addressed the deficit by adding supplemental PN to the EN being infused.[41]

Additional protocols were developed during this period to differentiate the concept of nutrition risk from that of malnutrition. Scoring systems such as the NUTRIC score (nutrition risk in the critically ill) and NRS 2002 (nutrition risk score) helped to show that nutritional risk is determined by both baseline nutritional status and degree of disease severity, differentiating it from malnutrition, which is determined primarily by anthropometric indices of a patient's current nutritional status alone.[15,42]

PERSONALIZED NUTRITION AND REDEFINING GOALS OF NUTRITION THERAPY

The decade beginning in 2010 saw a shift toward "personalized nutrition," with individualized feeding plans based on patient-specific needs and conditions. Design of the nutrition regimen was driven by patient metabolism, energy expenditure, and individual tolerances, with EN or PN (or both in combination) being used interchangeably after newer studies reported equivalence in outcomes between the 2 routes of feeding populations in ICU.[43,44] The concept of personalized nutrition dictated that precise measurements of caloric expenditure by indirect calorimetry and protein requirements by nitrogen balance studies (or by equations derived from bioelectric impedance) be made daily, and that exact requirements need to be met by the nutrition therapeutic regimen. Such practice was supported by data from 2 out of 3 meta-analyses showing a reduction in mortality from the use of indirect calorimetry (compared to the use of weight-based predictive equations alone).[45–47]

Other studies refuted this practice, such as the EAT-ICU trial (early goal-directed nutrition in ICU patients) showing that nutrition therapy based on precise measurements had similar outcomes to therapy directed by weight-based predictive equations.[48] Furthermore, meeting exact requirements invariably necessitated the addition of supplemental PN.[48] Early in this decade, Greet van de Berge published a classic paper from the EPaNIC trial, where patients on EN were randomized to either early (at 3 days) or late (at 8 days) supplemental PN.[49] Those patients receiving early supplemental PN had significantly higher complication rates and slower recovery.[49] Eventually, out of a total of 7 randomized trials comparing full feeds (EN plus supplemental PN) versus EN alone, only one study by Gao showed significant positive outcome benefits from the combination full feeds.[50]

More physiologic, better balanced PN became available during this period. Pure soy-based IVLEs were rapidly being replaced after Food and Drug Administration approval in 2016 of a more physiologic IVLE containing soy oil, medium chain triglycerides, olive oil and fish oil.[51] These mixed lipid IVLEs were available over most of the globe earlier than their introduction into the United States and already had an excellent safety profile.[52]

Ironically during the same decade that saw the emergence of personalized nutrition, different studies were beginning to show that pushing an aggressive nutrition regimen to attain 100% of goal energy and protein needs (to meet requirements) might not be in the best interest of the patient.[53] Todd Rice in a landmark study comparing trophic feeds at 25% of goal to full goal feeds in medical patients in ICU reported equivalent outcomes between the 2 groups.[53] Soon after, additional trials by Arabi, Charles, and others reported similar findings.[54] Similarly, aggressive regimens pushing protein delivery to meet or exceed requirements was thought to benefit patients in the ICU by overcoming anabolic resistance. Subsequent studies failed to show a benefit from this strategy (EFFORT trial - Effect of Higher Portein Dosing in Critically Ill Patients), and such high doses of protein, particularly in patients on steroids or in renal failure, could cause an increase in the urea/creatinine ratio creating an environment that was actually toxic to skeletal muscle.[55]

FOCUS ON THE INTESTINAL MICROBIOME AND OBJECTIVE MEASURES OF ENTERAL NUTRITION TOLERANCE

In the decade beginning in 2010, the focus of nutrition therapy again shifted toward possible methods by which to control the intestinal microbiome in order to maintain a stable population of commensal bacteria and prevent the conversion to a virulent pathobiome.[56] John Alverdy published trials that clearly delineated the rapid and detrimental changes that take place in the patient microbiome upon admission to an ICU, where greater than 90% of the commensal organisms disappear and diversity is greatly diminished from greater than 5 major phyla to just 1 or 2 remaining.[57] The complexity of this process is great and current understanding is poor, such that attempts to favorably manipulate the microbiome for patients in the ICU have shown mixed results.[57] A strategy that shows some promise includes influencing the "cues" released by the host to the microbiome that impact refaunation of the commensal organisms following insult or injury, such as limiting use of opioids and antibiotics, maintaining gut perfusion, and providing fermentable carbohydrate-soluble fiber substrates yielding butyrate and other beneficial short chain fatty acids.[57] Maintaining microbial diversity in the patient in ICU is a start, but defining the ideal community of intestinal microbes for a patient in the ICU remains elusive.

Also during this decade, sustained efforts were made to establish objective measures or monitors of tolerance of enteral feeding.[58] While specific definitions of intolerance or intestinal failure have been difficult to determine, studies have focused on a combination of findings involving symptoms (nausea, vomiting, abdominal pain, diarrhea, cessation of passing gas, or stool) and physical findings (hypoactive bowel sounds, abdominal distention, GI bleeding, intra-abdominal hypertension).[58] Scoring systems comprised components of these signs and symptoms have been linked to adverse outcomes (including mortality), suggesting a correlation that the greater the disease severity of the patient, the more likely that intolerance to enteral feeding will be seen. Unfortunately, these signs and symptoms do not represent a continuous spectrum of increasing intestinal failure. The occurrence of intra-abdominal hypertension has nearly been eliminated through the adoption of goal-directed volume resuscitation. Diarrhea has its own differential independent of tolerance, being most commonly related in the ICU to pharmacologic agents (sorbitol mixing agent, cathartic drugs initiated as a bowel prep) or infection (*Clostridioides difficile*). In the absence of risk factors for ischemic bowel, GI bleeding in the ICU occurs most commonly from stress gastritis, a condition that represents an indication for continued delivery of EN, not a sign of intolerance that should lead to cessation.

EVOLVING EVIDENCE TO SUPPORT A "LESS IS MORE" STRATEGY

In the decade beginning in 2020, the previous trend of providing early trophic enteral feeding during the acute phases of critical illness gained further support from international studies. In 2 large studies from France, the NUTRIREA-2 and NUTRIREA-3 trials, Reignier showed that patients with sepsis on pressor support and mechanical ventilation given aggressive full dose enteral feeding within 2 days of being admitted to the ICU (vs PN or low-dose trophic EN) resulted in a significant increase in bowel ischemia.[44,59] Most importantly in the NUTRIREA-3 trial, low-dose trophic EN (at 25% of calorie and protein requirements) significantly reduced time to discharge alive, duration of mechanical ventilation, ICU length of stay, and GI complications compared to full feeding.[59] The rationale for the benefit of trophic feedings in critical illness relates to minimizing the chance for overfeeding (when nutrients infused enterally are added to circulating glucose from hepatic gluconeogenesis), reducing risk of ischemic bowel and refeeding syndrome, decreasing demand on dysfunctional mitochondria, supporting autophagy, and promoting tolerance to the EN.[60,61]

Review of these trials suggests that the benefit of early enteral feeding for improving clinical outcomes in the ICU represents a bell-shaped curve based on disease severity.[62] Nutritional therapy is less likely to change outcome in patients with mild-to-moderate disease severity and in those patients who may be preterminal with the greatest severity of critical illness. In between there may be a "sweet spot" where patients are moderately severely ill and appropriate nutritional therapy is most likely to favorably alter outcomes. This concept is supported by the Merker study (a post hoc analysis of the EFFORT trial) that showed that a step-wise protocol in nutritional support compared to hospital food reduced mortality in patients with mild-to-moderate inflammation, but not in patients with the highest level of inflammation.[63] In contrast, for patients with a markedly severe degree of critically illness, the likelihood of causing harm from early enteral feeding represents a U-shaped curve based on the volume of feeding delivered (as a percentage of requirements).[62] If no EN is provided, harm to the patient in ICU may be increased due to loss of gut barrier defense, dysbiosis, and emergence of a pathobiome. Over a span of feeding from 20% to 50% of requirements, the curve may be flat with little change in harm. But as the volume of feeding delivered increases toward 70% to 80% of requirements or more, the chance of harm may increase significantly for a group of patients who already have the least likelihood for improvement in outcomes from the nutrition regimen.[62] This latter concept is supported by the Eden-Omega, PERMIT, and NUTRIREA-3 trials.

SUMMARY

The history of critical care nutrition is marked by continuous advancements with occasional setbacks, but the growing understanding of the important role that nutrition plays in patient in ICU outcomes is apparent. From the rudimentary methods of the 1950s to the sophisticated and personalized approaches of the 2020s, the field has evolved significantly, driven by innovation, research, and a commitment to improving the care of critically ill patients. These contributions discussed earlier have collectively advanced the field of critical care nutrition, improving the management and outcomes of critically ill patients. The integration of digital health technologies, including electronic health records, decision support systems, and now artificial intelligence, will continue to help streamline the management of PN and EN. Ongoing research focuses on the use of novel lipid formulations and the impact of micronutrient supplementation on patient outcomes. The development of personalized PN solutions based on genetic and metabolic profiles represents an exciting frontier for the future of critical care nutrition. Additional research continues to focus on optimizing the timing, composition, and delivery methods of nutrition support to enhance recovery and outcomes for critically ill patients.

CLINICS CARE POINTS

- Selecting the correct level of caloric delivery must be based on the patient's disease severity, phase of critical illness, and ability to utilize the delivered energy.

- Patient physiology and response to catabolic/metabolic insults can be beneficially or detrimentally altered by type and dose of specific nutrients (eg, the type and quantity of lipids).

- The benefit of early enteral feeding for improving clinical outcomes in the ICU represents a bell-shaped curve based on disease severity, with the greatest benefit seen in patients with moderately severe (but not preterminal) critical illness.

- If no EN is provided, detrimental outcomes to the patient in ICU may be increased due to loss of gut barrier defense, immune dysregulation, and dysbiosis with emergence of a pathobiome. On the other hand, delivery of excess EN becomes detrimental to the host by increasing intolerance, risk for gut ischemia, and duration of ICU length of stay.

DISCLOSURE

No funders of this manuscript and none of authors have research in this area of the article. No disclosures for this manuscript by any of authors.

REFERENCES

1. Kelly FE, Fong K, Hirsch N, et al. Intensive care medicine is 60 years old: the history and future of the intensive care unit. Clin Med (Lond) 2014;14(4):376–9.
2. Dudrick SJ, Palesty JA. Historical highlights of the development of total parenteral nutrition. Historical article. Surg Clin 2011;91(3):693–717.
3. Dudrick SJ, Wilmore DW, Vars HM, et al. Long-term total parenteral nutrition with growth, development, and positive nitrogen balance. Surgery 1968;64(1):134–42.
4. Mirtallo JM, Ayers P, Boullata J, et al. ASPEN lipid injectable emulsion safety recommendations, part 1: background and adult considerations. Nutr Clin Pract 2020;35(5):769–82.
5. Driscoll DF. Pharmaceutical and clinical aspects of lipid injectable emulsions. JPEN J Parenter Enter Nutr 2017;41(1):125–34.
6. Hurt RT, Steiger E. Early history of home parenteral nutrition: from hospital to home. Nutr Clin Pract 2018;33(5):598–613.
7. Gow KW, Tapper D, Hickman RO. Between the lines: the 50th anniversary of long-term central venous catheters. Am J Surg 2017;213(5):837–48.
8. Copeland EM, MacFadyen BV Jr, MacComb WS, et al. Intravenous hyperalimentation in patients with head and neck cancer. Cancer 1975;35(3):606–11.
9. Lindor KD, Fleming CR, Abrams A, et al. Liver function values in adults receiving total parenteral nutrition. JAMA 1979;241(22):2398–400.
10. Goldmann DA, Maki DG. Infection control in total parenteral nutrition. JAMA 1973;223(12):1360–4.
11. Moore FA, Moore EE, Jones TN, et al. TEN versus TPN following major abdominal trauma–reduced septic morbidity. J Trauma 1989;29(7):916–22 [discussion 922-3].
12. Moore EE, Jones TN. Benefits of immediate jejunostomy feeding after major abdominal trauma–a prospective, randomized study. J Trauma 1986;26(10):874–81.
13. Kudsk KA, Croce MA, Fabian TC, et al. Enteral versus parenteral feeding. Effects on septic morbidity after blunt and penetrating abdominal trauma. Ann Surg 1992;215(5):503–11 [discussion 511-3].
14. Braunschweig CL, Levy P, Sheean PM, et al. Enteral compared with parenteral nutrition: a meta-analysis. Am J Clin Nutr 2001;74(4):534–42.
15. McClave SA, DiBaise JK, Mullin GE, et al. ACG clinical guideline: nutrition therapy in the adult hospitalized patient. Am J Gastroenterol 2016;111(3):315–34 [quiz 335].
16. McDonald WS, Sharp CW Jr, Deitch EA. Immediate enteral feeding in burn patients is safe and effective. Ann Surg 1991;213(2):177–83.
17. Stellato TA, Gauderer MW, Ponsky JL. Percutaneous endoscopic gastrostomy following previous abdominal surgery. Ann Surg 1984;200(1):46–50.
18. Delany HM, Carnevale N, Garvey JW, et al. Postoperative nutritional support using needle catheter feeding jejunostomy. Ann Surg 1977;186(2):165–70.
19. McClave SA, Taylor BE, Martindale RG, et al. Guidelines for the provision and assessment of nutrition support therapy in the adult critically ill patient: Society of Critical Care Medicine (SCCM) and American Society for Parenteral and Enteral Nutrition (A.S.P.E.N.). JPEN J Parenter Enteral Nutr 2016;40(2):159–211.
20. Patel JJ, McClain CJ, Sarav M, et al. Protein requirements for critically ill patients with renal and liver failure. Nutr Clin Pract 2017;32(1_suppl):101S–11S.

21. Malone AM. The use of specialized enteral formulas in pulmonary disease. Nutr Clin Pract 2004;19(6):557–62.
22. Daly JM, Lieberman MD, Goldfine J, et al. Enteral nutrition with supplemental arginine, RNA, and omega-3 fatty acids in patients after operation: immunologic, metabolic, and clinical outcome. Surgery 1992;112(1):56–67.
23. Bower RH, Cerra FB, Bershadsky B, et al. Early enteral administration of a formula (Impact) supplemented with arginine, nucleotides, and fish oil in intensive care unit patients: results of a multicenter, prospective, randomized, clinical trial. Crit Care Med 1995;23(3):436–49.
24. Wernerman J. Clinical use of glutamine supplementation. J Nutr 2008;138(10):2040s–4s.
25. Heyland D, Muscedere J, Wischmeyer PE, et al. A randomized trial of glutamine and antioxidants in critically ill patients. N Engl J Med 2013;368(16):1489–97.
26. McCarthy MS, Martindale RG. Immunonutrition in critical illness: what is the role? Nutr Clin Pract 2018;33(3):348–58.
27. McClave SA, Hurt RT. Clinical guidelines and nutrition therapy: better understanding and greater application to patient care. Crit Care Clin 2010;26(3):451–66, viii.
28. Hurt RT, McClave SA. Gastric residual volumes in critical illness: what do they really mean? Crit Care Clin 2010;26(3):481–90, viii-ix.
29. McClave SA, Lukan JK, Stefater JA, et al. Poor validity of residual volumes as a marker for risk of aspiration in critically ill patients. Crit Care Med 2005;33(2):324–30.
30. Montejo JC, Miñambres E, Bordejé L, et al. Gastric residual volume during enteral nutrition in ICU patients: the REGANE study. Intensive Care Med 2010;36(8):1386–93.
31. Bolgeo T, Di Matteo R, Gallione C, et al. Intragastric prepyloric enteral nutrition, bolus vs continuous in the adult patient: a systematic review and meta-analysis. Nutr Clin Pract 2022;37(4):762–72.
32. Heffernan AJ, Talekar C, Henain M, et al. Comparison of continuous versus intermittent enteral feeding in critically ill patients: a systematic review and meta-analysis. Crit Care 2022;26(1):325.
33. Huang DX, Wu ZH, Wu ZG. The all-in-one nutrient solution in parenteral nutrition. Clin Nutr 1992;11(1):39–44.
34. Banko D, Rosenthal N, Chung J, et al. Comparing the risk of bloodstream infections by type of parenteral nutrition preparation method: a large retrospective, observational study. Clin Nutr ESPEN 2019;30:100–6.
35. Pontes-Arruda A, Zaloga G, Wischmeyer P, et al. Is there a difference in bloodstream infections in critically ill patients associated with ready-to-use versus compounded parenteral nutrition? Clin Nutr 2012;31(5):728–34.
36. Darouiche RO, Raad II, Heard SO, et al. A comparison of two antimicrobial-impregnated central venous catheters. Catheter Study Group. N Engl J Med 1999;340(1):1–8.
37. Marik PE, Zaloga GP. Early enteral nutrition in acutely ill patients: a systematic review. Crit Care Med 2001;29(12):2264–70.
38. Villet S, Chiolero RL, Bollmann MD, et al. Negative impact of hypocaloric feeding and energy balance on clinical outcome in ICU patients. Clin Nutr 2005;24(4):502–9.
39. McClave SA, Saad MA, Esterle M, et al. Volume-based feeding in the critically ill patient. JPEN J Parenter Enter Nutr 2015;39(6):707–12.

40. Yeh DD, Ortiz LA, Lee JM, et al. PEP uP (enhanced protein-energy provision via the enteral route feeding protocol) in surgical patients-a multicenter pilot randomized controlled trial. JPEN J Parenter Enter Nutr 2020;44(2):197–204.

41. Kutsogiannis J, Alberda C, Gramlich L, et al. Early use of supplemental parenteral nutrition in critically ill patients: results of an international multicenter observational study. Crit Care Med 2011;39(12):2691–9.

42. Cattani A, Eckert IC, Brito JE, et al. Nutritional risk in critically ill patients: how it is assessed, its prevalence and prognostic value: a systematic review. Nutr Rev 2020;78(12):1052–68.

43. Harvey SE, Parrott F, Harrison DA, et al. Trial of the route of early nutritional support in critically ill adults. N Engl J Med 2014;371(18):1673–84.

44. Reignier J, Boisramé-Helms J, Brisard L, et al. Enteral versus parenteral early nutrition in ventilated adults with shock: a randomised, controlled, multicentre, open-label, parallel-group study (NUTRIREA-2). Lancet 2018;391(10116):133–43.

45. Watanabe S, Izumino H, Takatani Y, et al. Effects of energy delivery guided by indirect calorimetry in critically ill patients: a systematic review and meta-analysis. Nutrients 2024;16(10). https://doi.org/10.3390/nu16101452.

46. Pertzov B, Bar-Yoseph H, Menndel Y, et al. The effect of indirect calorimetry guided isocaloric nutrition on mortality in critically ill patients-a systematic review and meta-analysis. Eur J Clin Nutr 2022;76(1):5–15.

47. Duan JY, Zheng WH, Zhou H, et al. Energy delivery guided by indirect calorimetry in critically ill patients: a systematic review and meta-analysis. Crit Care 2021;25(1):88.

48. Singer P, Pichard C, Rattanachaiwong S. Evaluating the TARGET and EAT-ICU trials: how important are accurate caloric goals? Point-counterpoint: the pro position. Curr Opin Clin Nutr Metab Care 2020;23(2):91–5.

49. Casaer MP, Mesotten D, Hermans G, et al. Early versus late parenteral nutrition in critically ill adults. N Engl J Med 2011;365(6):506–17.

50. Gao X, Liu Y, Zhang L, et al. Effect of early vs late supplemental parenteral nutrition in patients undergoing abdominal surgery: a randomized clinical trial. JAMA Surg 2022;157(5):384–93.

51. Mundi MS, Martindale RG, Hurt RT. Emergence of mixed-oil fat emulsions for use in parenteral nutrition. review. JPEN J Parenter Enter Nutr 2017;41(1_suppl):3S–13S.

52. Hurt RT, Mundi MS. Use of mixed-oil fat emulsion to improve intestinal failure-associated liver disease in long-term home parenteral nutrition: a case report. JPEN J Parenter Enter Nutr 2017;41(1_suppl):17S–9S.

53. Rice TW, Wheeler AP, Thompson BT, et al, National Heart, Lung, and Blood Institute Acute Respiratory Distress Syndrome (ARDS) Clinical Trials Network. Initial trophic vs full enteral feeding in patients with acute lung injury: the EDEN randomized trial. JAMA 2012;307(8):795–803.

54. Marik PE, Hooper MH. Normocaloric versus hypocaloric feeding on the outcomes of ICU patients: a systematic review and meta-analysis. Intensive Care Med 2016;42(3):316–23.

55. Heyland DK, Patel J, Compher C, et al. The effect of higher protein dosing in critically ill patients with high nutritional risk (EFFORT protein): an international, multicentre, pragmatic, registry-based randomised trial. Lancet 2023;401(10376):568–76.

56. Gilbert JA, Blaser MJ, Caporaso JG, et al. Current understanding of the human microbiome. Nat Med 2018;24(4):392–400.

57. Guyton K, Alverdy JC. The gut microbiota and gastrointestinal surgery. Nat Rev Gastroenterol Hepatol 2017;14(1):43–54.
58. Reintam BA, Preiser JC, Fruhwald S, et al. Gastrointestinal dysfunction in the critically ill: a systematic scoping review and research agenda proposed by the Section of Metabolism, Endocrinology and Nutrition of the European Society of Intensive Care Medicine. Crit Care 2020;24(1):224.
59. Reignier J, Plantefeve G, Mira JP, et al. Low versus standard calorie and protein feeding in ventilated adults with shock: a randomised, controlled, multicentre, open-label, parallel-group trial (NUTRIREA-3). Lancet Respir Med 2023;11(7): 602–12.
60. Patel JJ, Hurt RT, McClave SA, et al. Critical care nutrition: where's the evidence? Crit Care Clin 2017;33(2):397–412.
61. McClave SA, Wischmeyer PE, Miller KR, et al. Mitochondrial dysfunction in critical illness: implications for nutritional therapy. Curr Nutr Rep 2019;8(4):363–73.
62. Patel JJ, Lopez-Delgado JC, Stoppe C, et al. Enteral nutrition in septic shock: a call for a paradigm shift. Curr Opin Crit Care 2024;30(2):165–71.
63. Merker M, Felder M, Gueissaz L, et al. Association of baseline inflammation with effectiveness of nutritional support among patients with disease-related malnutrition: a secondary analysis of a randomized clinical trial. JAMA Netw Open 2020; 3(3):e200663.

Early Feeding in Critical Care - Where Are We Now?

Mette M. Berger, MD, PhD[a],*, Annika Reintam Blaser, MD, PhD[b,c], Orit Raphaeli, PhD[d], Pierre Singer, MD[e,f]

KEYWORDS

- Enteral nutrition • Target • Gastrointestinal dysfunction • Gastric residual volume
- Refeeding syndrome • Endogenous glucose production

KEY POINTS

- The critical illness journey is characterized by different phases with predominance of catabolism during the first days, which progressively shifts over to anabolism when inflammation fades: feeding tolerance is low during this phase.
- Full early feeding is deleterious whatever the route of feeding (enteral or parenteral).
- Enteral feeding intolerance (EFI), most often defined as increased gastric residual volumes (GRV), has repeatedly been shown to be associated with adverse patient-relevant outcomes that may justify continuing the measurements of GRV during initiation of enteral nutrition (EN), unless replaced by ultrasound or new technologies.
- Machine learning may be helpful to identify the risk of EFI and predict complications of EN.
- Early recognition of at-risk patients is a step toward personalized intensive care unit (ICU) nutrition that has the potential to improve outcomes across ICU patient journey.

INTRODUCTION

Medical nutrition therapy (MNT) has evolved considerably over the last 2 decades[1,2]; several high-quality trials were published, generating the need for a practical revision of the European guidelines.[3] The term MNT encompasses oral nutritional supplements, enteral nutrition (EN), and parenteral nutrition (PN). Despite recent studies having shown that PN is not inferior to EN when similar doses of nutrients are administered,[4,5] EN is still considered the next most physiologic after the oral intake,

[a] Faculty of Biology & Medicine, Lausanne University, Lausanne, Switzerland; [b] Department of Anaesthesiology and Intensive Care, University of Tartu, Tartu, Estonia; [c] Department of Intensive Care Medicine, Lucerne Cantonal Hospital, Lucerne, Switzerland; [d] Department of Industrial Engineering and Management, Ariel University, Ariel, Israel; [e] Department of Anesthesia and Intensive Care, Faculty for Medical and Health Sciences, Tel Aviv University, Herzlia Medical Center; [f] General Intensive Care Department, Beilinson Hospital, Rabin Medical Center, Petah Tikva 49100, Israel
* Corresponding author.
E-mail address: mette.berger@unil.ch

Crit Care Clin 41 (2025) 213–231
https://doi.org/10.1016/j.ccc.2024.09.002
0749-0704/25/© 2024 Elsevier Inc. All rights reserved, including those for text and data mining, AI training, and similar technologies.
criticalcare.theclinics.com

leaving the PN at the end of the "feeding hierarchy" in the critically ill in the most recent guidelines.[1,3,6] But in the 2019 guidelines of the European Society for Clinical Nutrition and Metabolism (ESPEN), for the first time, the existence of different metabolic phases of critical illness was recognized,[1] underlining the importance of dose rather than route, as the key player in the early MNT, explaining the results of randomized controlled trials (RCTs).

Accordingly, a question arises: is this strong encouragement of early EN really optimal in the sickest patients? Next to overall negative effect of full dose nutrition in the early acute phase of critical illness, recent evidence has outlined rare but life-threatening complications related specifically to early full EN, such as mesenteric ischemia and Ogilvie's syndrome,[5,7] and showed association of the commonly occurring enteral feeding intolerance (EFI) with impaired outcome.[8] It is not entirely clear what are the associated metabolic changes and mechanisms worsening the clinical outcome related to early full feeding.

Hereafter, we will explore the different trials that have investigated the impact of different feeding strategies on outcome, discuss possible mechanisms behind the findings, and address aspects that have not been studied sufficiently. We discuss definitions of EFI as a reflection of gastrointestinal (GI) dysfunction during acute illness and respective management of EFI.

RECENT HISTORY OF NUTRITIONAL INTERVENTIONS IN THE CRITICALLY ILL

The "enteral nutrition mantra" became dominant after the demonstration in the late 1980s that 5 days of PN compared to EN in healthy subjects resulted in an exacerbated inflammatory response to an endotoxin injection.[9] And indeed, the lipid emulsions used in PN were limited to n-6 fatty acids, which were proinflammatory.[10] Further overfeeding was the rule at that time, the first name of PN being "hyperalimentation." EN could only be better: thus an intense controversy resulted,[11] with authors writing articles entitled "Death by parenteral nutrition."[12] But the strong encouragement of EN as the "only accepted feeding route" has also potentially resulted in iatrogenic malnutrition.[13,14]

Importance of Energy Balance

Twenty years ago, 2 prospective observational studies using the same methodology[13,14] showed in 100 critically ill patients that growing negative energy balances caused by insufficient EN were linked to increasing number of complications. Both studies also showed that a modest energy deficit generated by the progressive feeding strategy was well tolerated: a cumulated deficit of −4'000 kcal (−50 kcal/kg) had no consequence. But with the progression of the deficit beyond −8'000 kcal (−100 kcal/kg) assumably malnutrition-related complications increased, affecting 100% of patients when −10'000 kcal (−130 kcal/kg) were reached. The complications presented as ventilator-associated pneumonia (VAP), wound dehiscence and infection, sepsis, pressure sores, and renal failure. Similarly Faisy and colleagues[15] showed that a *large negative energy balance (based on predictive equation)* during the first 14 days of the intensive care unit (ICU) stay was an independent determinant of mortality in a very sick medical oncological population with prolonged mechanical ventilation and ICU stay: the threshold for increasing mortality was 5021 kJ/d (−1200 kcal/d). A few years later, Yeh and colleagues[16] confirmed these data, showing in 213 surgical ICU patients that those who had negative energy balances exceeding −6'000 kcal were 3 times less likely to be discharged to home. More recently, similar consequences were shown in children: energy deficit, low serum albumin, and elevated C-reactive protein (CRP) were also associated with length of mecahnical ventilations and length of stay.[17] A pro-spective cohort study in 100 ICU patients identified a critical cutoff for complications of 480 kcal/d, which was present in 72% of patients, and was associated with higher mortality ($P = .03$).[18] Both energy and protein deficits increased the length of hospital stay, and protein deficit greater than 20 g/d was an independent factor for ICU mortality.[18]

Negative energy balances also impact the type of microorganisms causing infection, as shown by Faisy and colleagues.[19] In their second study, they first confirmed the link between deficit and severe infections. Then they showed that the largest cumulated energy deficits were associated with a higher incidence of *Staphylococcus aureus* ventilator associated pneumonia (VAP) than those with VAP caused by other pathogens ($-10,275 \pm 4211$ kcal vs -7376 ± 4013 kcal from ICU admission to the day of balance, $P < .01$). Taken together, information from these observational studies and physiologic rationale provided a base for RCTs comparing targeted (higher) versus nontargeted (or targeted lower) provision of energy and protein in critically ill to improve outcomes.

Randomized Controlled Trials on Early Nutrition

Having demonstrated the link between growing energy deficit and outcome,[13,14] early full feeding using a combination of EN and PN was considered the best preventive approach, but proved wrong.

Several "negative trials" attempted immediate full feeding from day 1 by EN, PN, or a combination. The randomized trials EPaNIC[20] and PEPaNIC[21] were conducted with similar protocols in adults and in children. The studies compared early supplemental PN within 24 hours of ICU admission introduced to a fixed target of 25 kcal/kg from day 01 on, or to receive PN after 7 days (late): EN was initiated during the first weeks in both groups, and insulin was infused to achieve normoglycemia. The higher insulin requirements in the early PN group likely reflected overfeeding. Both trials showed no mortality difference, but a higher rate of infectious complications, with prolonged mechanical ventilation, and delayed ICU and hospital discharge.[22]

The randomized EDEN trial compared initial "trophic" feeding with full feeding for up to 6 days, in patients with acute lung injury (ALI)[23] to test the hypothesis that trophic enteral feeding would be better. The trophic strategy did not improve ventilator-free days, 60 day mortality, or infectious complications but was associated with less GI intolerance.

The randomized INTACT study tested intensive feeding (ie, provision of >75% of estimated energy [25–30 kcal/kg]) and protein needs from ICU admission for ALI to hospital discharge compared with standard nutrition.[24] A significantly higher mortality (40% vs 16%, $P = .02$) in the early full feeding group was observed with first deaths occurring on day 4, and the study was stopped for futility. Of note the early full feeding group had been in hospital with poor/nil feeding for 8 days before ICU admission. While no phosphate data were available, the likeliness of a refeeding syndrome ranks high among possible causes of death.

In summary, no RCT has shown benefit from early full feeding in critically ill patients, and several studies have even shown potential harm. Accordingly, early full feeding by any route is clearly not advocated anymore.[1,3] The progressive delivery of enteral feeds with an individual adjustment of targets seems to be the safe way but the optimal timing, dose, and slope of progression for individual patient remain unclear.

The Swiss randomized supplemental PN trials, SPN1[25] and SPN2[26] used an individualized strategy while targeting a measured energy target only from day 4 of the ICU admission, addressing the question of tolerable energy deficit. Eligibility criterion was to be a patient on EN who was not receiving 60% of the initially prescribed target on day 3 (mean cumulated deficit −4000 kcal). The energy expenditure (EE) was measured by indirect calorimetry (IC) to adjust the feeding target. The intervention patients received SPN to complete the measured EE value, while control patients continued on EN only. The individually optimized energy completion with SPN starting on day 4 was associated with a significant reduction of nosocomial infections and reduced inflammatory response (TNF-α tumor necrosis factor-α).[26] That there might be a maximal of 3 to 4 days before energy deficit becomes deleterious is also supported by a surgical study[27]: in 230 major abdominal surgery patients with identified high nutritional risk and poor EN tolerance, early SPN, that is, introduced by day 3 versus day 7, resulted in higher energy delivery (26.5 ± 7.4 vs 15.1 ± 4.8 kcal/kg daily), and fewer nosocomial infections (10 out of 115 [8.7%] vs 21 out of 114 [18.4%]; $P = .04$). In the TICACOS International study,[28] energy target was guided by daily IC measurements. When compared to standard therapy using predictive equations, the study group received significantly more energy, despite measured and estimated energy targets being similar, and showed a trend to decrease in the infection rate and the mortality rate without reaching significance. A meta-analysis of studies comparing energy targeted using IC and standard therapy found a significantly improved short-time survival without differences in other outcomes.[28]

Importantly, underfeeding is even more difficult to detect at bedside as compared to overfeeding. There is a relevant risk that recent evidence on the harm of early full feeding will cause feeding practices worldwide switching from early overfeeding to prolonged underfeeding. Therefore, careful interpretation of available studies and possible mechanisms for harm is needed. It will be a big challenge to design the next relevant and meaningful large study on nutrition, and it would thereby be important to avoid a research question "when is a lower energy delivery not enough during early and later phases?"

METABOLIC CONSEQUENCES OF THE EARLY FULL FEEDING

The metabolic consequences of achieving a full energy target determined by a predictive equation faces four types of risks that may explain their disappointing and even negative results: (1) the risk of early overfeeding due to the low metabolic rate during shock phase, and the persistence of the endogenous substrate production as long as the inflammatory response persists; (2) the risk of refeeding syndrome in patients who had low or nil intakes for several days before the ICU admission[29]; (3) the suppression of adaptive mechanisms that are evolutionary developed to cope with severe illness (autophagy and ketogenesis); and (4) aggravating GI dysfunction by high feed volumes with EN.

Overfeeding

Providing excessive amounts of energy is deleterious but is an easily modifiable factor. Mainly 2 mechanisms cause it: prescribing feeds higher than needs and not respecting adaptive mechanisms to disease. A delivery of feeds in excess of the EE is a consequence of the full feeding strategy[30]: it is frequent with predictive equations,[31] and the IC is useful.[32] However, in the early phase, the elevated endogenous glucose production (EGP), which is present during the acute phase of inflammation is not quantified by IC and is not repressed by feeding.[33] EGP cannot be measured at the bedside (measure requires isotopic methods), but it is indirectly reflected by high insulin requirements and high VCO_2.[34] Full coverage of estimated energy requirements with feeding in addition to an elevated EGP is potentially deleterious as it generates overfeeding.[30] In young patients with major trauma, starved by day 3 for undue reasons,

Tappy and colleagues[35] showed that EGP generated the 3.1 mg/kg/min of glucose, equivalent of 1200 kcal/d: this occurred at the expense of protein catabolism, amino acids being used for gluconeogenesis. Similar results were observed in partially fed 65 year old patients: the mean amount of EGP by day 4 was still 180 g/d glucose (720 kcal/d).[26]

The metabolic processes leading to nonsuppressible EGP and clinical harm from more energy in the early phase are not entirely understood. The purpose of EGP is to provide a continuous glucose supply to the glucose-dependent organs (brain, blood cells, and kidney medulla) to enable ATP production, while not preventing the consequences of persisting energy deficit. By providing too much extrinsic energy, that is, feeding, we disturb some protective adaptive mechanisms developed during evolution. The progressive feeding strategy has the advantage of not overwhelming the organism.

This early phase is generally characterized by an intense inflammation during which there is resistance to nutrition.[36] Intramuscular inflammation and altered substrate utilization have been shown to be present during the first week of critical illness,[37] potentially impeding beneficial effects of nutrition and exercise. Accordingly, inflammation markers (even the simple CRP) may provide an interesting research tool in fine-tuning of nutritional interventions as well as exercising in the ICU.

Refeeding Syndrome

The transition from fasting to eating is a physiologic process that can malfunction,[38] and early full feeding is a major risk factor: a small intake of glucose from feeding or drug dilution is sufficient to initiate it. When nutrition begins, insulin not only transports glucose but also moves potassium and phosphate to intracellular space. Glucose oxidation increases the demand for thiamine and phosphate, resulting in hypokalemia, hypophosphatemia, hypomagnesemia and may lead to fatal arrhythmias, muscle weakness, congestive heart failure, lactic acidosis, and acute abdominal symptoms. Prevention resides in a progressive delivery of feeding (whatever the route), and in case of development of hypophosphatemia (Pi < 0.65 mmol/L for ESPEN[3] and for Doig and colleagues,[39] or a 0.16 mmol/L decrease for the latter),[39] to slow down the process by temporary reduction of feeding.[3]

Impact on Mitochondrial Adaptive Mechanisms

Mitochondrial function is strongly altered in the early phases of shock.[40] These functions include the production of ATP by oxidative phosphorylation, regulation of programmed cell death, calcium homeostasis, and the generation and control of reactive oxygen species.[41] In vitro their morphology changes in response to metabolic inputs. Mitochondrial fragmentation occurs in response to nutrient excess and cellular dysfunction, and it has been observed in cardiovascular and neuromuscular disorders, cancer, and obesity. It facilitates the autophagic clearance of mitochondria and allows the adaption to physiologic demands.[41]

Autophagy is a housekeeping mechanism,[42] a catabolic process induced under conditions of cellular stress, which prevents cell damage and promotes survival in the event of energy or nutrient shortage[43]: it is deregulated in the context of various human pathologies including critical illness. It serves to eliminate large protein aggregates and as a survival mechanism in starvation for generating energy (ATP) and promoting protein synthesis to maintain cell structure.[44] The effect of feeding on autophagy is complex, poorly understood, and difficult to predict.[45,46] Some authors consider that early PN and proteins might inhibit autophagy.[47] However, the argument to withhold feeding to preserve autophagy is poorly substantiated.[42]

Ketogenesis

Starvation initiates an integrated metabolic response to prevent hypoglycemia and energy depletion, and the generation of ketone bodies (ketone-3-hydroxybutyrate and acetoacetate) by the liver is the normal response to fasting in healthy subjects. The nonesterified fatty acids released during lipolysis triggered by fasting are degraded through β-oxidation within liver mitochondria, resulting in the production of acetyl-CoA, which is then either incorporated into the tricarboxylic acid cycle or channelled into the ketogenesis pathway.[48] Insulin typically inhibits ketogenesis as does full feeding.

In critical illness utilization of glucose and fatty acids is impaired, which may contribute to organ dysfunction. A pilot study including 29 critically ill patients randomized them to either ketogenic (n = 14) versus standard enteral feeding for 10 days[49]: the ketogenic high lipid diet proved to be safe and well tolerated and resulted in a modest but significant ketosis in all patients. This was associated with lower insulin requirements, fewer hypoglycemic events, but more diarrhea. The interest of this strategy remains to be confirmed.

Overloading the Gastrointestinal Tract

The impact of early EN on the GI tract is described in "Obstacles to Enteral Feeding" and "Impact of EFI on Clinical Outcomes" sections. Overloading with EN may result in gastric overfilling, intestinal dilatation and/or diarrhea, all with potentially severe consequences. In a study including 278 patients and 1595 patient-days, diarrhea was observed in 38 patients (14%) and 83 patient-days.[50] Diarrhea risk factors were EN covering greater than 60% of energy target (relative risk, 1.75 [1.02–3.01]), antibiotics, and antifungal drugs.

ENTERAL FEEDING INTOLERANCE AND GASTROINTESTINAL DYSFUNCTION
Definitions

There is no unique consensus definition available for EFI, with different approaches being proposed.[51–53] A systematic review[53] largely confirmed the results of an earlier review[54] with still the same wide variation of definitions being used in studies. Different studies have measured EFI by assessing gastric residual volumes (GRV), a variety of GI signs and symptoms (eg, vomiting, abdominal distension, and diarrhea) including or excluding GRV, or the amount of EN received compared to an estimated full energy target:[53,54]

- GRV alone is of limited use due to different cutoffs[53,54] and measurement strategies[55] with some ICUs not using this technique at all. Moreover, gastric intolerance may not be clinically as significant as postpyloric intolerance that may remain undetected or even mismanaged with focusing solely on GRV.[51,52,56]
- GI signs and symptoms may reflect GI dysfunction caused or aggravated by EFI, but the assessment is observer dependent. Studies suggest that number of concomitant symptoms is important and considering different aspects necessitate a complex scoring system.[57]
- The amount of energy target reached with EN. Practically, EFI indeed means that EN cannot be administered in a planned amount due to GI dysfunction. However, several other definitions and decisions influence the amount of EN (**Fig. 1**).[56]

GRV and IAP are the only numerical variables on the list of variables possibly reflecting GI dysfunction, but their respective value is disputed.[51,53] A broad approach covering all different mechanisms of EFI is advocated by the third group of authors.[52]

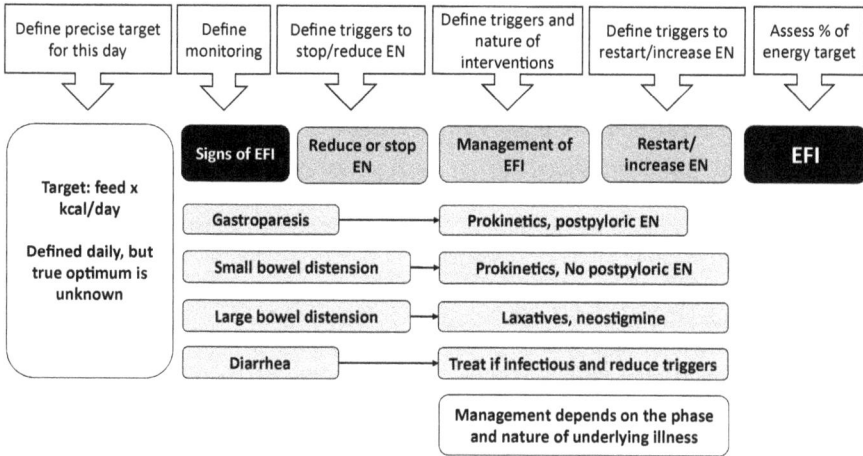

Fig. 1. Definitions and decisions before using the proportion of energy target as definition for EFI.[56] (Reproduced with permission.[56])

The latter is complicated and includes several observer-dependent features but is supported by the evidence showing that inclusion of all available aspects of GI dysfunction results in better prediction of mortality.[57] A recent consensus process on daily monitoring of GI function (Core Outcome Set of daily MOnitoring of GastroIntestinal function in critically ill patients—https://cosmogi.site) united researchers and physicians worldwide for a joint effort in this area. McClave and colleagues[51] importantly pointed out that a new definition of EFI is probably not helpful if it does not lead to a correct therapy, or even leads to a wrong therapy.

The main difference between EFI and GI dysfunction is application of EN, considering EFI as worsening of GI dysfunction in response to EN, whereas GI dysfunction can also occur without application of EN. Current assessment of GI dysfunction is limited to mainly signs of GI dysmotility, not enabling accurate measurement of digestion and absorption, endocrine, immunologic, and barrier functions. Accordingly, while clinical assessment can be used in the absence of biomarkers,[51,52,58] search for biomarkers, mainly focusing on absorption of nutrients and on barrier function, needs to be continued. In the future, a score of GI dysfunction should ideally enable the identification of patients with a greater likelihood for EFI upon initiation of EN and, at the same time, enable the identification of patients at an increased risk for adverse outcomes related to EFI.[51]

Obstacles to Enteral Feeding

Multiple obstacles to achieve enteral feeding targets have been observed in different studies.[59] They include inadequate tube position, missing energy target due to unadjusted time, speed or body position, nutrition interruptions due to investigations and interventions, GI complications, and missing protocols. Nasogastric tube malposition is relatively common: around 24,000 cases of pulmonary malposition occurred for 1.2 million nasogastric tubes inserted in the United States.[60] This complication may induce around 5000 pulmonary complications and increase length of stay and hospital costs.[61] A small study in 61 patients showed 115 EN interruptions occurring mainly due to a computed tomography scan (n = 27), gastric paresis with high GRV (n = 19), nasogastric tube dysfunction (n = 16), and planned extubation (n = 10). Most interruptions occur within the first 3 days of ICU admission, lasting the longest in case of tube malfunction.[62,63] A nurse-driven study in 87 patients showed that the main reasons for not introducing and progressing EN were recent GI surgery, shock, and large GRV.[64]

Impact of Enteral Feeding Intolerance on Clinical Outcomes

EFI has repeatedly been shown to be associated with adverse patient-relevant outcomes.[8,53,54,65,66] The most recent and largest study including 15,918 patients used a broad approach identifying EFI as interruption of EN due to either high GRV, increased abdominal girth, distension, subjective discomfort, emesis, or diarrhea.[8] One-quarter of patients developed EFI, and adjusted hazard of death increased by 1.5 (95% CI 1.4–1.6) after the development of EFI. High GRV increased the risk of having another day with EFI compared to patients in whom EFI was diagnosed without high GRV.[8] Another large study observed a GRV of 250 mL or greater in 46% of patients, more often in patients receiving energy-dense feeds, and an increase in adjusted 90 days mortality in patients presenting with high GRV.[66] It is not clear whether this finding should be attributed to a different composition (energy density) of the EN causing EFI or rather supports the hypothesis that higher energy dose provided by EN results in both more EFI and worse outcome. Prevalence and mortality of EFI are obviously highly dependent on the definition of EFI that is applied.[53,54,67]

Measuring GRV is a matter of discussion since Reignier and colleagues demonstrated that not measuring GRV contributed to improve feed delivery[68] without increasing the incidence of VAP in medical ICU patients receiving full EN.[69] However, 3 large observational studies showed its association with adverse outcomes,[8,66,70] suggesting that measurements should not be abandoned without a robust substitute for monitoring gastric feeding intolerance. Two large RCTs compared full EN versus PN initiated within 24 to 36 hours of ICU admission: the CALORIES trial with 2400 patients (target 25 kcal/d),[4] and the NUTRIREA-2 trial with 2410 patients (20–25 kcal/kg/d).[5] In both studies, more GI complications and increased use of prokinetics were shown in the EN group.

The question whether EFI is reflecting severity of illness and the applied organ support therapies rather than the result of GI dysfunction or inappropriate EN, is matter of debate.[51,52] Clearly, EFI occurs more often in more severely ill patients, who also receive more treatments potentially causing or aggravating GI dysfunction such as vasopressors, opioids, sedatives, mechanical ventilation, and broad-spectrum antibiotics. However, recent studies using adjusted analyses suggest that GI dysfunction itself may influence patient-relevant outcomes independently.[8,57,65,66]

Why EFI or its management may impact outcomes has not been widely studied and discussed. Assessment of EFI is performed at the bedside by ICU health care professionals without robust monitoring tools and also decisions to manage EFI are subjective and probably widely variable. When considering definition of EFI based on achieved energy target via EN, this obviously may include several interventions to increase provision of EN, which potentially may have impact on outcome beyond the effect of EFI itself.

Dose of Enteral Nutrition as a Target of Nutritional Intervention

Recent evidence suggesting harm from full energy dose provided in the early phase[7,71] supports the hypothesis that EFI may be an adaptive mechanism. Indeed, earlier studies comparing EN versus PN consistently showed worse outcomes in patients with PN: more recent knowledge attributes this effect to the lower energy administered with EN and higher with PN, leading to overfeeding in the latter. Accordingly,

EFI might be seen as a protective mechanism against overfeeding. EN may result in specific complications, leading to not only a higher number of GI symptoms but also potentially life-threatening conditions such as Ogilvie's syndrome and acute mesenteric ischemia, as shown in studies administering an early full dose of EN, especially in patients receiving vasopressors.[5,7,71] On one hand, this may appear logical because EFI can occur only in patients receiving EN. On the other hand, the provision of EN would be expected to have positive effects on GI motility, enterocyte function, intestinal mucosal integrity, and microbiome.[72–74]

The effect of difference in dosing between EN and PN was only realized more recently.[75] This hypothesis, may have important implications for feeding practices, suggesting that EFI should, maybe, not always be "aggressively" treated, but that a reduction of EN might be a more appropriate intervention. With this concern, the recent update of ESPEN guidelines already revised the suggestion to treat EFI with reasonable measures, instead of maximizing EN.[3]

Some important questions remain:

- Does early trophic EN exhibit beneficial effects on GI motility, enterocyte function, mucosal integrity, and microbiome, while balanced against potential negative metabolic effects of nutrients in the early acute phase, and accordingly, should early trophic EN be aimed in majority of patients?
- How to differentiate negative effect of too much nutrition from negative effect of GI dysfunction, and accordingly, how large energy deficit should be accepted before SPN becomes indicated?

The hypothesis that EFI might be adaptive at some stages of critical illness, but become maladaptive with time, if left untreated, similar to many other adaptive mechanisms (eg, tachycardia and tachypnea), requires validation. Future studies assessing different dose and progression of EN should also integrate assessment of GI dysfunction and possibly treatment of EFI.

Achievement of nutrition targets via EN should probably not be seen as an alone-standing treatment goal and is rather not a patient-relevant outcome. The strategy is summarized in **Fig. 2**. As the first attempt to combine nutrition targets with assessment of GI function and its management, a recent single-center RCT demonstrated that progressive targets of EN were more appropriately reached with a novel system allowing automated regulation of the dosage of EN with concomitant reflux control.[76] Whether this translates to improved patient-relevant outcomes remains to be clarified.

PERSONALIZED NUTRITION WITH NEW TECHNOLOGIES AND ARTIFICIAL INTELLIGENCE
Machine-Learning Models to Predict Enteral Feeding Response

Machine learning (ML), a subfield of artificial intelligence (AI), uses statistical analysis and computational technologies to learn from experience and detect patterns from datasets[77]. ML is valuable when predictors are numerous and/or their effects are complex and nonlinear. Studies have applied ML to predict clinical outcomes and complications in the ICU, including identifying nutrition-related issues (**Table 1**). Wang and colleagues[77] created a model to identify ICU populations needing EN by applying 6 ML algorithms to a dataset of 53,150 patients. The eXtreme Gradient Boosting (XGBoost) algorithm had the best performance with an Area Under the Receiver Operating Characteristic Curve (AUROC) of 0.90 (95% CI 0.89–0.91). Key predictors were sepsis, Sequential Organ Failure Assessment (SOFA) score, and acute kidney injury.

Early feeding strategy

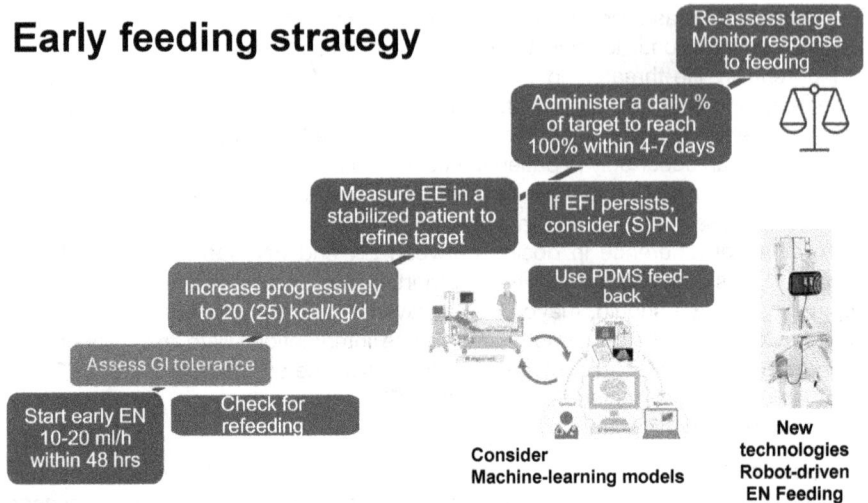

Fig. 2. In critically ill patients, the feeding strategy should be individualized from start: proceed stepwise over the first days, while carefully monitoring intestinal and metabolic responses, and adapting to those responses. Protein delivery should be monitored, but it will progress according to your available feeding products. EFI, enteral feeding intolerance; EE, energy expenditure; PN, parenteral nutrition; SPN, supplemental PN; PDMS, patient data management system.

Lu and colleagues[78] developed a clinical prediction model for EFI risk in ICU patients receiving EN using a cohort of 203 patients. A logistic regression algorithm achieved an AUROC of 0.70 (95% CI 0.63–0.77), with age, GI disease, and early feeding as important predictors. Hu and colleagues[79] validated a model to predict EFI in ICU patients with sepsis using a dual-center, retrospective, case–control study of 195 patients. The artificial neural network algorithm had an AUROC of 0.79 (95% CI 0.68–0.89), with respiratory infections, peptide EN, and shock as the main factors. Raphaeli and colleagues[70] examined EFI markers during early ICU in a retrospective single-center study, using seven ML algorithms on data from 1584 patients. The gradient boosting algorithm had the highest predictive value with an AUROC of 0.71 (95% CI 0.67–0.74), with BMI, high GRV on day 2, and high SOFA on day 1 as the main factors for early EN failure. Choi and colleagues[80] used an ML model to identify patients at risk for refeeding syndrome in a study of 806 patients. The XGBoost algorithm had an AUROC of 0.95 (95% CI 0.92–0.97), with low initial phosphate, recent weight loss, and high creatinine as the main factors to predict refeeding syndrome. Overall, these studies show ML can support nutritional therapy decisions, but methodological differences in designs, endpoint definitions, and risk factors limit generalization. More research is needed to improve ML model generalization.

New Technologies

A large gap between EN prescription and delivery has been described in numerous observational studies,[81] the most efficient centers achieving 80% of the prescribed value.[82,83] Computerized information systems can or are customized to enable visualization of nutrition quantity being delivered.[61] Technological help to monitor the actual feeding in an individual patient has been available since a while, but it is still rarely requested/used.

Table 1
Main characteristics of machine learning-based predictive models of enteral nutrition response

Study	N patients	Primary Endpoint	ML Algorithms Compared	Best Algorithm	Main Predictors
Wang et al,[77] 2023	N = 53,150, n = 7210 (13.5%) initiated EN at early phase	EN initiation	XGBoost, SVM, KNN, RF, LR, and DT	XGBoost	Sepsis, SOFA score, AKI, and body temperature
Lu et al,[78] 2022	N = 203, n = 77 (37.9%) with EFI	EFI	LR	LR	Age, GI disease, early feeding, mechanical ventilation before EN started, and abnormal serum sodium
Hu et al,[79] 2022	N = 195, n = 86 (44.1%) with EFI	EFI	ANN, GB, RF, LR, and NB	ANN	Infection of the lower respiratory tract, peptide EN, and shock
Raphaeli et al,[70] 2023	N = 1584, n = 1019 (64.3%) with early EN failure	Early EN failure	GB, KNN, DT, RF, XGBoost, LR, and AdaBoost	GB	BMI, high GRV (>250 mL) on second day of ICU admission, SOFA, and age
Choi et al,[80] 2021	N = 806, n = 367 (45.5%) with hypophosphatemia	Refeeding syndrome	XGBoost, LR, L1, and L2	XGBoost	Low initial phosphate, recent weight loss, high creatinine, diabetes mellitus with insulin use, low HbA1c, furosemide use, ICU admission, blood urea nitrogen level of 19–65 mmol/L, PN, magnesium below or above the normal range, low potassium, and older age

Abbreviations: AdaBoost, Adaptive Boosting; ANN, artificial neural networks; DT, decision tree; GB, gradient boosting; KNN, K-nearest neighbor; L1, lasso regression; L2, ridge regression; LR, logistic regression; ML, machine learning; NB, Naïve Bayes; RF, random forest; SVM, support vector machines; XGBoost, eXtreme Gradient Boosting.

Intragastric balloon monitoring

A technique to assess gastric motility by measuring the pressure in a low-volume intragastric balloon mounted on a gastric feeding tube was presented by Goelen and colleagues.[84–86] This device might serve to detect GI motility disorders but requires validation in ICU patients.

An integrative platform

A new platform to improve feeding has been developed aiming at overcoming frequent problems of EN,[76] called smART+ (ART Medical, Netanya, Israel): its originality resides in the integration of tube positioning confirmation, reflux and gastric residual volume monitoring using a nasogastric tube equipped with sensors, and EE calculation from an integrated VCO_2 measurement.[87,88] Accordingly, the system should facilitate achieving the EN target. EN is administered or stopped according to the detection of refluxes, ensuring a high feeding efficiency in case of the absence of refluxes and safety in case of presence of refluxes, accordingly.[76] It may confirm Reignier's hypothesis[69] that gastroesophageal reflux is independent of the actual GRV.

The performance of this platform was compared with conventional feeding. The EE was calculated from VCO_2 in the intervention group versus measured by IC in the controls—the latter patients having a higher prescribed energy target (2030 vs 1725 kcal). Kagan and colleagues[76] showed close to a 100% feeding efficiency (ie, reaching prescribed value), overfeeding, defined as exceeding of estimated and prescribed needs was avoided and underfeeding minimalized (**Fig. 3, Table 2**). The prescribed target was reached only in 34% of control patients. Whether the targets, set in a progressive way with starting low and not exceeding 70% of targets, were entirely appropriate for each individual patient considering EGP and refeeding, is not known. However, adjusted length of stay and length of ventilation were significantly reduced (by 3 or more days) in the intervention group, supporting a benefit.[76] Whether this benefit might have occurred largely due to the prevention of regurgitation remains to be answered. In a post hoc analysis, most feeding interruptions (80%) were related to diagnostic/therapeutic interventions.[89] These results are promising and must be confirmed in further studies including cost–benefit analysis and nurse acceptance.

This integrative platform and the use of AI are tools to personalize EN in critically ill patients.[90] Whereas the guideline recommendations[3] suggest using the gastric route, to determine energy and protein target, to administer EN continuously and only react to GI intolerance and vomiting, AI might become a tool enabling prediction of EN success and preventing complications.

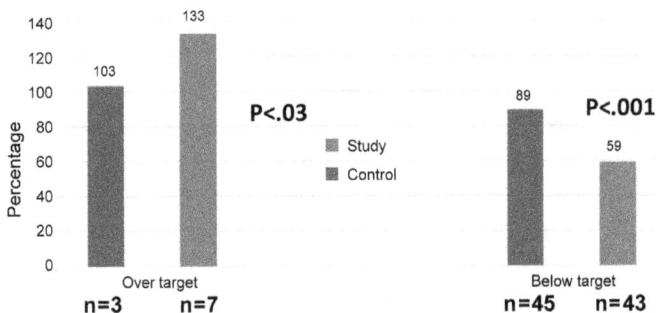

Fig. 3. Average deviation from 100% feeding efficacy defined as reaching prescribed target using a robot-guided enteral feeding system.[76]

Table 2
Main differences observed in 100 critically ill patients between enteral standard therapy and the use of the integrative platform.[76]

	Standard Therapy	Integrative Platform[76]	Pro/con
NGT position	Intermittent by radiography[59,60]	Continuously by sensors	NGT misplacement is easier recognized with platform: Sensors are alerting for misplacement and radiography is not required
Energy target determination	By predictive equation and calculation	Target based on EE calculated from VCO_2[87,88]	Automatic adjustment according to VCO_2 with progressive targets facilitates planning and delivery of EN
Choice of the formula	Dietician (or by protocol in many ICUs)	Computerized[a] according to the energy requirements and the hospital availability	Facilitates the dietician work but is more expensive
GI intolerance (reflux)	Not detected except vomiting, or if GRV is measured	Sensors detecting massive and minor refluxes	Reflux is difficult to detect clinically, and small reflux has been shown to be frequent. The tool could potentially replace GRV measurements
Energy target reached	Around 70% of the target[83]	Around 90% of the target	Progressive energy targets difficult to reach without automatization
Interruptions	Not compensated[32]	Compensated	Automatic compensation enables to nearly reach the target
Nonnutritional energy intake	Often not measured	Integrated manually[b] in the calculation of the energy target	May prevent overfeeding

Abbreviations: NGT, nasogastric tube; GRC, gastric residual volume.
[a] The platform enables customization of locally available formula, including special formula.
[b] The platform is not yet connected to the data management system or to pumps.

SUMMARY

After 3 decades of controversies regarding the feeding route and timing, a more physiologic approach to MNT is emerging. The recognition of different phases of critically illness is paramount for understanding apparently contradictory evidence. Critical illness in its early phase is associated with catabolism and inability to use nutrients for anabolism, and aggressive achievement of energy targets during this period may worsen GI dysfunction, delay recovery, and worsen outcome. PN is a decent alternative to EN in presence of EFI, whereas the main challenge remains to identify the appropriate dynamic targets avoiding overfeeding, refeeding, and underfeeding. It is possible and even likely that strong recommendations in favor of EN including aggressive treatment of EFI might be softened in future guidelines.

CLINICS CARE POINTS

- Education of staff (residents and registrars, nurses) regarding the complex nutritional needs of critically ill patients should be embedded into hospital orientation for ICU, and wards.
- Early assessment of the patient should be included the ICU protocols, and the specific tasks be precisely assigned to the different caregiver types.
- While an early progressive initiation of EN is desirable, the high incidence of EFI should be particularly emphasized in the teaching, as it informs about the severity of the metabolic alterations.
- Reporting of the indicators of intestinal function and indicators of feeding tolerance should belong to the medical visit.
- Collaborative multidisciplinary research is required to ensure appropriate delivery and monitoring of nutrition therapy.

DISCLOSURE

M.M. Berger received speaker honoraria from Abbott, Baxter, Fresenius Kabi, Nestlé Health; Support for attending meetings from Baxter and Fresenius Kabi Int. A. Reintam Blaser received speaker fees from Nutricia Danone and consultancy fee from VIPUN Medical and is holding a grant from the Estonian Research Council (Grant PRG1255). O. Raphaeli: declares no COI. P. Singer received Honoraria for lectures from Abbott, Baxter, Fresenius Kabi, Nestlé Health; Support for attending meetings from Baxter, Nestle Health and Fresenius Kabi Int.; Research grant to institution from Baxter, United States, Fresenius Kabi, Germany, Nestle, Switzerland, ART MEDICAL. Advisory board: Fresenius Kabi, ART MEDICAL.

REFERENCES

1. Singer P, Reintam-Blaser A, Berger MM, et al. ESPEN guideline on clinical nutrition in the intensive care unit. Clin Nutr 2019;38:48–79.
2. McClave SA, Taylor BE, Martindale RG, et al. Guidelines for the provision and assessment of nutrition support therapy in the adult critically ill patient: society of critical care medicine (SCCM) and American Society for parenteral and enteral nutrition (A.S.P.E.N.). JPEN - J Parenter Enter Nutr 2016;40:159–211.
3. Singer P, Reintam Blaser A, Berger MM, et al. ESPEN practical and partially revised guideline: clinical nutrition in the intensive care unit. Clin Nutr 2023;42: 1671–89.

4. Harvey SE, Parrott F, Harrison DA, et al. Trial of the route of early nutritional support in critically ill adults - calories Trial. N Engl J Med 2014;371:1673–84.
5. Reignier J, Boisrame-Helms J, Brisard L, et al. Enteral versus parenteral early nutrition in ventilated adults with shock: a randomised, controlled, multicentre, open-label, parallel-group study (NUTRIREA-2). Lancet 2018;391:133–43.
6. Compher C, Bingham AL, McCall M, et al. Guidelines for the provision of nutrition support therapy in the adult critically ill patient: the American Society for Parenteral and Enteral Nutrition. JPEN - J Parenter Enter Nutr 2022;46:12–41.
7. Reignier J, Plantefeve G, Mira JP, et al. Low versus standard calorie and protein feeding in ventilated adults with shock: a randomised, controlled, multicentre, open-label, parallel-group trial (NUTRIREA-3). Lancet Respir Med 2023;11:602–12.
8. Heyland DK, Ortiz A, Stoppe C, et al. Incidence, risk factors, and clinical consequence of enteral feeding intolerance in the mechanically ventilated critically ill: an analysis of a multicenter, multiyear database. Crit Care Med 2021;49:49–59.
9. Fong YM, Marano MA, Braber A, et al. Total parenteral nutrition and bowel rest modify the metabolic response to endotoxin in humans. Ann Surg 1989;210:449–57.
10. Calder PC. Hot topics in parenteral nutrition. Rationale for using new lipid emulsions in parenteral nutrition and a review of the trials performed in adults. Proc Nutr Soc 2009;68:252–60.
11. Jeejeebhoy KN. Total parenteral nutrition: potion or poison? Am J Clin Nutr 2001;74:160–3.
12. Marik PE, Pinsky M. Death by parenteral nutrition. Intensive Care Med 2003;29:867–9.
13. Villet S, Chioléro RL, Bollmann MD, et al. Negative impact of hypocaloric feeding and energy balance on clinical outcome in ICU patients. Clin Nutr 2005;24:502–9.
14. Dvir D, Cohen J, Singer P. Computerized energy balance and complications in critically ill patients: an observational study. Clin Nutr 2006;25:37–44.
15. Faisy C, Lerolle N, Dachraoui F, et al. Impact of energy deficit calculated by a predictive method on outcome in medical patients requiring prolonged acute mechanical ventilation. Br J Nutr 2009;101:1079–87.
16. Yeh DD, Fuentes E, Quraishi SA, et al. Adequate nutrition may get you home: effect of caloric/protein deficits on the discharge destination of critically ill surgical patients. JPEN - J Parenter Enter Nutr 2016;40:37–44.
17. Carvalhal FB, Ferreira Peres WA, Fontes Lima GC, et al. Impact of energy deficit during hospitalization and biomarkers at admission on clinical outcomes in critically ill children: a longitudinal study. Clin Nutr ESPEN 2019;32:70–5.
18. Siqueira-Paese MC, Dock-Nascimento DB, De Aguilar-Nascimento JE. Critical energy deficit and mortality in critically ill patients. Nutr Hosp 2016;33:253.
19. Faisy C, Llerena M, Savalle M, et al. Early ICU energy deficit is a risk factor for Staphylococcus aureus ventilator-associated nneumonia. Chest 2011;140:1254–60.
20. Casaer MP, Mesotten D, Hermans G, et al. Early versus late parenteral nutrition in critically ill adults. N Engl J Med 2011;365:506–17.
21. Vanhorebeek I, Verbruggen S, Casaer MP, et al. Effect of early supplemental parenteral nutrition in the paediatric ICU: a preplanned observational study of post-randomisation treatments in the PEPaNIC trial. Lancet Respir Med 2017;5:475–83.
22. Casaer MP, Wilmer A, Hermans G, et al. Role of disease and macronutrient dose in the randomized controlled EPaNIC trial: a post hoc analysis. Am J Respir Crit Care Med 2013;187:247–55.

23. Rice TW, Wheeler AP, Thompson BT, et al. Initial trophic vs full enteral feeding in patients with acute lung injury: the EDEN randomized trial. JAMA 2012;307:795–803.

24. Braunschweig CL, Freels S, Sheean PM, et al. Role of timing and dose of energy received in patients with acute lung injury on mortality in the Intensive Nutrition in Acute Lung Injury Trial (INTACT): a post hoc analysis. Am J Clin Nutr 2017;105: 411–6.

25. Heidegger CP, Berger MM, Graf Set al, et al. Optimisation of energy provision with supplemental parenteral nutrition in critically ill patients: a randomised controlled clinical trial. Lancet 2013;381:385–93.

26. Berger MM, Pantet O, Jacquelin-Ravel Net al, et al. Supplemental parenteral nutrition improves immunity with unchanged carbohydrate and protein metabolism in critically ill patients: the SPN2 randomized tracer study. Clin Nutr 2019;38:2408–16.

27. Gao X, Liu Y, Zhang L, et al. Effect of early vs late supplemental parenteral nutrition in patients undergoing abdominal surgery: a randomized clinical trial. JAMA Surg 2022;157:384–93.

28. Duan JY, Zheng WH, Zhou H, et al. Energy delivery guided by indirect calorimetry in critically ill patients: a systematic review and meta-analysis. Crit Care 2021; 25:88.

29. Koekkoek WAC, Van Zanten ARH. Is refeeding syndrome relevant for critically ill patients? Curr Opin Clin Nutr Metab Care 2018;21:130–7.

30. Oshima T, Berger MM, De Waele E, et al. Indirect calorimetry in nutritional therapy. A position paper by the ICALIC study group. Clin Nutr 2017;36:651–62.

31. Zusman O, Kagan I, Bendavid I, et al. Predictive equations versus measured energy expenditure by indirect calorimetry: a retrospective validation. Clin Nutr 2019;38:1206–10.

32. Page A, Langan A, Wan YI, et al. Association between energy surplus and intensive care unit length of stay in critically ill patients: a retrospective cohort study. JPEN - J Parenter Enter Nutr 2024;48:206–14.

33. Wolfe RR. Sepsis as a modulator of adaptation to low and high carbohydrate and low and high fat intakes. Eur J Clin Nutr 1999;53(Suppl 1):S136–42.

34. Udin I, Habisreutinger M, Tappy L, et al. Magnitude of gluconeogenesis and endogenous glucose production: are they predictable in clinical settings? Clin Nutr 2021;40:3807–14.

35. Tappy L, Schwarz JM, Schneiter P, et al. Effects of isoenergetic glucose-based or lipid-based parenteral nutrition on glucose metabolism, de novo lipogenesis, and respiratory gas exchanges in critically ill patients. Crit Care Med 1998;26:860–7.

36. Merker M, Felder M, Gueissaz L, et al. Association of baseline inflammation with effectiveness of nutritional support among pPatients with disease-related malnutrition: a secondary analysis of a randomized clinical trial. JAMA Netw Open 2020;3:e200663.

37. Jameson TSO, Caldow MK, Stephens F, et al. Inflammation and altered metabolism impede efficacy of functional electrical stimulation in critically ill patients. Crit Care 2023;27:428.

38. van Zanten ARH. Nutritional support and refeeding syndrome in critical illness. Lancet Respir Med 2015;3:904–5.

39. Doig GS, Simpson F, Heighes PTet al, et al. Restricted versus continued standard caloric intake during the management of refeeding syndrome in critically ill adults: a randomised, parallel-group, multicentre, single-blind controlled trial. Lancet Respir Med 2015;3:943–52.

40. Singer M. Mitochondrial function in sepsis: acute phase versus multiple organ failure. Crit Care Med 2007;35:S441–8.

41. Wai T, Langer T. Mitochondrial dynamics and metabolic regulation. Trends Endocrinol Metab 2016;27:105–17.
42. McClave SA, Weijs PJ. Preservation of autophagy should not direct nutritional therapy. Curr Opin Clin Nutr Metab Care 2015;18:155–61.
43. Dikic I, Elazar Z. Mechanism and medical implications of mammalian autophagy. Nat Rev Mol Cell Biol 2018;19:349–64.
44. Glick D, Barth S, Macleod KF. Autophagy: cellular and molecular mechanisms. J Pathol 2010;221:3–12.
45. Wesselink E, Koekkoek WAC, Grefte S, et al. Feeding mitochondria: potential role of nutritional components to improve critical illness convalescence. Clin Nutr 2019;38:982–95.
46. Abate M, Festa A, Falco M, et al. Mitochondria as playmakers of apoptosis, autophagy and senescence. Semin Cell Dev Biol 2020;98:139–53.
47. Wernerman J, Christopher KB, Annane D, et al. Metabolic support in the critically ill: a consensus of 19. Crit Care 2019;23:318.
48. Fukao T, Lopaschuk GD, Mitchell GA. Pathways and control of ketone body metabolism: on the fringe of lipid biochemistry. Prostaglandins Leukot Essent Fatty Acids 2004;70:243–51.
49. McNelly A, Langan A, Bear DE, et al. A pilot study of alternative substrates in the critically Ill subject using a ketogenic feed. Nat Commun 2023;14:8345.
50. Thibault R, Graf S, Clerc A, et al. Diarrhoea in the intensive care unit: respective contribution of feeding and antibiotics. Crit Care 2013;17:R153.
51. McClave SA, Gualdoni J, Nagengast A, et al. Gastrointestinal dysfunction and feeding intolerance in critical illness: do we need an objective scoring system? Curr Gastroenterol Rep 2020;22:1.
52. Reintam Blaser A, Deane AM, Preiser JC, et al. Enteral feeding intolerance: updates in definitions and pathophysiology. Nutr Clin Pract 2021;36:40–9.
53. Jenkins B, Calder PC, Marino LV. A systematic review of the definitions and prevalence of feeding intolerance in critically ill adults. Clin Nutr ESPEN 2022;49:92–102.
54. Reintam Blaser A, Starkopf J, Kirsimagi U, et al. Definition, prevalence, and outcome of feeding intolerance in intensive care: a systematic review and meta-analysis. Acta Anaesthesiol Scand 2014;58:914–22.
55. Lindner M, Padar M, Mandul M, et al. Current practice of gastric residual volume measurements and related outcomes of critically ill patients: a secondary analysis of the intestinal-specific organ function assessment study. JPEN - J Parenter Enter Nutr 2023;47:614–23.
56. Reintam Blaser A, Bachmann KF, Deane AM. Gastrointestinal function in critically ill patients. Curr Opin Clin Nutr Metab Care 2023;26:463–9.
57. Reintam Blaser A, Padar M, Mandul M, et al. Development of the Gastrointestinal Dysfunction Score (GIDS) for critically ill patients - a prospective multicenter observational study (iSOFA study). Clin Nutr 2021;40:4932–40.
58. Jenkins B, Calder PC, Marino LV. A scoping review considering potential biomarkers or functional measures of gastrointestinal dysfunction and enteral feeding intolerance in critically ill adults. Clin Nutr ESPEN 2022;52:331–9.
59. Hoffmann M, Schwarz CM, Furst S, et al. Risks in management of enteral nutrition in intensive care units: a literature review and narrative synthesis. Nutrients 2020;13.
60. Motta APG, Rigobello MCG, Silveira Rccp, et al. Nasogastric/nasoenteric tube-related adverse events: an integrative review. Rev Lat Am Enfermagem 2021;29:e3400.

61. de Aguilar-Nascimento JE, Kudsk KA. Clinical costs of feeding tube placement. JPEN - J Parenter Enter Nutr 2007;31:269–73.
62. van Nieuwkoop MM, Ramnarain D, Pouwels S. Enteral nutrition interruptions in the intensive care unit: a prospective study. Nutrition 2022;96:111580.
63. Onuk S, Ozer NT, Savas N, et al. Enteral nutrition interruptions in critically ill patients: a prospective study on reasons, frequency and duration of interruptions of nutritional support during ICU stay. Clin Nutr ESPEN 2022;52:178–83.
64. Kuslapuu M, Jogela K, Starkopf J, et al. The reasons for insufficient enteral feeding in an intensive care unit: a prospective observational study. Intensive Crit Care Nurs 2015;31:309–14.
65. Gungabissoon U, Hacquoil K, Bains C, et al. Prevalence, risk factors, clinical consequences, and treatment of enteral feed intolerance during critical illness. JPEN - J Parenter Enter Nutr 2015;39:441–8.
66. Arunachala Murthy T, Chapple LS, Lange K, et al. Gastrointestinal dysfunction during enteral nutrition delivery in intensive care unit (ICU) patients: risk factors, natural history, and clinical implications. A post-hoc analysis of the Augmented versus Routine approach to Giving Energy Trial (TARGET). Am J Clin Nutr 2022;116: 589–98.
67. Reintam Blaser A, Starkopf L, Deane AM, et al. Comparison of different definitions of feeding intolerance: a retrospective observational study. Clin Nutr 2015;34: 956–61.
68. Poulard F, Dimet J, Martin-Lefevre L et al, et al. Impact of not measuring residual gastric volume in mechanically ventilated patients receiving early enteral feeding: a prospective before-after study. JPEN - J Parenter Enter Nutr 2010;34:125–30.
69. Reignier J, Mercier E, Le Gouge A et al, et al. Effect of not monitoring residual gastric volume on risk of ventilator-associated pneumonia in adults receiving mechanical ventilation and early enteral feeding: a randomized controlled trial. JAMA 2013;309:249–56.
70. Raphaeli O, Statlender L, Hajaj C, et al. Using machine-learning to assess the prognostic value of early enteral feeding intolerance in critically ill patients: a retrospective study. Nutrients 2023;15.
71. Pardo E, Lescot T, Preiser JC, et al. Association between early nutrition support and 28-day mortality in critically ill patients: the FRANS prospective nutrition cohort study. Crit Care 2023;27:7.
72. Nguyen NQ, Besanko LK, Burgstad C, et al. Delayed enteral feeding impairs intestinal carbohydrate absorption in critically ill patients. Crit Care Med 2012; 40:50–4.
73. Piton G, Le Gouge A, Brule N, et al. Impact of the route of nutrition on gut mucosa in ventilated adults with shock: an ancillary of the NUTRIREA-2 trial. Intensive Care Med 2019;45:948–56.
74. Ralls MW, Demehri FR, Feng Y, et al. Enteral nutrient deprivation in patients leads to a loss of intestinal epithelial barrier function. Surgery 2015;157:732–42.
75. Elke G, van Zanten AR, Lemieux M, et al. Enteral versus parenteral nutrition in critically ill patients: an updated systematic review and meta-analysis of randomized controlled trials. Crit Care 2016;20:117.
76. Kagan I, Hellerman-Itzhaki M, Bendavid I, et al. Controlled enteral nutrition in critical care patients - a randomized clinical trial of a novel management system. Clin Nutr 2023;42:1602–9.
77. Wang YX, Li XL, Zhang LH, et al. Machine learning algorithms assist early evaluation of enteral nutrition in ICU patients. Front Nutr 2023;10:1060398.

78. Lu XM, Jia DS, Wang R, et al. Development of a prediction model for enteral feeding intolerance in intensive care unit patients: a prospective cohort study. World J Gastrointest Surg 2022;14:1363–74.

79. Hu K, Deng XL, Han L, et al. Development and validation of a predictive model for feeding intolerance in intensive care unit patients with sepsis. Saudi J Gastroenterol 2022;28:32–8.

80. Choi TY, Chang MY, Heo S, et al. Explainable machine learning model to predict refeeding hypophosphatemia. Clin Nutr ESPEN 2021;45:213–9.

81. Alberda C, Gramlich L, Jones N, et al. The relationship between nutritional intake and clinical outcomes in critically ill patients: results of an international multicenter observational study. Intensive Care Med 2009;35:1728–37.

82. Soguel L, Revelly JP, Schaller MD, et al. Energy deficit and length of hospital stay can be reduced by a two-step quality improvement of nutrition therapy: the intensive care unit dietitian can make the difference. Crit Care Med 2012;40:412–9.

83. Ridley EJ, Davies AR, Hodgson CL, et al. Delivery of full predicted energy from nutrition and the effect on mortality in critically ill adults: a systematic review and meta-analysis of randomised controlled trials. Clin Nutr 2018;37:1913–25.

84. Goelen N, Tack J, Janssen P. Erythromycin stimulates phasic gastric contractility as assessed with an isovolumetric intragastric balloon pressure measurement. Neuro Gastroenterol Motil 2021;33:e13991.

85. Raymenants K, Huang IH, Goelen N, et al. Clinical validation of the VIPUN gastric monitoring system versus manometry for the evaluation of gastric motility. Neuro Gastroenterol Motil 2024;e14783.

86. Goelen N, de Hoon J, Morales JF, et al. Codeine delays gastric emptying through inhibition of gastric motility as assessed with a novel diagnostic intragastric balloon catheter. Neuro Gastroenterol Motil 2020;32:e13733.

87. Stapel SN, de Grooth HJ, Alimohamad H, et al. Ventilator-derived carbon dioxide production to assess energy expenditure in critically ill patients: proof of concept. Crit Care 2016;19:370.

88. Kagan I, Zusman O, Bendavid I, et al. Validation of carbon dioxide production (VCO(2)) as a tool to calculate resting energy expenditure (REE) in mechanically ventilated critically ill patients: a retrospective observational study. Crit Care 2018;22:186.

89. Kagan I, Hellerman Isthaki M, Singer P. Evaluation and compensation of patient related and diagnostic/therapeutic related interruptions of enteral nutrition using the smART + platform. a post hoc computerized analysis. Clin Nutr ESPEN 2024; 63:980.

90. Wischmeyer PE, Bear DE, Berger MM, et al. Personalized nutrition therapy in critical care: 10 expert recommendations. Crit Care 2023;27:261.

Protein Delivery in Critical Care- What Have Recent Trials Shown Us?

Michelle Carmen Paulus, MD[a,b],
Arthur Raymond Hubert van Zanten, MD, PhD[a,b],*

KEYWORDS

- Protein • Intensive care unit • Nutrition • Critically ill • Endotyping • Phenotyping
- Anabolic resistance • UCR

KEY POINTS

- Critically ill patients may experience adverse effects if their protein intake falls below the recommended target, yet they often fail to achieve these protein recommendations.
- According to recent trials, it is not advisable to recommend a protein intake lower than 1.0 g/kg/day or a higher protein intake than 1.6 g/kg/day.
- Due to proteins' time-dependent effect, it is recommended that protein intake be gradually increased during the first 4 to 5 days of intensive care unit (ICU) stay.
- Utilizing individualized protein dosing based on phenotyping and endotyping is recommended instead of a one-size-fits-all approach.
- Nutritional interventional studies for post-ICU patients are needed as patients frequently fail to meet their goals.

INTRODUCTION

To effectively manage critically ill patients, ensuring that the timing and dosage of proteins are precisely calibrated is paramount. The rapid loss of muscle protein during critical illness, which can result in reductions of muscle mass of up to 18% within the first 10 days of intensive care unit (ICU) admission, highlights this approach's significance.[1] The 2016 American Society for Parenteral and Enteral Nutrition (ASPEN) guidelines recommend a daily protein intake of 1.2 to 2.0 g/kg during critical illness. For patients with burns, obesity, and trauma, a higher amount is recommended.[2] The revised 2022 version retained these recommendations due to a need for more

[a] Department of Intensive Care Medicine & Research, Gelderse Vallei Hospital, Willy Brandtlaan 10, 6716 RP Ede, The Netherlands; [b] Division of Human Nutrition and Health, Nutritional Biology, Wageningen University & Research, HELIX (Building 124), Stippeneng 4, 6708 WE Wageningen, The Netherlands
* Corresponding author.
E-mail addresses: zantena@zgv.nl; arthur.vanzanten@wur.nl

Crit Care Clin 41 (2025) 233–246
https://doi.org/10.1016/j.ccc.2024.09.003
0749-0704/25/© 2024 Elsevier Inc. All rights reserved, including those for text and data mining, AI training, and similar technologies.
criticalcare.theclinics.com

high-quality evidence.[3] According to the European Society for Clinical Nutrition and Metabolism (ESPEN) 2019 guideline, a protein equivalent intake of 1.3 g/kg per day is advised.[4] The revised guideline recommends achieving this target progressively, rather than within the first 48 to 72 hours, to avoid overnutrition.[5] Studies have shown that meeting dietary recommendations during critical illness is possible with high-intact-protein formulas or enteral supplemental protein.[6,7] Despite evidence demonstrating the feasibility of achieving protein targets, critically ill patients frequently fail to meet protein targets.[8–11] It is evident from daily practice that the prescribed amount of protein internationally falls below the recommended targets (1.2 g/kg/day), with the average protein intake being even lower and only 0.6 g/kg/day.[9] Achieving the recommended protein targets has been associated with several positive outcomes, including improved survival,[12–17] attenuated muscle loss, and slight improvement in activities of daily living.[18,19] The adequacy of recommended protein intakes is currently a topic of growing interest. This review aims to provide an overview of recent trials investigating protein dosing for critically ill patients.

RISKS OF LOW PROTEIN INTAKE

Failure to achieve the recommended targets can adversely affect the critically ill patient. In the retrospective PROTINVENT study involving ICU patients requiring prolonged ventilation, an overall low protein intake (<0.8 g/kg/day) was associated with the highest ICU, in-hospital, and 6-month mortality.[20] Similarly, a protein intake of <0.5 g/kg/day on the seventh day of critical illness is a risk factor for 28-day mortality.[21] On the contrary, a protein intake closer to the recommended targets has been linked with a reduced incidence of mortality.[22–25] A cohort study of critically ill patients who survived hospitalization found that the peak daily protein intake was only 0.32 g/kg, with a 17% reduction in 90-day post-discharge mortality observed for every 1 g/kg increase in daily protein intake.[22] Modeling conducted in an international database also indicated that a late standard protein diet (median 0.99 g/kg/d) was associated with lower in-hospital mortality compared with a low-protein-only diet (median 0.49 g/kg).[23] Additionally, a post-hoc analysis from a large randomized controlled multicenter study (NEED trial)[24] revealed that in patients with an ICU stay of at least 7 days and exclusive enteral nutrition, the median daily protein delivery was 0.6 g/kg. Each 0.2 g/kg increase was associated with mortality reduction.[25] Nevertheless, this only applied to patients with lactate concentrations of up to 2 mmol/L.[25]

Beyond mortality risk, critically ill patients receiving a low protein intake (<1.0 g/kg/d) compared to those with high protein intake (>1.0 g/kg/d) exhibit weaker muscle strength upon ICU discharge and a slower recovery rate to independent walking before hospital discharge.[26]

Whether the protein targets set by the ASPEN and ESPEN guidelines are essential or a slightly lower target can be pursued remains a question. A recent meta-analysis of Lee and colleagues showed that a protein dosage of 0.9 g/kg compared to 1.3 g/kg during critical illness did not improve clinical or patient-centered outcomes.[27] Thus, a minimum daily intake of 0.9 to 1.0 g/kg should be targeted, as a lower protein intake may harm ICU patients.

ARE HIGHER PROTEIN TARGETS NEEDED?

Recent research has extensively investigated attaining higher protein targets in critically ill patients. A recent update of Lee and colleagues's meta-analysis included 23 randomized controlled trials (RCTs) comparing protein delivery of 0.92 g/kg/day to 1.49 g/kg/day.[28] They found higher protein delivery was not associated with overall mortality rates or other clinical outcomes. Another meta-analysis from Ruijven and colleagues[29] conducted in 2023 compared 29 studies of all designs of ICU patients with protein intakes of $\geq$1.2 g/kg compared to <1.2 g/kg. Protein intakes greater than 1.2 g/kg improved nitrogen balance, resulted in short-run muscle mass changes, and likely reduced 60-day mortality.[29] However, no differences were found in other clinical endpoints such as ICU and hospital mortality, 6-month mortality, ICU and hospital length of stay, duration of mechanical ventilation, gastrointestinal symptoms, overall infections, physical performance, and psychological status.[29] The EFFORT trial is a recent trial investigating higher protein doses.[30] This study was conducted in 85 ICUs across 16 countries in which mechanically ventilated patients were randomly assigned to receive either a high dose of protein ($\geq$2.2 g/kg per day) or a usual dose of protein ($\leq$1.2 g/kg per day). The actual mean intake of patients was 1.6 g/kg in the high-dose group and 0.9 g/kg in the usual-dose group. The results showed no significant difference in time to discharge from the hospital or 60-day mortality between the high-dose and the usual-dose protein groups. Post-hoc analysis revealed that higher protein doses did not improve clinical outcomes in obese patients (>30 kg/m^2), including those with nutritional or frailty risk.[31] Additionally, high-protein treatment, with or without pre-existing malnutrition, was not associated with time to discharge alive.[32]

The potential harm of high protein intake emerges from one of the post-hoc analyses of the aforementioned NEED trial,[24] indicating that both the low protein intake cohort (mean 0.38 g/kg) and the high-protein intake cohort (mean 1.68 g/kg) exhibited elevated 28-day mortality rates in comparison to the medium protein intake cohort (mean 0.8 g/kg).[33] Subsequent adjustment for energy intake suggests that this association remains significant solely within the high-protein intake group.[33] The recently published PRECISe trial, a double-blind, multicenter, randomized controlled study, compared higher enteral protein intake (2.0 g/kg per day) to standard protein intake (1.3 g/kg per day) in mechanically ventilated, critically ill patients.[34] The primary outcome, measured using the EuroQol 5-Dimension 5-level (EQ-5D-5 L) health utility score over 180 days post-randomization, showed a lower health-related quality of life in the high-protein group compared to the standard-protein group. Additionally, post-hoc analysis revealed a significant increase in time-to-discharge-alive for patients receiving high protein compared to those on standard protein. Based on the current body of conducted studies, it appears undesirable to aim for the higher end of the ASPEN guidelines. It may be more prudent to adhere to the lower end of the ASPEN and ESPEN guidelines (**Fig. 1**).

COMBINED ROLE FOR PROTEINS AND PHYSICAL EXERCISE?

Furthermore, a growing interest is in integrating protein intake and physical exercise programs. An extensive systematic review and meta-analysis in non-critically ill adult patients demonstrated that the effectiveness of protein supplementation to increase lean body mass diminished once intake exceeded 1.3 g/kg body weight per day.[35] However, resistance training significantly mitigated this decline.[35] Similarly, positive outcomes have been observed in critically ill patients.[28] The impact of protein intake on early physical rehabilitation in critically ill patients is investigated in the meta-analysis by Lee and colleagues,[28] showing from small studies that there is no difference in overall mortality. However, a trend is observed toward improved self-reported quality of life and physical function at day 90. The ExPrES study[36] implemented a combined mobility and strength rehabilitation program, neuromuscular electrical stimulation, and high-protein dietary supplements (prescription 1.75 g/kg/ day) and compared it to standardized ICU care. This combined program reduced

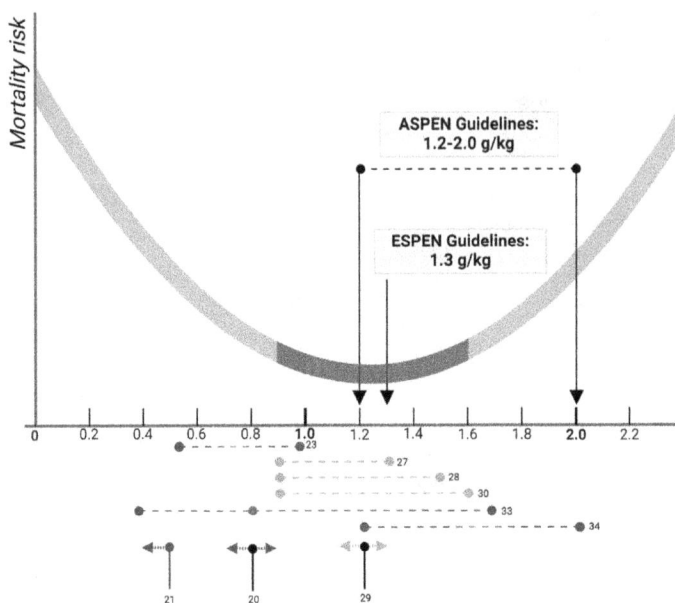

Fig. 1. Suggested protein dosage range for critically ill patients. Based on the limited studies conducted, the figure suggests a safe range of achievable protein goals in critically ill patients. Achieving a protein intake between 0.9 and 1.6 g/kg/day is advisable, additional caution should be exercised with high-protein doses in patients with high disease acuity (Sequential Organ Failure Assessment [SOFA]>9) and acute kidney injury without renal replacement therapy. A dashed line between 2 dots signifies a comparison between the 2 protein doses represented by the dots. A single dot with arrows pointing both left and right indicates a comparison between a lower (*arrow pointing left*) or higher (*arrow pointing right*) dose than the dose indicated by the dot. Red indicates a higher mortality rate, green indicates a lower mortality rate, and orange indicates an equal mortality rate. The numbers below the graph correspond to the reference numbers. Although mortality was not the primary outcome in the PRECISe trial, it was included in the figure, as preplanned sensitivity and exploratory analyses showed an elevated hazard ratio for overall mortality (1.24, 95% CI 0.99–1.55; $P = .063$) in the high-protein group.[34] (Created with BioRender.com.)

lower extremity muscle loss, but there were no differences in length of stay or mortality. Combining protein intake with physical activity yields benefits, although this area remains under-researched to date.

TIMING OF PROTEIN INTAKE

In addition to focusing on protein dosage, the optimal timing of protein supplementation for critically ill patients is becoming increasingly relevant. Early commencement of nutrition is beneficial for the critically ill patient. Starting with early enteral nutrition within 3 days of mechanical ventilation is associated with reduced hospital mortality, increased likelihood of discharge to home, decreased ICU and hospital length of stay, and mechanical ventilation duration.[37] This effect also applies to the early introduction of proteins, as evidenced by a retrospective study demonstrating that early administration of protein (>0.7 g/kg/day) was associated with improved survival compared to patients who achieved less than 0.7 g/kg/day in the first 3 days.[38] However, a randomized controlled trial (RCT) of ICU patients (EAT-ICU RCT) assigned to either early goal-directed nutrition or standard care, with increased protein intake from 0.5 g/kg/day to 1.47 g/kg/day, found no difference in physical quality of life at 6 months.[39] In addition, there were no discernible differences in other clinical outcomes, including mortality, incidence of organ failure, intensive care unit infections, length of ICU or hospital stay, or days alive without life support.[39]

Early administration of an excessive amount of protein may also be harmful. The recently conducted RCT NUTRIREA-3[40] found that for patients receiving invasive mechanical ventilation and vasopressor support for shock, early nutrition (within 24 hours after intubation) with low calorie and protein intake (energy 6 kcal/kg/day and protein 0.2 g/kg/day) was associated with a shorter duration of invasive mechanical ventilation and fewer gastrointestinal and hepatic complications compared to standard calorie and protein intake (energy 25 kcal/kg/day and protein 1.0–1.3 g/kg/day), without difference in all-cause mortality. Although difficult to ascertain, the observed differences in favor of early calorie-protein restriction group could be attributed to the possible harmful effect of high dose of proteins and energy administration in the usual care group. A systematic review showed the lack of benefit of early parenteral nutrition for critically ill patients.[41] This finding was further illustrated by the randomized multicenter ePANIC trial, which found that early parenteral nutrition (<48 hours after ICU admission) was associated with delayed recovery and more complications compared to late initiation (>8 days).[42] A post-hoc analysis of the EPaNIC revealed that delayed recovery might be associated with cumulative protein/amino acid dose administered early during the ICU stay rather than cumulative glucose dose.[43] Another post-hoc analysis of the EPaNIC trial suggests that early parenteral nutrition led to increased suppression of autophagy and an increased risk of weakness.[44] Tentative conclusions can be drawn that proteins may also play a role in suppressing autophagy, and caution may be warranted regarding excessive protein doses in the early stages of critical illness. This time-dependent effect of protein is also found in other studies. The aforementioned PROTINVENT study shows that the lowest 6-month mortality occurred when protein intake was increased from less than 0.8 g/kg/day on days 1 to 2 to 0.8 to 1.2 g/kg/day on days 3 to 5 and above 1.2 g/kg/day after day 5.[20] In another retrospective study of mechanically ventilated patients, early high (>1.2 g/kg/day) and late low (<0.8 g/kg/day) protein intakes were associated with higher 6-month mortality compared with low and high intakes, respectively, in non-sepsis patients but not in sepsis patients.[45] Based on recent studies, it is increasingly recognized that while the early introduction of protein after ICU admission is crucial, there is a growing emphasis on gradually increasing protein intake over the first days.[4,46,47]

TOWARD INDIVIDUALIZED PROTEIN STRATEGIES

Personalized nutrition therapy has emerged as a promising strategy to avoid a one-size-fits-all approach (**Fig. 2**).[48] Basing protein intake on actual total body weight, as recommended in the guidelines, is debatable, as there are differences in lean body mass between patients with the same body weight.[49] This assumption is evidenced by the finding that early high protein intake (1.2 g/kg/day) was associated with lower mortality in critically ill patients with low skeletal muscle area and density but not in patients with normal skeletal muscle area on admission.[50] Phenotyping becomes crucial when dosing nutritional proteins for critically ill patients who are not at their ideal weight. Body composition makers like lean body mass (LBM) or fat-free-mass (FFM) could be utilized for protein dosing instead of actual body weight.[51] Body composition can be estimated through computed tomography (CT) scans, muscle ultrasound, and bioelectric impedance analyses. In the absence of these

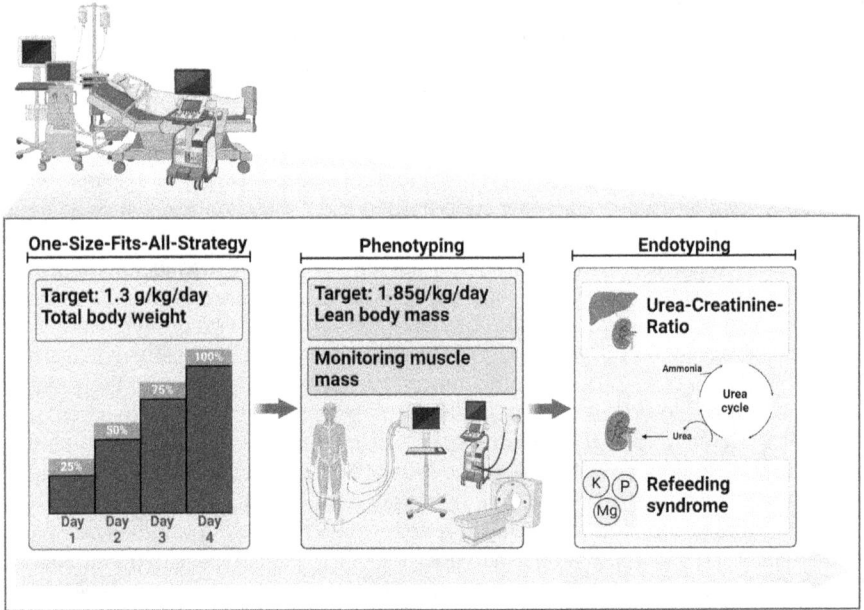

Fig. 2. A shift away from a one-size-fits-all approach to personalized nutrition. Personalized nutrition therapy represents an alternative to the one-size-fits-all approach, which typically involves basing protein dosing on total body weight and gradually increasing intake. Phenotyping involves thoroughly considering body composition, allowing protein dosing based on lean body mass. Additionally, it is crucial to monitor muscle mass using tools such as bioimpedance analysis, ultrasound, or CT scan. Endotyping also plays a significant role in identifying the stage of critical illness via monitoring the urea-creatinine ratio and detecting the occurrence of refeeding syndrome expressed by refeeding hypophosphatemia. (Created with BioRender.com.)

methods, a formula that tends to overestimate LBM or FFM is preferred to minimize the risk of underdosing.[4,49] Meeting FFM-based protein targets (1.85 g/kg FFM/day) has reduced mortality rates for critically ill coronavirus disease 2019 patients.[52] The current guidelines do not recommend basing the protein target on individualised body composition. Nevertheless, the ESPEN guidelines recommend that protein supplementation monitoring be based on urinary nitrogen losses or lean body mass for specific patient groups, such as obese hospitalized patients.[4]

In addition to body composition, other factors must be considered when determining the appropriate protein dose for critically ill patients. The ESPEN and ASPEN guidelines already include adjusted targets for elderly, obese, trauma, burn, and acute kidney injury (AKI) patients. However, limited RCT data are available on dosages.[3,4,53] Previously, it was stated that there was no justification for reducing protein targets in patients with AKI to prevent elevated urea levels.[53] However, a recent meta-analysis has shown that higher protein intake (mean 1.49 g/kg) compared to lower protein intake (mean 0.92 g/kg) was associated with higher mortality in critically ill patients with AKI.[27] In the EFFORT trial, higher doses of protein were shown to be harmful to patients with AKI and higher organ failure scores (Sequential Organ Failure Assessment [SOFA] score ≥ 9) at baseline on both time-to-discharge-alive and 60-day mortality.[30] This suggests that high-protein dosing in AKI patients should be evaluated carefully, particularly if kidney replacement therapy is not used, as continuous renal replacement therapy (CRRT) seems to abolish the adverse effects.[54] In the case of CRRT, providing 10 to 20 g more protein to compensate for the amino acids lost through the membrane during ultrafiltration is advised.[53,55] For patients with burns and trauma, the ESPEN guidelines[4] recommend additional doses of glutamine (GLN) for the first 5 days of enteral nutrition. This is advised to reduce infection risk in burn patients[56] and compensate for the additional protein loss in trauma patients.[57] However, a recent large RCT has shown no benefit of glutamine in burn patients.[58] For this reason, the ESPEN guidelines will be updated, and changes in recommendations for GLN may be expected.[59]

Protein targets during ICU stay should also be adjusted according to the stage of critical illness. Endotyping can assist in this process by mapping disease-related mechanisms and metabolic biomarkers to determine the body's ability to process proteins. Growing evidence shows that metabolic phenotyping pathways in critically ill patients can exhibit disturbances in specific amino acid pathways.[60] Excess amino acids administered are converted into ammonia in the liver, which is then converted into urea for excretion. The urea-creatinine ratio (UCR) may reflect whether amino acids are being utilized for muscle protein synthesis, oxidized for energy, or metabolized into urea.[48] In the randomized controlled REDOXS trial, it was found that high-dose glutamine was associated with higher mortality rates among critically ill patients with multiple organ failure.[61] The recent post-hoc analyses revealed that catabolic phenotypes, as indicated by an increased UCR, were correlated with an increased risk of death during extended ICU stays.[62] The adverse effects of administering high-dose glutamine in the REDOXS study were mainly seen among patients with high UCR.[62] Furthermore, the association of UCR with mortality was also identified from a reanalysis of the EFFORT trial.[63] Elevated risk of death was observed among patients who received higher protein doses when UCR was higher in the first week of ICU stay, reflecting the inability to utilize proteins (anabolic resistance).[63] The UCR presents a promising marker of catabolism and a potential target for adjusting protein targets.[62] In addition, monitoring the occurrence of refeeding syndrome (eg, by monitoring phosphate levels) during critical illness is recommended in the ESPEN guideline.[4,5] A high-protein dose in patients with refeeding hypophosphatemia, rather than carbohydrate or lipid dose, during the first 3 days of ICU admission was associated with higher 6-month mortality.[64] Thirdly, monitoring the nitrogen balance, which indicates the balance between protein consumption and excretion (mainly via urinary urea), can be a helpful approach.[51,65]

It is necessary to move away from protein dosing based solely on total body weight and emphasize the importance of phenotyping, for example, bedside bioelectrical impedance analysis (BIA)-derived body composition (LBM or FFM) and endotyping using metabolic biomarkers, such as UCR, to transition toward a personalized protein strategy.[48]

PROTEINS IN POST-INTENSIVE CARE UNIT PATIENTS

There are no formal recommendations or guidelines regarding protein intake for post-ICU patients at this stage. However, considering the average post-ICU patient is older and frail, previous literature suggests an intake of 1.5 to 2.5 g/kg/day due to higher anabolic thresholds for protein synthesis (anabolic resistance).[47] Adequate protein intake remains important after critical illness, as patients may experience persistent weight loss up to 3 months after ICU admission.[66] A recent review shows that in patients discharged from the ICU and given solely oral nutrition on the regular ward, only 27% to 74% of their protein goals were achieved,[67] contributing to the already emerging protein deficit during ICU admission. Furthermore, the ordered proteins may occasionally fail to accurately reflect the actual intake. The PROSPECT-I study revealed that post-ICU patients ordered less protein than recommended but also consumed less protein than they ordered after removal of the feeding tube.[68] The findings from Mitchell and colleagues corroborate that protein goals are not met after ICU discharge. However, their study demonstrates that these goals can be significantly improved by using high-protein enteral formulas and protein supplements.[69] High-protein oral supplements containing beta-hydroxy-beta-methylbutyrate (HMB) also reduced 90-day mortality for malnourished older adults (>65 years).[70] Beyond nutritional support, there is growing interest in combined physical and nutritional rehabilitation programs. A combined study offering physical and nutritional rehabilitation to post-ICU patients showed no significant difference in physical function or health-related quality of life compared to usual care.[71] Conversely, a rehabilitation program combined with an amino acid supplement drink improved physical recovery.[72] Also, in elderly patients, combining collagen peptide and resistance training improved body composition by increasing fat-free mass and muscle strength.[73] The limited number of studies highlights the ongoing need for research on nutritional interventions in post-ICU patients.[74]

UPCOMING PROTEIN STUDIES IN INTENSIVE CARE UNIT PATIENTS

The TARGET Protein Trial[75] investigates the impact of increasing dietary protein in ICU patients using a double cross-over design in 8 ICUs in Australia and New Zealand. It aims to determine if higher protein enteral nutrition (1.2–2.0 g/kg/day) improves patient outcomes compared to standard practice, with primary outcome assessment focusing on days free of the index hospital and survival at day 90. The EFFORT-X trial[76] is a 2-arm, parallel-group, RCT investigating the effect of a combined high-protein diet and early resistance exercise intervention compared to usual care in mechanically ventilated critically ill patients. The primary focus is to assess the impact of this intervention on muscle mass, quality, and strength. Additionally, the trial will evaluate clinical outcomes, functional capacity, and health-related quality of life in this patient population. The NEXIS trial[77] is a multicenter, RCT that compares the effects of a combined intervention of intravenous amino acid supplementation and in-bed cycle ergometry exercise with usual care in critically ill patients suffering from acute respiratory failure who require mechanical ventilation in an ICU. The Amino Acid Nutrition in the Critically-ill (AA-ICU) study[78] investigates if providing intravenous amino acids to ICU patients can improve their metabolic state.

UPCOMING PROTEIN STUDIES IN POST INTENSIVE CARE UNIT PATIENTS

The INTENT trial[79] has been conducted in 23 hospitals across Australia and New Zealand. It examines the feasibility and efficacy of a comprehensive whole-hospital nutrition intervention compared to standard care in critically ill patients. The primary outcome evaluation focuses on daily energy delivery from nutrition therapy, while secondary outcomes include factors such as duration of ventilation, bloodstream infection rate, and length of hospital stay. The CONFUCIUS trial[80] investigates whether a daily protein supplement for 6 weeks post-ICU improves physical function in ICU patients with moderate ICU-acquired weakness, compared to a control isocaloric control group.

The new studies on high protein intake versus standard intake during ICU stay and after ICU discharge will give us better insight into the optimal protein dose during the initial phase in ICU and recovery.

SUMMARY

The stated objectives of ESPEN and ASPEN are frequently not being met in practice. Failure to meet the targets may have adverse consequences for critically ill patients. Trials that have used higher protein doses than the current targets have not shown beneficial effects on relevant clinical endpoints. Additionally, this approach may negatively impact quality of life,[34] and in patients with high disease acuity (SOFA score >9) and AKI without renal replacement therapy, it could increase the risk of mortality.[30,54] Based on recent studies, the authors recommend a protein intake of 1.3 g/kg/day (range 1.0–1.5 g/kg/day). Timing is also essential and protein intake should be gradually increased during the first 4 to 5 days after ICU admission. Personalized protein dosing based on phenotyping and endotyping could help to optimize nitrogen balance, prevent muscle wasting, and improve clinical outcomes in critically ill patients[48] while avoiding the detrimental effects of excessive protein intake. Muscle ultrasound or BIA measurements during ICU stay could help monitor individual high-risk patients. In addition, future studies should indicate whether dosing based on fat-free mass is better than dosing based on total body weight. In post-ICU patients, nutritional trials are warranted to address optimal targets and ways to better meet the targets set. More research could be performed on the combined effect of protein and exercise programs.

CLINICS CARE POINTS

- Recent trials have indicated that recommending a protein intake below 0.9 g/kg/day or above 1.6 g/kg/day is not advisable. However, it is crucial to ensure that the optimal protein target is achieved. The results of ongoing trials will inform the need to adjust the current guidelines.

- It is important to note that critically ill patients may experience adverse effects if their protein intake falls below the recommended targets or is markedly above the targets. A more U-shaped association between protein dose and outcome is likely. Moreover, it is challenging for critically ill patients to meet these recommendations and keep them in the safe zone.

- Given proteins' time-dependent effect on outcomes, it can be recommended that protein intake be gradually increased during the first 4 to 5 days. Subsequently, efforts should be made to meet the recommended targets, with close monitoring to ensure goal attainment.

- Rather than a uniform approach, a more effective strategy would be to employ a personalized protein dosing regimen based on phenotyping and endotyping. This approach should consider several factors, including body composition, monitoring parameters (UCR), and the occurrence of refeeding syndrome (phosphate). Concerning individualized protein dosing, a daily protein intake of 1.85 g/kg FFM may be considered after the progression phase.

- It is evident that nutritional intervention studies for patients who have undergone ICU treatment are warranted to find the optimal target and ways to improve the attainment of nutritional goals.

DISCLOSURES

Prof. Dr A.R H. van Zanten reported receiving honoraria for advisory board meetings, lectures, research, and travel expenses from AOP Pharma, Abbott, Baxter, Cardinal Health, Danone-Nutricia, DIM3, Dutch Medical Food, Fresenius Kabi, GE Healthcare, InBody, Mermaid, Rousselot, and Lyric. The other author has nothing to declare.

REFERENCES

1. Puthucheary ZA, Rawal J, McPhail M, et al. Acute skeletal muscle wasting in critical illness. JAMA 2013;310(15):1591–600.
2. McClave SA, Taylor BE, Martindale RG, et al. Guidelines for the provision and assessment of nutrition support therapy in the adult critically ill patient: Society of Critical Care Medicine (SCCM) and American Society for Parenteral and Enteral Nutrition (ASPEN). JPEN J Parenter Enteral Nutr 2016;40(2):159–211.
3. Compher C, Bingham AL, McCall M, et al. Guidelines for the provision of nutrition support therapy in the adult critically ill patient: the American Society for Parenteral and Enteral Nutrition. JPEN J Parenter Enteral Nutr 2022;46(1):12–41.
4. Singer P, Blaser AR, Berger MM, et al. ESPEN guideline on clinical nutrition in the intensive care unit. Clin Nutr 2019;38(1):48–79.
5. Singer P, Blaser AR, Berger MM, et al. ESPEN practical and partially revised guideline: clinical nutrition in the intensive care unit. Clin Nutr 2023;42(9): 1671–89.
6. O'Keefe GE, Shelton M, Qiu Q, et al. Increasing enteral protein intake in critically ill trauma and surgical patients. Nutr Clin Pract 2019;34(5):751–9.
7. van Zanten AR, Petit L, De Waele J, et al. Very high intact-protein formula successfully provides protein intake according to nutritional recommendations in overweight critically ill patients: a double-blind randomized trial. Crit Care 2018;22:1–12.
8. Lee-anne SC, Deane AM, Heyland DK, et al. Energy and protein deficits throughout hospitalization in patients admitted with a traumatic brain injury. Clin Nutr 2016;35(6):1315–22.
9. Alberda C, Gramlich L, Jones N, et al. The relationship between nutritional intake and clinical outcomes in critically ill patients: results of an international multicenter observational study. Intensive Care Med 2009;35:1728–37.
10. Peterson SJ, Tsai AA, Scala CM, et al. Adequacy of oral intake in critically ill patients 1 week after extubation. J Am Diet Assoc 2010;110(3):427–33.
11. Heyland DK, Dhaliwal R, Wang M, et al. The prevalence of iatrogenic underfeeding in the nutritionally 'at-risk'critically ill patient: results of an international, multicenter, prospective study. Clin Nutr 2015;34(4):659–66.
12. Nicolo M, Heyland DK, Chittams J, et al. Clinical outcomes related to protein delivery in a critically ill population: a multicenter, multinational observation study. JPEN J Parenter Enteral Nutr 2016;40(1):45–51.
13. Song JH, Lee HS, Kim SY, et al. The influence of protein provision in the early phase of intensive care on clinical outcomes for critically ill patients on mechanical ventilation. Asia Pac J Clin Nutr 2017;26(2):234–40.
14. Zusman O, Theilla M, Cohen J, et al. Resting energy expenditure, calorie and protein consumption in critically ill patients: a retrospective cohort study. Crit Care 2016;20:1–8.
15. Weijs PJ, Looijaard WG, Beishuizen A, et al. Early high protein intake is associated with low mortality and energy overfeeding with high mortality in non-septic mechanically ventilated critically ill patients. Crit Care 2014;18:1–10.
16. Silvah JH, de Lima CMM, Nicoletti CF, et al. Protein provision and lower mortality in critically ill patients with COVID-19. Clin Nutr ESPEN 2021;45:507–10.
17. Tsai J-R, Chang W-T, Sheu C-C, et al. Adequacy of prescribed caloric and protein intake and reduction of mortality in critically ill patients with body mass indices< 30 kg/m2. Nutrition 2022;94:111529.

18. Ferrie S, Allman-Farinelli M, Daley M, et al. Protein requirements in the critically ill: a randomized controlled trial using parenteral nutrition. JPEN J Parenter Enteral Nutr 2016;40(6):795–805.
19. Nakanishi N, Matsushima S, Tatsuno J, et al. Impact of energy and protein delivery to critically ill patients: a systematic review and meta-analysis of randomized controlled trials. Nutrients 2022;14(22):4849.
20. Koekkoek WK, van Setten CC, Olthof LE, et al. Timing of PROTein INtake and clinical outcomes of adult critically ill patients on prolonged mechanical VENTilation: the PROTINVENT retrospective study. Clin Nutr 2019;38(2):883–90.
21. Zhong M, Qiu Y, Pan T, et al. Improving enteral nutrition tolerance and protein intake maybe beneficial to intensive care unit patients. Sci Rep 2023;13(1):21614.
22. Weijs PJ, Mogensen KM, Rawn JD, et al. Protein intake, nutritional status and outcomes in ICU survivors: a single center cohort study. J Clin Med 2019;8(1):43.
23. Hartl WH, Kopper P, Bender A, et al. Protein intake and outcome of critically ill patients: analysis of a large international database using piece-wise exponential additive mixed models. Crit Care 2022;26:1–12.
24. Ke L, Lin J, Doig GS, et al. Actively implementing an evidence-based feeding guideline for critically ill patients (NEED): a multicenter, cluster-randomized, controlled trial. Crit Care 2022;26(1):46.
25. Chen Y, Liu Z, Wang Q, et al. Enhanced exclusive enteral nutrition delivery during the first 7 days is associated with decreased 28-day mortality in critically ill patients with normal lactate level: a post hoc analysis of a multicenter randomized trial. Crit Care 2024;28(1):26.
26. Matsushima S, Yoshida M, Yokoyama H, et al. Effects on physical performance of high protein intake for critically ill adult patients admitted to the intensive care unit: a retrospective propensity-matched analysis. Nutrition 2021;91:111407.
27. Lee Z-Y, Yap CSL, Hasan MS, et al. The effect of higher versus lower protein delivery in critically ill patients: a systematic review and meta-analysis of randomized controlled trials. Crit Care 2021;25:1–15.
28. Lee Z-Y, Dresen E, Lew CCH, et al. The effects of higher versus lower protein delivery in critically ill patients: an updated systematic review and meta-analysis of randomized controlled trials with trial sequential analysis. Crit Care 2024;28(1):15.
29. van Ruijven IM, Abma J, Brunsveld-Reinders AH, et al. High protein provision of more than 1.2 g/kg improves muscle mass preservation and mortality in ICU patients: a systematic review and meta-analyses. Clin Nutr 2023;42(12):2395–403.
30. Heyland DK, Patel J, Compher C, et al. The effect of higher protein dosing in critically ill patients with high nutritional risk (EFFORT Protein): an international, multicentre, pragmatic, registry-based randomised trial. Lancet 2023;401(10376):568–76.
31. Tweel LE, Compher C, Bear DE, et al. A comparison of high and usual protein dosing in critically ill patients with obesity: a post hoc analysis of an international, pragmatic, single-blinded, randomized clinical trial. Crit Care Med 2024;52(4):586–95.
32. Lew CCH, Lee Z-Y, Day AG, et al. The association between malnutrition and high protein treatment on outcomes in critically ill patients: a post hoc analysis of the EFFORT protein randomized trial. Chest 2024;165(6):1380–91.
33. Lin J, Chen W, Ye X, et al. Trajectories of protein intake and 28-day mortality in critically ill patients: a secondary analysis of a cluster-randomized controlled trial. Clin Nutr 2022;41(8):1644–50.

34. Bels JLM, Thiessen S, van Gassel RJJ, et al. Effect of high versus standard protein provision on functional recovery in people with critical illness (PRECISe): an investigator-initiated, double-blinded, multicentre, parallel-group, randomised controlled trial in Belgium and The Netherlands. Lancet 2024;404(10453): 659–69. https://doi.org/10.1016/s0140-6736(24)01304-7.

35. Tagawa R, Watanabe D, Ito K, et al. Dose–response relationship between protein intake and muscle mass increase: a systematic review and meta-analysis of randomized controlled trials. Nutr Rev 2021;79(1):66–75.

36. Verceles AC, Serra M, Davis D, et al. Combining exercise, protein supplementation and electric stimulation to mitigate muscle wasting and improve outcomes for survivors of critical illness—the ExPrES study. Heart Lung 2023;58:229–35.

37. Haines KL, Ohnuma T, Grisel B, et al. Early enteral nutrition is associated with improved outcomes in critically ill mechanically ventilated medical and surgical patients. Clin Nutr ESPEN 2023;57:311–7.

38. Bendavid I, Zusman O, Kagan I, et al. Early administration of protein in critically ill patients: a retrospective cohort study. Nutrients 2019;11(1):106.

39. Allingstrup MJ, Kondrup J, Wiis J, et al. Early goal-directed nutrition versus standard of care in adult intensive care patients: the single-centre, randomised, outcome assessor-blinded EAT-ICU trial. Intensive Care Med 2017;43:1637–47.

40. Reignier J, Plantefève G, Mira J-P, et al. Low versus standard calorie and protein feeding in ventilated adults with shock: a randomised, controlled, multicentre, open-label, parallel-group trial (NUTRIREA-3). Lancet Respir Med 2023;11(7): 602–12.

41. Bost RB, Tjan DH, van Zanten AR. Timing of (supplemental) parenteral nutrition in critically ill patients: a systematic review. Ann Intensive Care 2014;4:1–13.

42. Casaer MP, Mesotten D, Hermans G, et al. Early versus late parenteral nutrition in critically ill adults. N Engl J Med 2011;365(6):506–17.

43. Casaer MP, Wilmer A, Hermans G, et al. Role of disease and macronutrient dose in the randomized controlled EPaNIC trial: a post hoc analysis. Am J Respir Crit Care Med 2013;187(3):247–55.

44. Hermans G, Casaer MP, Clerckx B, et al. Effect of tolerating macronutrient deficit on the development of intensive-care unit acquired weakness: a subanalysis of the EPaNIC trial. Lancet Respir Med 2013;1(8):621–9.

45. de Koning MSLY, Koekkoek WAC, Kars JCN, et al. Association of protein and caloric intake and clinical outcomes in adult septic and non-septic ICU patients on prolonged mechanical ventilation: the PROCASEPT Retrospective Study. JPEN J Parenter Enteral Nutr 2020;44(3):434–43.

46. Koekkoek W, van Zanten A. Primum non nocere in early nutrition therapy during critical illness: balancing the pros and cons of early very high protein administration. Clin Nutr 2019;38(4):1963–4.

47. van Zanten ARH, De Waele E, Wischmeyer PE. Nutrition therapy and critical illness: practical guidance for the ICU, post-ICU, and long-term convalescence phases. Crit Care 2019;23:1–10.

48. van Zanten AR. Personalized nutrition therapy in critical illness and convalescence: moving beyond one-size-fits-all to phenotyping and endotyping. Curr Opin Crit Care 2023;29(4):281–5.

49. Moonen HP, Hermans AJ, Jans I, et al. Protein requirements and provision in hospitalised COVID-19 ward and ICU patients: agreement between calculations based on body weight and height, and measured bioimpedance lean body mass. Clin Nutr ESPEN 2022;49:474–82.

50. Looijaard WG, Dekker IM, Beishuizen A, et al. Early high protein intake and mortality in critically ill ICU patients with low skeletal muscle area and-density. Clin Nutr 2020;39(7):2192–201.
51. Wischmeyer PE, Bear DE, Berger MM, et al. Personalized nutrition therapy in critical care: 10 expert recommendations. Crit Care 2023;27(1):261.
52. Melchers M, Hermans AJH, Hulsen SB, et al. Individualised energy and protein targets achieved during intensive care admission are associated with lower mortality in mechanically ventilated COVID-19 patients: the COFEED-19 study. Clin Nutr 2023;42(12):2486–92.
53. Singer P. Protein metabolism and requirements in the ICU. Clin Nutr ESPEN 2020; 38:3–8.
54. Stoppe C, Patel JJ, Zarbock A, et al. The impact of higher protein dosing on outcomes in critically ill patients with acute kidney injury: a post hoc analysis of the EFFORT protein trial. Crit Care 2023;27(1):399.
55. Chua HR, Baldwin I, Fealy N, et al. Amino acid balance with extended daily diafiltration in acute kidney injury. Blood Purif 2012;33(4):292–9.
56. Lin J-J, Chung X-J, Yang C-Y, et al. A meta-analysis of trials using the intention to treat principle for glutamine supplementation in critically ill patients with burn. Burns 2013;39(4):565–70.
57. Cheatham ML, Safcsak K, Brzezinski SJ, et al. Nitrogen balance, protein loss, and the open abdomen. Crit Care Med 2007;35(1):127–31.
58. Heyland DK, Wibbenmeyer L, Pollack J, et al. A randomized trial of enteral glutamine for treatment of burn injuries. N Engl J Med 2022;387(11):1001–10.
59. van Zanten AR, Singer P. Response to letter to the editor clinical nutrition. Clin Nutr 2024;43(1):297.
60. Deutz NE, Singer P, Wierzchowska-McNew RA, et al. Comprehensive metabolic amino acid flux analysis in critically ill patients. Clin Nutr 2021;40(5):2876–97.
61. Heyland D, Muscedere J, Wischmeyer PE, et al. A randomized trial of glutamine and antioxidants in critically ill patients. N Engl J Med 2013;368(16):1489–97.
62. Haines RW, Fowler AJ, Wan YI, et al. Catabolism in critical illness: a reanalysis of the REducing Deaths due to OXidative Stress (REDOXS) Trial. Crit Care Med 2022;50(7):1072–82.
63. Haines RW, Prowle JR, Day A, et al. Association between urea trajectory and protein dose in critically ill adults: a secondary exploratory analysis of the effort protein trial (RE-EFFORT). Crit Care 2024;28(1):24.
64. Slingerland-Boot R, Rooijakkers E, Koekkoek K, et al. Macronutrient intake and outcomes of ICU patients with refeeding hypophosphatemia. Clin Nutr ESPEN 2023;55:191–9.
65. Kim TJ, Park S-H, Jeong H-B, et al. Optimizing nitrogen balance is associated with better outcomes in neurocritically ill patients. Nutrients 2020;12(10):3137.
66. Chapple L-AS, Deane AM, Williams LT, et al. Longitudinal changes in anthropometrics and impact on self-reported physical function after traumatic brain injury. Crit Care Resusc 2017;19(1):29–36.
67. Moisey LL, Merriweather JL, Drover JW. The role of nutrition rehabilitation in the recovery of survivors of critical illness: underrecognized and underappreciated. Crit Care 2022;26(1):270.
68. Slingerland-Boot R, van der Heijden I, Schouten N, et al. Prospective observational cohort study of reached protein and energy targets in general wards during the post-intensive care period: the PROSPECT-I study. Clin Nutr 2022;41(10): 2124–34.

69. Mitchell A, Clemente R, Downer C, et al. Protein provision in critically ill adults requiring enteral nutrition: are guidelines being met? Nutr Clin Pract 2019; 34(1):123–30.
70. Deutz NE, Matheson EM, Matarese LE, et al. Readmission and mortality in malnourished, older, hospitalized adults treated with a specialized oral nutritional supplement: a randomized clinical trial. Clin Nutr 2016;35(1):18–26.
71. Walsh TS, Salisbury LG, Merriweather JL, et al. Increased hospital-based physical rehabilitation and information provision after intensive care unit discharge: the RECOVER randomized clinical trial. JAMA Intern Med 2015;175(6):901–10.
72. Jones C, Eddleston J, McCairn A, et al. Improving rehabilitation after critical illness through outpatient physiotherapy classes and essential amino acid supplement: a randomized controlled trial. J Crit Care 2015;30(5):901–7.
73. Zdzieblik D, Oesser S, Baumstark MW, et al. Collagen peptide supplementation in combination with resistance training improves body composition and increases muscle strength in elderly sarcopenic men: a randomised controlled trial. Br J Nutr 2015;114(8):1237–45.
74. Latronico N, Herridge M, Hopkins RO, et al. The ICM research agenda on intensive care unit-acquired weakness. Intensive Care Med 2017;43:1270–81.
75. Summers MJ, Lee-anne SC, Bellomo R, et al. Study protocol for TARGET protein: the effect of augmented administration of enteral protein to critically ill adults on clinical outcomes: a cluster randomised, cross-sectional, double cross-over, clinical trial. Crit Care Resusc 2023;25(3):147–54.
76. ClinicalTrials.gov. The effect of high protein and early resistance exercise versus usual care in critically ill patients (EFFORT-X). Available at: https://classic.clinicaltrials.gov/ct2/show/NCT04261543.
77. Heyland DK, Day A, Clarke GJ, et al. Nutrition and Exercise in Critical Illness Trial (NEXIS Trial): a protocol of a multicentred, randomised controlled trial of combined cycle ergometry and amino acid supplementation commenced early during critical illness. BMJ Open 2019;9(7):e027893.
78. ClinicalTrials.gov. Amino acid nutrition in the critically-ill (AA-ICU). Available at: https://classic.clinicaltrials.gov/ct2/show/NCT02865408.
79. Ridley EJ, Bailey M, Chapman M, et al. Protocol summary and statistical analysis plan for Intensive Nutrition Therapy comparEd to usual care iN criTically ill adults (INTENT): a phase II randomised controlled trial. BMJ Open 2022;12(3):e050153.
80. Boelens YF, Strookappe B, Vasse E, et al. The effect of an intervention of porcine protein versus maltodextrin supplement on CONvalescence of FUnCtional outcomes after IcU Stay (CONFUCIUS): study protocol for a randomized controlled, single-center, double-blind trial. Clin Nutr ESPEN 2022;52:86–93.

Why One-Size-Fits-All Doesn't Work in Intensive Care Unit Nutrition?

Danielle E. Bear, PhD, MRes, BHealthSci (Nutr&Diet)[a,*],
Kate J. Lambell, PhD, MNutrDiet, BHSc, PhD[b],
Christian Stoppe, MD, PhD[c,d]

KEYWORDS

- Critical illness • Nutrition • Nutrition therapy • Energy • Protein • Biomarker

KEY POINTS

- Critically ill patients are heterogenous in terms of patient characteristics and clinical conditions, which may influence the response to nutrition therapy.
- Current trials of nutrition therapy do not adequately take into consideration important patient differences when calculating energy and protein targets, which may impact outcome.
- Biomarkers may provide a tool to monitor and individualize nutrition therapy in the future.

INTRODUCTION

Advances in medical treatment over the recent decades have led to increased rates of survival.[1] However, it is well documented that survival from critical illness is complicated by prolonged recovery periods, with persistent and potentially irreversible, physical, functional, and cognitive disability.[2] The myriad of features experienced by survivors of critical illness is termed 'Post-Intensive Care Syndrome', and nutrition therapy may play an important role in the prevention and management of this debilitating syndrome.[2]

The decline in mortality from critical illness has led to difficulties in demonstrating the impact of single interventions to alter this outcome.[3] This is particularly true for trials of nutrition therapy undertaken within the intensive care unit (ICU) and may have contributed to the neutral results of several large, randomized controlled trials (RCTs).[4–7] Importantly, harm from early enhanced nutrition and particular interventions

[a] Department of Nutrition & Dietetics, St Thomas' Hospital, Westminster Bridge Road, London SE1 7EH, UK; [b] Department of Nutrition and Dietetics, Alfred Health, Melbourne, Australia; [c] Department of Anaesthesiology, Intensive Care, Emergency and Pain Medicine, Universitätsklinikum Würzburg, Oberdürrbacher Str. 6, 97080 Würzburg, Germany; [d] Department of Cardiac Anesthesiology and Intensive Care Medicine, Charité Berlin, Berlin, Germany
* Corresponding author. Department of Nutrition and Dietetics, St Thomas' Hospital, 3rd Floor, B-Block South Wing, Westminster Bridge Road, London, SE1 7EH, UK
E-mail address: Danielle.Bear@gstt.nhs.uk
Twitter: @danni_dietitian (D.E.B.)

Crit Care Clin 41 (2025) 247–262
https://doi.org/10.1016/j.ccc.2024.09.008
criticalcare.theclinics.com
0749-0704/25/Crown Copyright © 2024 Published by Elsevier Inc. All rights reserved, including those for text and data mining, AI training, and similar technologies.

in certain subgroups of patients has also been demonstrated,[4,6,8] improving our understanding of the complexity of nutrition interventions. These results have encouraged the critical care nutrition community to reconsider the biological underpinnings of nutrition therapy in the critically ill to allow more individualized approaches and to shift focus toward more patient-centered outcomes, such as physical function and quality of life[9] whilst balancing these with the potential for harm.

Nutrition therapy is a complex intervention with several underlying considerations that may influence effectiveness which, although yet to be studied, underpin the rationale for more individualized interventions moving away from a 'one-size-fits-all' approach. Considerations include the mechanism of action of the intervention and the patient phenotype, including sex, ethnicity, body composition, and nutritional status.

This article will discuss the evidence underpinning the rationale for more individualized nutrition interventions in the critically ill, specifically considering the metabolic response to illness, energy and protein dosing, how body composition and nutritional status may influence nutrition prescription and interventions, and the role that biomarkers may play in the future.

MECHANISMS UNDERPINNING THE RATIONALE FOR INDIVIDUALIZED NUTRITION INTERVENTIONS IN THE CRITICALLY ILL

Critical illness is known to trigger inflammation, oxidative stress, and significant metabolic alterations, which frequently lead to alterations in energy expenditure, protein metabolism, and nutrient utilization.[10] These changes in metabolism can vary over the course of critical illness and may determine the patients' readiness to start feeding and tolerance to medical nutritional therapy. An inadequate consideration of the phases of illness and patients' inflammatory status have been discussed as potential explanations for the discrepancies between the neutral[5–7] or even harmful findings[4,8,11–13] in several multicenter RCTs and promising effects, which have been observed in smaller observational studies.[14,15] The individual metabolic demands during critical illness are known to be associated with muscle wasting, impaired immune function, and delayed wound healing,[16] indicating an urgent need to identify a 'metabolic trajectory' of individual patients, and to detect changes in metabolism that alter responsiveness to nutrition interventions. This conceptual framework can be expressed in terms of phases of critical illness and their potential impacts on metabolic homeostasis; for example, in the early acute phase, individual patients may fail to properly use dietary substrates for anabolic purposes. In this context, recent data indicated that patients displaying a high inflammatory status[17,18] or those with severe organ dysfunction do not benefit from, or even might be harmed by a nutrition therapy.[4,13,19] Further, nutrient availability or use can be altered by enteric absorption,[20,21] utilization,[22] and alterations in cellular adaptive processes such as autophagy.[23] Potential sources of variability include metabolic or even genetic drivers of disease susceptibility and progression, as well as the underlying etiology of illness (eg, surgery, trauma and sepsis) and severity of organ dysfunction,[24] which all needs better recognition in daily clinical practice. Guidelines emphasize the consideration of the different phases of critical illness and recommend a progressive and individualized nutrition strategy for critical illness,[25] yet it remains an ongoing challenge to transfer this theoretic model to clinical practice.

ENERGY EXPENDITURE AND DELIVERY

International guidelines for clinical nutrition in the ICU differ significantly in their recommendations for energy targets in early critical illness, with the European guidelines recommending hypocaloric feeding (<70% of measured target) in the first 72 hours of ICU admission (considered the early acute phase) with the aim of avoiding over-feeding, which may be exacerbated by the endogenous production of glucose in this early phase.[25] When following these guidelines, the balance between avoiding harm from overfeeding in the early phase needs to be balanced with the likely negative impact of prolonged underfeeding.[26] In contrast, the American guidelines recommend a range of energy targets (12–25 kcal/kg/day), but to advance toward goal as quickly as tolerated in patients at high nutrition risk.[27,28] These differences reflect the conflict-ing available evidence and highlight the complexities of providing a 'one-size-fits-all' approach.

Measuring energy expenditure using indirect calorimetry (IC) is recommended in both the European and American guidelines,[25,27] although this is not routinely used in clinical practice and instead clinicians often rely on predictive equations. In the absence of IC, predictive equations provide an estimate of energy expenditure and several equations have been developed for use in the critically ill.[29] The most com-mon equation used in clinical practice and in RCTs is a weight-based equation with 20 kcal/kg recommended in early acute critical illness, increasing to 25 kcal/kg following the acute phase.[25] Interestingly, there are no data detailing the initial devel-opment and validation of this equation for critically ill patients. Several issues are evident when considering the standardized use of a weight-based equation for all critically ill patients. First, energy expenditure is not static and will fluctuate over the course of ICU admission and recovery depending on the clinical condition of the patient.[30–32] Second, a majority of ICU patients will not have their weight measured on admission to the ICU, and estimations are often used. Further, skeletal muscle mass is the biggest driver of energy expenditure and level of muscularity is influenced by a range of factors, including age, sex, ethnicity, nutritional status, and level of physical activity.[33] Weight alone does not account for muscle mass, so using a basic weight-based equation will inevitably result in inaccuracies in pre-dicting the energy expenditure. No studies have investigated the most appropriate weight to use for patients, which may be problematic for those at the extreme ends of body mass index (BMI) categories (ie, underweight and obese),[34] meaning that standardization of the equation is impossible. It is therefore not surprising that the comparison of - based equations with measured energy expenditure leads to wide limits of agreement both during[29] and following an ICU admission.[35] Taking these points together, patients may remain on the same energy provision for the en-tirety of their ICU and hospital stay, which, hypothetically, may negatively impact their recovery.

Despite the limitations associated with using a weight-based predictive equation, studies on targeted nutrition based on measured energy expenditure using IC compared to 25 kcal/kg, have not shown benefits for outcomes such as infection rate, mortality, length of stay, and physical quality of life.[36–39] These studies highlight an important barrier to the consistent use of IC on a group and individual level, which is the exclusion associated with its use. For example, patients requiring high Fio_2, high positive end expiratory pressure and those with leaks via chest drains are all excluded from IC. Indeed, patients in the EAT-ICU trial had a median of only 2 measurements each for the duration of the trial.[38] Further, the tight calorie control study International was stopped short of the recruitment target because of slow recruitment as a result of lack of eligible patients due to IC exclusions.[37] This has also been demonstrated in a study of patients following ICU admission with lesser than 20% of eligible patients measured.[40] However, given the known inaccuracies with estimating energy expendi-ture using weight-based equations and clear fluctuations in energy expenditure over the course of illness and recovery (and likely corresponding energy under- and/or over-feeding), further research is warranted to determine the impact of using IC to target energy delivery across the continuum of care on both clinical and patient-centered outcomes.

Given the limitations associated with IC, most studies investigating the impact of hypocaloric or full energy provision on outcome in the critically ill have used various predictive equations including weight-based in various formats,[8,13] such as using corrected ideal body weight,[8] (Penn State and Ireton Jones).[5] Different patient groups have been studied over various durations and unsurprisingly, outcomes have varied between trials. Additionally, patients may be receiving differing amounts of nonnutritional calories from propofol, intravenous glucose and regional citrate anticoagulation, which all need to be considered within the context of an individualized nutrition intervention.

All of these factors provide a strong argument against using a one-size-fits-all approach for the calculation of energy expenditure and delivery of energy to patients both in and after an ICU admission. The use of IC should be considered where large errors in estimation are likely, such as in patients at the extremes of BMI. When IC is not available and predictive equations are used, consideration should be given to the time point in the ICU admission (eg, the phases of critical illness), individual patient characteristics (eg, severity of illness, how do they compare to those in published studies, BMI) and provision of nonnutritional calories (**Figs. 1** and **2**).

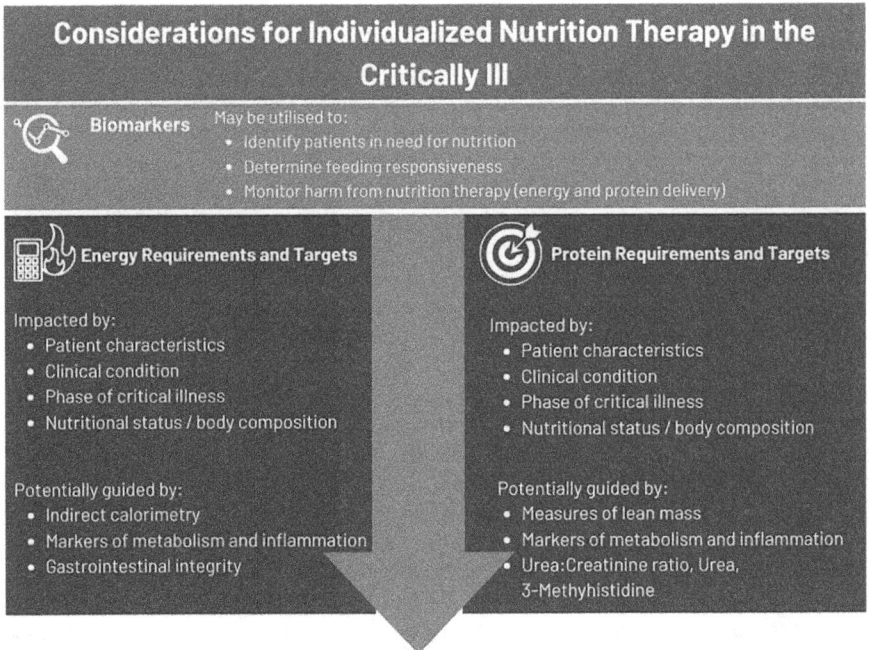

Fig. 1. Considerations for individualized nutrition therapy in the critically ill. This figure describes the potential role that biomarkers may play in the decision to start nutrition therapy, determine response to feeding and monitor harm when delivering energy and protein. It also describes the variables that may impact energy and protein requirements and targets and methods that may be used to guide these interventions.

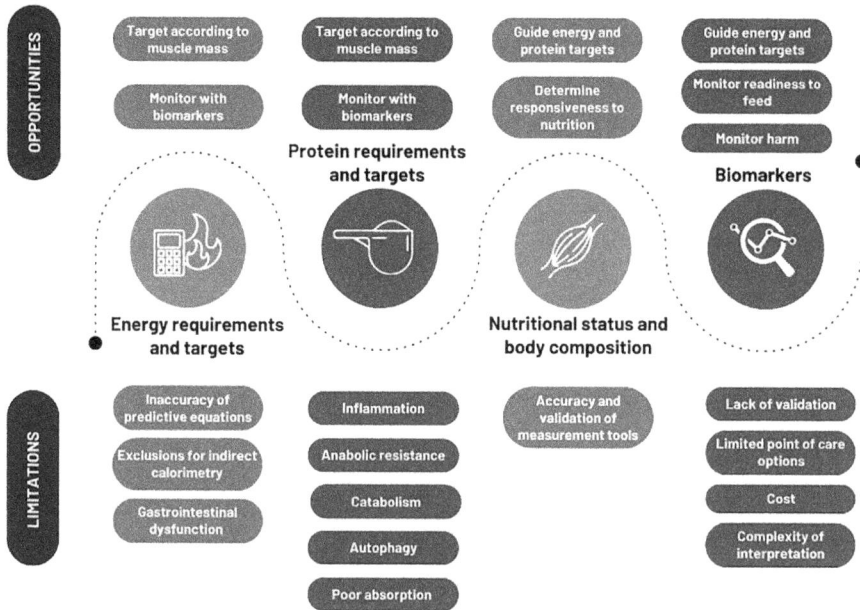

Fig. 2. Opportunities and limitations of individualized nutrition therapy. This figure describes the opportunities and limitations of individualizing protein and energy targets and using nutrition status, body composition, and biomarkers to guide individualized nutrition therapy.

PROTEIN TARGETS AND DELIVERY

Critically ill patients experience a profound loss of muscle mass,[41] which impacts negatively on their recovery.[42] Altered protein metabolism is evident resulting in a net catabolic balance.[41] Further, critically ill patients have 60% less uptake of protein into their muscle compared with healthy comparators.[22] Protein (amino acids) is essential to maintain the balance between muscle protein synthesis and muscle protein breakdown.[43] Protein is also essential for maintaining good health by optimizing body defense mechanisms. Therefore, it is reasonable to suggest that protein delivery is an important component of nutrition therapy both during and following critical illness.

Similar to energy expenditure, equations are used to estimate protein requirements in the critically ill. Given the alterations in protein homeostasis leading to increased muscle protein breakdown, it has generally been accepted that these patients have higher protein requirements than their healthy counterparts, with guidelines recommending between 1.3 to 2.0 g/kg/day depending on the phase of critical illness and clinical condition of the patients (eg, those requiring continuous renal replacement therapy or with burn injuries).[25,28] However, few RCTs have investigated the optimal protein dose in the critically ill and no evidence exists supporting the most appropriate weight to use when calculating the dose (eg, actual, ideal, or adjusted bodyweight).[34] Protein dosing is therefore also subject to inaccuracies associated with the lack of weights taken at ICU admission and during hospitalization, and patients may remain on the same dose for the duration of their admission. Further, using a calculation of lean mass rather than actual body weight to calculate protein dose has been suggested.[44]

Studies investigating different protein doses in the critically ill have, overall, shown no benefits on clinical outcomes, but there may be some benefit to higher doses on outcomes such as muscle mass,[45,46] especially when provided in conjunction with exercise interventions.[47] Acknowledgment must be given to the smaller sample size of studies investigating muscle mass as an outcome, and importantly, this benefit must be balanced with the potential harm on clinical outcomes demonstrated in recent large RCTs in certain subgroups of patients.[4,13,19] For example, the EFFORT Protein Trial, investigating greater than 2.2 g/kg/day versus lesser than 1.2 g/kg/day protein, in mechanically ventilated, nutritionally at-risk patients, found a longer time-to-discharge-alive and 60-day mortality in patients with acute kidney injury and higher organ failure at admission when receiving the higher protein dose.[4] This study underscores the importance of considering patient characteristics when determining protein dose in the critically ill as providing a one-size-fits-all dosing strategy may result in harm in some patients.

Although harm has been demonstrated in certain subgroups, patients who may benefit from higher protein doses are not yet evident. Although, those with additional protein losses, such as patients receiving continuous renal replacement therapy, with severe burn injuries, and/or with wounds[27,48] should be considered candidates for more individualized, higher protein strategies. Additionally, recent work has shown that sex differences may play a role in the metabolism of amino acids and future work should explore this further.[49]

The timing of different doses of protein may also be relevant when considering outcome. In a retrospective observational study, The PROTINVENT study found that low protein intake (<0.8 g/kg/day) before day 3 and high protein intake (>0.8 g/kg/day) after day 3 was associated with lower 6-month mortality.[50] The relevance and importance of the timing of protein delivery was confirmed recently in the NUTRIREA-3 RCT. NUTRIREA-3, investigating low versus standard calorie and protein feeding commenced within 24 hours of ICU admission and continued for 7 days (6 kcal/kg/day and 0.2–0.4 g/kg/day protein or 25 kcal/kg/day, and 1.0–1.3 g/kg/day protein) in ventilated adults with shock, found a 1-day shorter readiness to ICU discharge in the group receiving lower energy and protein targets.[13]

All of these studies point toward consideration of individualized approaches to protein dosing, but this is complicated by a lack of available assessment and monitoring tools (see **Figs. 1** and **2**). For example, there is currently no way to determine the point at which an 'anabolic switch' occurs, but biological markers such as Urea to Creatinine Ratio[51] and Urea levels[52] have been proposed and may provide a means to individualize the protein levels delivered and avoid harm. These will be discussed below.

WHAT ROLE DOES UNDERLYING NUTRITIONAL STATUS PLAY?

As stated earlier, within critically ill populations, there is significant heterogeneity in admission characteristics such as age, severity of illness, comorbidities, nutritional status, and body composition. Preexisting conditions such as malnutrition and obesity present different challenges, with both groups having complex metabolic requirements that require specific considerations in targeting and monitoring nutrition therapy.[25] It is evident that weight and BMI alone are poor indicators of nutritional status, and international clinical guidelines recommend that nutrition screening and a comprehensive nutrition assessment for those at high risk should be conducted early in the ICU admission;[25,53] ideally, this should include an assessment of body composition, which comes with its own challenges in the critically ill population, as will be discussed below.

Internationally, the reported prevalence of malnutrition in critically ill populations is highly variable, ranging from 38% to 78%.[54] The wide range in prevalence is, in part, because of the various populations studied and the use of different diagnostic tools. Key criterion in most malnutrition diagnostic methods involves an assessment of weight and diet history, nutrition impact symptoms, and muscle mass assessment (to identify muscle depletion).[55] However, obtaining an accurate history is often challenging in critically ill patients if they are sedated and mechanically ventilated. Furthermore, traditional methods of bedside muscle assessment (eg, subjective physical assessment, arm and calf circumference, and bioimpedance analysis) are not well validated to identify patients with lower-than-normal muscularity at ICU admission when compared with reference methods,[56] with fluid likely masking muscle depletion. Other methods such as computed tomography (CT) image analysis and ultrasound show promise to provide estimates of whole-body muscularity and to identify muscle depletion, although standardized assessment protocols and cutpoints are yet to be developed and cannot yet be recommended for use in routine clinical practice.[57]

Despite the challenges in performing a nutritional assessment in the ICU setting, an assessment of nutritional status using the information available (eg, weight, BMI, weight history, duration of admission, severity of illness, and age) along with a physical assessment is an important foundation and ongoing monitoring tool of individualized nutrition therapy and can help guide clinical judgment for nutrition practices that may be harmful (see **Figs. 1** and **2**). For example, patients that are premorbidly malnourished may be at risk of refeeding syndrome. Clinical guidelines recommend a progressive increase of nutrition in those who are severely malnourished on admission.[25] For patients presenting with refeeding hypophosphatemia (0.16 mmol/L), restricting energy delivery for 48 hours before increasing is recommended, along with close monitoring and replacement of electrolytes 2 to 3 times/day.[25] These recommendations are supported by an RCT in patients with hypophosphataemia, which showed protocoled caloric restriction for 48 hours improved survival.[58]

International clinical guidelines also recognize the impact that nutrition status may play on clinical outcomes, recommending consideration of early parenteral nutrition (before day 7) in patients who are malnourished or have low muscle mass.[28] However, there is a paucity of data to support these recommendations, with the American guidelines recommending that future studies include the Global Leadership Initiative of Malnutrition (GLIM) to diagnose malnutrition to facilitate meta-analysis and to measure the impact of nutrition interventions on clinical outcomes according to nutritional status.[28] One of the first studies to do this was a recent post hoc analysis of the EFFORT Protein trial, which investigated the association between malnutrition at ICU admission (using GLIM) and time-to-discharge alive, and whether high protein delivery influenced this association.[59] In the primary study, 1,301 patients were enrolled, and the average protein delivery in the high versus usual treatment groups was 1.6 g/kg per day vs 0.9 g/kg per day over the first 28 days of admission. The prevalence of preexisting malnutrition was 43.8% and this was independently associated with a slower time-to-discharge alive, but high protein delivery did not modify the association.[59] Only clinical outcomes were investigated in this study and the association between nutritional status, nutrition interventions, and outcomes such as muscle mass, physical function, and quality of life remain unknown. Indeed, critically ill patients demonstrate impaired ability for the body to use proteins for muscle protein synthesis and anabolic recovery in the context of inflammation as observed in recent mechanistic studies.[22] However, further powered studies are required to assess the impact of enhanced nutrition interventions on outcomes in patients with preexisting malnutrition and levels of obesity including whether these interventions prevent further progression of malnutrition and known associated outcomes.[54]

On the other end of the spectrum, the number of patients admitted to ICUs with obesity is increasing (prevalence of ~20% in ICUs internationally), and contributes to increased resource usage, with these patients often experiencing longer hospital length of stay and increased risk of respiratory and cardiovascular complications.[60] Obesity is associated with several other comorbidities including type 2 diabetes, cardiovascular diseases, dyslipidemia, fatty liver disease, mood disorders, and physical disabilities, all requiring consideration of these when planning nutrition interventions during critical illness.[60] There are conflicting recommendations in clinical guidelines for delivering nutrition to patients with obesity in critical illness, because of the limited and low-level evidence in this subpopulation. Specifically, the Americans recommend hypocaloric, high protein feeding,[53] and the Europeans recommend isocaloric, high protein feeding.[25] As described earlier, both guidelines acknowledge that estimation of energy expenditure is especially challenging in patients with obesity because of the difficulties assessing metabolically active tissue, and recommend using IC to target energy needs.[25,53] A recent systematic review demonstrated this, finding significant variation in measured energy expenditure (MEE) in patients with obesity admitted to ICU (range 12–32 kcal/kg).[61] Additionally, there was poor agreement between MEE and predicted energy requirements using clinical guideline recommendations, with predictive equations most commonly underestimating energy needs.[61] As such, wherever possible, it is important that clinicians prioritize the use of IC to target energy needs in patients with obesity and ensure appropriate monitoring for both under- and over-feeding with particular attention to biochemistry including blood glucose levels and triglycerides.[25,53] In terms of nutrition interventions in this population, few studies have been undertaken. In a post hoc analysis of the EFFORT Protein trial, higher protein doses did not improve clinical outcomes in patients with different levels of obesity.[62] However, similar to the discussion on malnutrition above, only clinical outcomes were investigated and the impact on muscle mass, physical function, and quality of life remain unknown.

CAN BIOMARKERS BE USED TO GUIDE INDIVIDUALIZED NUTRITION PRACTICE?

Biomarkers can be measured accurately and reproducibly and play a critical role as either prognostic, predictive, or diagnostic markers in clinical practice. Biomarkers may further reflect the effects of nutrient intake or a lack thereof and in certain cases, they can also act as an intermediate biomarker that reflect the biological response or which indicates intolerances or the potential risk of developing complications (**Table 1**). Whilst most markers remain either difficult to widely implement or have failed to fully reflect the biological mechanisms that predict susceptibility or physiologic responses to nutrition interventions,[63] understanding the relationship between measurable biological processes and clinical outcomes is vital to further individualize the nutrition therapy in critically ill patients.[64]

Several studies have appraised the clinical significance of different biomarkers in the field of ICU nutrition (see **Table 1**), whereas most studies are based on smaller and often single center studies, meaning no clear recommendations yet exist for daily use in critically ill patients. The measurement of muscle protein synthesis and breakdown currently reflects the most robust method to estimate the nutrient absorption in the body,[65] and an increase in protein balance and promotion of anabolism was demonstrated to be induced by energy intake and enteral feeding in critically ill patients.[66,67] However, this method is complex, costly, and impractical in clinical

Table 1
Biomarker candidates to guide individualized nutrition support in critically ill patients

	Biomarker	Description	Proposed Use and Considerations for Clinical Practice
Markers of inflammation	CRP, IL6	Clinical markers of inflammation.	May guide 'readiness to feed' or responsiveness to nutrition support. Not validated for this use.
	Albumin, preAlbumin	Negative acute-phase protein	Proposed maker of nutritional status. Has failed to identify patients who will benefit from nutrition support due to being a negative acute-phase protein.
Markers of metabolism	Nitrogen loss	Indicator for nitrogen/protein loss	Used to assess the net balance between protein intake and loss. Complex, costly and has inaccuracies in the critically ill.
	Blood Urea	End product of the breakdown of nitrogen compounds (eg, amino acids)	High levels may indicate those who will be harmed from high protein dose. Not yet prospectively validated.
	Triglycerides	Triglycerides are a type of fats or lipids that circulate in the blood. They are composed of glycerin and fatty acids.	Used to guide a parenteral nutritional strategy. May be influenced by propofol co-administration and inflammation.
	Phosphate	Important biological functions in the energy metabolism of cells.	Used to identify and direct up-titration of nutrition support in patients with refeeding syndrome
	Insulin resistance	Need for high insulin doses to maintain recommended target blood glucose levels	Used to evaluate the metabolic tolerance to feeding. Used in current clinical practice as a potential indicator of overfeeding.

(continued on next page)

Table 1
(continued)

	Biomarker	Description	Proposed Use and Considerations for Clinical Practice
Gastrointestinal integrity	i-FABP	Released when enterocyte integrity is lost	May detect acute intestinal ischemia and therefore likely nutrient absorption. Limited evidence to identify enteral nutrition failure
	D-la	D-la is produced by colonic bacteria such as *Escherichia coli*	May indicate mucosal injury and therefore nutrient absorption. Limited clinical studies performed to date
	Citrulline	May reflect enterocyte mass and function	Decreased levels may indicated gastrointestinal dysfunction Limited evidence to identify enteral nutrition failure
Others	3-methylhistidine	Indicates protelysis of myofibrils	May guide transition to anabolic state. Difficult to measure in routine clinical practice and limited studies performed to date
	Urea–Creatinine ratio	Potential biomarker of critical illness-associated catabolism	May indicate those who will be harmed from high protein dose and guide transition to anabolic state. Not yet prospectively validated

Abbreviations: CRP, C-reactive protein; IL6, interleukin-6.

practice. The calculation of nitrogen balance allows estimation about the net difference between protein synthesis and breakdown but demonstrated significant variability and limitations in critically ill patients.[68,69] The monitoring of catabolism in critically ill patients is further challenging as there is no routinely available biomarker with acceptable sensitivity and specificity. Among potential candidates, the assessment of circulating blood levels of 3-methylhistidine seems promising but extends beyond routine measurements.[70,71] More recently, the urea to creatinine ratio and urea have been proposed as potential biological signatures of harm from protein dose and may be able to detect the switch from catabolism to anabolism.[51,52] However, neither marker has been studied prospectively.

The use of albumin, prealbumin, retinal binding protein, transthyretin, and transferrin has been discussed as potential markers to characterize the nutritional status, substrate availability, and metabolism.[64,72–75] However, their use is limited by the negative impact of inflammation on blood levels, and their use has not been demonstrated to be specifically influenced by nutritional interventions.[76–78]

Biomarkers of gastrointestinal function such as Citrulline, D-lactate (D-la), and Intestinal fatty acid–binding protein (i-FABP) have also been tested to monitor the efficacy of nutrient delivery or absorption. However, they are costly to perform and limited evidence supports their clinical significance, therefore limiting their use in clinical practice.[79,80]

Table 1 provides an overview of proposed potential biomarkers to individualize nutrition support during critical illness and considerations for their use in clinical practice. Some of these markers are already frequently used in clinical practice, but prospective validations are missing.

In summary, biomarkers reflect the patients' metabolic response mechanisms and may help to identify patients that benefit from a nutritional intervention and guide the initiation and monitoring of nutritional support and tolerance. Especially in the complex setting of critical illness, biomarkers may support the assessment of nutritional status, to monitor metabolic processes, and guide interventions to further optimize patient outcomes (see **Figs. 1** and **2**). Point of care methods at the bedside, which allow a timely assessment of these markers, would further facilitate these more personalized nutritional interventions in the complex setting of critical care medicine.

SUMMARY

Critically ill patients display heterogenous characteristics, which may not lend themselves to a one-size-fits-all approach to nutrition therapy. This includes differences in clinical condition, age, sex, premorbid nutritional status, body composition, and individual biological responses to interventions. Individualizing elements of nutrition therapy such as energy and protein targets may provide benefits but have not yet been widely studied. Biomarkers may present an avenue for such individualization and should be explored.

CLINICS CARE POINTS

- Individualized nutrition therapy during critical illness may be important for improving clinical and functional outcomes.
- Preexisting nutrition status, phase of critical illness and severity of organ injury are important considerations for energy and protein dosing to prevent harm in the early phase of critical illness.

- Estimating energy targets has limitations that may lead to significant over or underfeeding of individual patients, but measuring energy expenditure in all patients is not possible.
- Protein dosing is limited by inaccurate estimations, anabolic resistance, and the potential for causing harm in certain patient subgroups with high doses.
- Biomarkers have the potential to guide nutrition therapy and enable more individualized approaches in daily clinical practice.

DISCLOSURES

D.E. Bear has received honoraria for speaking engagements from Fresenius Kabi and consulting fees from Nutricia and Baxter Healthcare. C. Stoppe received honoraria for speaking engagements and medical advisory board participation from BBRAUN, Baxter, and Fresenius. K.J. Lambell has no conflicts of interest.

REFERENCES

1. Herridge MS, Azoulay É. Outcomes after critical illness. N Engl J Med 2023; 388(10):913–24.
2. Needham DM, Davidson J, Cohen H, et al. Improving long-term outcomes after discharge from intensive care unit: report from a stakeholders' conference. Crit Care Med 2012;40(2):502–9.
3. Bear DE, Puthucheary ZA. Designing nutrition-based interventional trials for the future: addressing the known knowns. Crit Care 2019;23(1):53.
4. Heyland DK, Patel J, Compher C, et al. The effect of higher protein dosing in critically ill patients with high nutritional risk (EFFORT Protein): an international, multicentre, pragmatic, registry-based randomised trial. Lancet 2023;401(10376): 568–76.
5. Arabi YM, Aldawood AS, Haddad SH, et al. Permissive underfeeding or standard enteral feeding in critically ill adults. N Engl J Med 2015;372(25):2398–408.
6. Reignier J, Boisrame-Helms J, Brisard L, et al. Enteral versus parenteral early nutrition in ventilated adults with shock: a randomised, controlled, multicentre, open-label, parallel-group study (NUTRIREA-2). Lancet 2018;391(10116): 133–43.
7. Harvey SE, Parrott F, Harrison DA, et al. Trial of the route of early nutritional support in critically ill adults. N Engl J Med 2014;371(18):1673–84.
8. Casaer MP, Mesotten D, Hermans G, et al. Early versus late parenteral nutrition in critically ill adults. N Engl J Med 2011;365(6):506–17.
9. Davies TW, van Gassel RJJ, van de Poll M, et al. Core outcome measures for clinical effectiveness trials of nutritional and metabolic interventions in critical illness: an international modified Delphi consensus study evaluation (CONCISE). Crit Care 2022;26(1):240.
10. Dresen E, Pimiento JM, Patel JJ, et al. Overview of oxidative stress and the role of micronutrients in critical illness. JPEN J Parenter Enteral Nutr 2023;47(Suppl 1): S38–49.
11. Lamontagne F, Masse MH, Menard J, et al. Intravenous vitamin C in adults with sepsis in the intensive care unit. N Engl J Med 2022;386(25):2387–98.
12. Heyland D, Muscedere J, Wischmeyer PE, et al. A randomized trial of glutamine and antioxidants in critically ill patients. N Engl J Med 2013;368(16):1489–97.
13. Reignier J, Plantefeve G, Mira J-P, et al. Low versus standard calorie and protein feeding in ventilated adults with shock: a randomised, controlled, multicentre,

open-label, parallel-group trial (NUTRIREA-3). Lancet Respir Med 2023;11(7): 602–12.

14. Casaer MP, Van den Berghe G. Nutrition in the acute phase of critical illness. N Engl J Med 2014;370(25):2450–1.

15. Gunst J, Casaer MP, Preiser JC, et al. Toward nutrition improving outcome of critically ill patients: how to interpret recent feeding RCTs? Crit Care 2023;27(1):43.

16. van Gassel RJJ, Baggerman MR, van de Poll MCG. Metabolic aspects of muscle wasting during critical illness. Curr Opin Clin Nutr Metab Care 2020;23(2): 96–101.

17. Merker M, Felder M, Gueissaz L, et al. Association of baseline inflammation with effectiveness of nutritional support among patients with disease-related malnutrition: a secondary analysis of a randomized clinical trial. JAMA Netw Open 2020; 3(3):e200663.

18. Puthucheary ZA, Astin R, McPhail MJW, et al. Metabolic phenotype of skeletal muscle in early critical illness. Thorax 2018;73(10):926–35.

19. Stoppe C, Patel JJ, Zarbock A, et al. The impact of higher protein dosing on outcomes in critically ill patients with acute kidney injury: a post hoc analysis of the EFFORT protein trial. Crit Care 2023;27(1):399.

20. Chapman MJ, Fraser RJ, Matthews G, et al. Glucose absorption and gastric emptying in critical illness. Crit Care 2009;13(4):R140.

21. Ali Abdelhamid Y, Cousins CE, Sim JA, et al. Effect of critical illness on triglyceride absorption. JPEN J Parenter Enteral Nutr 2015;39(8):966–72.

22. Chapple LS, Kouw IWK, Summers MJ, et al. Muscle protein synthesis after protein administration in critical illness. Am J Respir Crit Care Med 2022;206(6): 740–9.

23. Vanhorebeek I, Casaer M, Gunst J. Nutrition and autophagy deficiency in critical illness. Curr Opin Crit Care 2023;29(4):306–14.

24. Zeisel SH. A conceptual framework for studying and investing in precision nutrition. Front Genet 2019;10:200.

25. Singer P, Blaser AR, Berger MM, et al. ESPEN practical and partially revised guideline: clinical nutrition in the intensive care unit. Clin Nutr 2023;42(9):1671–89.

26. Reintam Blaser A, Rooyackers O, Bear DE. How to avoid harm with feeding critically ill patients: a synthesis of viewpoints of a basic scientist, dietitian and intensivist. Crit Care 2023;27(1):258.

27. McClave SA, Taylor BE, Martindale RG, et al. Guidelines for the provision and assessment of nutrition support therapy in the adult critically ill patient: society of critical care medicine (SCCM) and American society for parenteral and enteral nutrition (A.S.P.E.N.). JPEN J Parenter Enteral Nutr 2016;40(2):159–211.

28. Compher C, Bingham AL, McCall M, et al. Guidelines for the provision of nutrition support therapy in the adult critically ill patient: the American Society for Parenteral and Enteral Nutrition. JPEN J Parenter Enteral Nutr 2022;46(1):12–41.

29. Zusman O, Kagan I, Bendavid I, et al. Predictive equations versus measured energy expenditure by indirect calorimetry: a retrospective validation. Clin Nutr 2019;38(3):1206–10.

30. Niederer LE, Miller H, Haines KL, et al. Prolonged progressive hypermetabolism during COVID-19 hospitalization undetected by common predictive energy equations. Clin Nutr ESPEN 2021;45:341–50.

31. Plank LD, Hill GL. Sequential metabolic changes following induction of systemic inflammatory response in patients with severe sepsis or major blunt trauma. World J Surg 2000;24(6):630–8.

32. Plank LD, Connolly AB, Hill GL. Sequential changes in the metabolic response in severely septic patients during the first 23 days after the onset of peritonitis. Ann Surg 1998;228(2):146–58.

33. Baumgartner RN, Waters DL, Gallagher D, et al. Predictors of skeletal muscle mass in elderly men and women. Mech Ageing Dev 1999;107(2):123–36.

34. Weijs PJ, Sauerwein HP, Kondrup J. Protein recommendations in the ICU: g protein/kg body weight - which body weight for underweight and obese patients? Clin Nutr 2012;31(5):774–5.

35. Rousseau AF, Fadeur M, Colson C, et al. Measured energy expenditure using indirect calorimetry in post-intensive care unit hospitalized survivors: a comparison with predictive equations. Nutrients 2022;14(19):3981.

36. Singer P, Anbar R, Cohen J, et al. The tight calorie control study (TICACOS): a prospective, randomized, controlled pilot study of nutritional support in critically ill patients. Intensive Care Med 2011;37(4):601–9.

37. Singer P, De Waele E, Sanchez C, et al. TICACOS international: a multi-center, randomized, prospective controlled study comparing tight calorie control versus Liberal calorie administration study. Clin Nutr 2021;40(2):380–7.

38. Allingstrup MJ, Kondrup J, Wiis J, et al. Early goal-directed nutrition versus standard of care in adult intensive care patients: the single-centre, randomised, outcome assessor-blinded EAT-ICU trial. Intensive Care Med 2017;43(11):1637–47.

39. Tatucu-Babet OA, Fetterplace K, Lambell K, et al. Is energy delivery guided by indirect calorimetry associated with improved clinical outcomes in critically ill patients? A systematic review and meta-analysis. Nutr Metab Insights 2020;13. 1178638820903295.

40. Ridley EJ, Parke RL, Davies AR, et al. What happens to nutrition intake in the post-intensive care unit hospitalization period? An observational cohort study in critically ill adults. JPEN J Parenter Enteral Nutr 2019;43(1):88–95.

41. Puthucheary ZA, Rawal J, McPhail M, et al. Acute skeletal muscle wasting in critical illness. JAMA 2013;310(15):1591–600.

42. Parry SM, El-Ansary D, Cartwright MS, et al. Ultrasonography in the intensive care setting can be used to detect changes in the quality and quantity of muscle and is related to muscle strength and function. J Crit Care 2015;30(5):1151, e9-14.

43. Atherton PJ, Smith K. Muscle protein synthesis in response to nutrition and exercise. J Physiol 2012;590(5):1049–57.

44. Wischmeyer PE, Bear DE, Berger MM, et al. Personalized nutrition therapy in critical care: 10 expert recommendations. Crit Care 2023;27(1):261.

45. Lee ZY, Dresen E, Lew CCH, et al. The effects of higher versus lower protein delivery in critically ill patients: an updated systematic review and meta-analysis of randomized controlled trials with trial sequential analysis. Crit Care 2024;28(1):15.

46. van Ruijven IM, Abma J, Brunsveld-Reinders AH, et al. High protein provision of more than 1.2 g/kg improves muscle mass preservation and mortality in ICU patients: a systematic review and meta-analyses. Clin Nutr 2023;42(12):2395–403.

47. Barth I, Beumeler LFE, Nahar-van Venrooij L, et al. The effect of protein provision and exercise therapy on patient-reported and clinical outcomes in intensive care unit survivors: a systematic review. J Hum Nutr Diet 2023;36(5):1727–40.

48. Singer P, Blaser AR, Berger MM, et al. ESPEN guideline on clinical nutrition in the intensive care unit. Clin Nutr 2019;38(1):48–79.

49. Deutz NEP, Singer P, Wierzchowska-McNew RA, et al. Females have a different metabolic response to critical illness, measured by comprehensive amino acid flux analysis. Metabolism 2023;142:155400.

50. Koekkoek W, van Setten CHC, Olthof LE, et al. Timing of PROTein INtake and clinical outcomes of adult critically ill patients on prolonged mechanical VENTilation: the PROTINVENT retrospective study. Clin Nutr 2019;38(2):883–90.
51. Haines RW, Fowler AJ, Wan YI, et al. Catabolism in critical illness: a reanalysis of the REducing deaths due to OXidative stress (REDOXS) trial. Crit Care Med 2022;50(7):1072–82.
52. Haines RW, Prowle JR, Day A, et al. Association between urea trajectory and protein dose in critically ill adults: a secondary exploratory analysis of the effort protein trial (RE-EFFORT). Crit Care 2024;28(1):24.
53. Taylor BE, McClave SA, Martindale RG, et al. Guidelines for the provision and assessment of nutrition support therapy in the adult critically ill patient: society of critical care medicine (SCCM) and American society for parenteral and enteral nutrition (A.S.P.E.N.). Crit Care Med 2016;44(2):390–438.
54. Lew CCH, Yandell R, Fraser RJL, et al. Association between malnutrition and clinical outcomes in the intensive care unit: a systematic review. JPEN J Parenter Enteral Nutr 2017;41(5):744–58 [Formula: see text].
55. Cederholm T, Jensen GL, Correia M, et al. GLIM criteria for the diagnosis of malnutrition - a consensus report from the global clinical nutrition community. Clin Nutr 2019;38(1):1–9.
56. Lambell KJ, Earthman CP, Tierney AC, et al. How does muscularity assessed by bedside methods compare to computed tomography muscle area at intensive care unit admission? A pilot prospective cross-sectional study. J Hum Nutr Diet 2021;34(2):345–55.
57. Paris M, Mourtzakis M. Assessment of skeletal muscle mass in critically ill patients: considerations for the utility of computed tomography imaging and ultrasonography. Curr Opin Clin Nutr Metab Care 2016;19(2):125–30.
58. Doig GS, Simpson F, Heighes PT, et al. Restricted versus continued standard caloric intake during the management of refeeding syndrome in critically ill adults: a randomised, parallel-group, multicentre, single-blind controlled trial. Lancet Respir Med 2015;3(12):943–52.
59. Lew CCH, Lee ZY, Day AG, et al. The association between malnutrition and high protein treatment on outcomes in critically ill patients: a post hoc analysis of the EFFORT protein randomized trial. Chest 2024;165(6):1380–91.
60. Schetz M, De Jong A, Deane AM, et al. Obesity in the critically ill: a narrative review. Intensive Care Med 2019;45(6):757–69.
61. Lambell KJ, Tatucu-Babet OA, Miller EG, et al. How do guideline recommended energy targets compare with measured energy expenditure in critically ill adults with obesity: a systematic literature review. Clin Nutr 2023;42(4):568–78.
62. Tweel LE, Compher C, Bear DE, et al. A comparison of high and usual protein dosing in critically ill patients with obesity: a post hoc analysis of an international, pragmatic, single-blinded, randomized clinical trial. Crit Care Med 2024;52(4):586–95.
63. Ware LB. Biomarkers in critical illness: new insights and challenges for the future. Am J Respir Crit Care Med 2017;196(8):944–5.
64. Stoppe C, Wendt S, Mehta NM, et al. Biomarkers in critical care nutrition. Crit Care 2020;24(1):499.
65. Millward DJ. Metabolic demands for amino acids and the human dietary requirement: millward and rRvers (1988) revisited. J Nutr 1998;128(12 Suppl):2563s–76s.
66. Liebau F, Wernerman J, van Loon LJ, et al. Effect of initiating enteral protein feeding on whole-body protein turnover in critically ill patients. Am J Clin Nutr 2015;101(3):549–57.

67. Berg A, Rooyackers O, Bellander BM, et al. Whole body protein kinetics during hypocaloric and normocaloric feeding in critically ill patients. Crit Care 2013; 17(4):R158.
68. Weijs PJ, Wischmeyer PE. Optimizing energy and protein balance in the ICU. Curr Opin Clin Nutr Metab Care 2013;16(2):194–201.
69. Allingstrup MJ, Esmailzadeh N, Wilkens Knudsen A, et al. Provision of protein and energy in relation to measured requirements in intensive care patients. Clin Nutr 2012;31(4):462–8.
70. Ferrie S, Tsang E. Monitoring nutrition in critical illness: what can we use? Nutr Clin Pract 2018;33(1):133–46.
71. Wandrag L, Brett SJ, Frost GS, et al. Exploration of muscle loss and metabolic state during prolonged critical illness: implications for intervention? PLoS One 2019;14(11):e0224565.
72. Bharadwaj S, Ginoya S, Tandon P, et al. Malnutrition: laboratory markers vs nutritional assessment. Gastroenterol Rep (Oxf) 2016;4(4):272–80.
73. Fuhrman MP, Charney P, Mueller CM. Hepatic proteins and nutrition assessment. J Am Diet Assoc 2004;104(8):1258–64.
74. Ingenbleek Y, Van Den Schrieck HG, De Nayer P, et al. The role of retinol-binding protein in protein-calorie malnutrition. Metabolism 1975;24(5):633–41.
75. Parent B, Seaton M, O'Keefe GE. Biochemical markers of nutrition support in critically ill trauma victims. JPEN J Parenter Enteral Nutr 2018;42(2):335–42.
76. Arabi YM, Aldawood AS, Al-Dorzi HM, et al. Permissive underfeeding or standard enteral feeding in high- and low-nutritional-risk critically ill adults. Post hoc analysis of the PermiT trial. Am J Respir Crit Care Med 2017;195(5):652–62.
77. Bretscher C, Buergin M, Gurzeler G, et al. Association between prealbumin, all-cause mortality, and response to nutrition treatment in patients at nutrition risk: secondary analysis of a randomized controlled trial. JPEN J Parenter Enteral Nutr 2023;47(3):408–19.
78. Bretschera C, Boesiger F, Kaegi-Braun N, et al. Admission serum albumin concentrations and response to nutritional therapy in hospitalised patients at malnutrition risk: secondary analysis of a randomised clinical trial. EClinicalMedicine 2022;45:101301.
79. Evennett NJ, Petrov MS, Mittal A, et al. Systematic review and pooled estimates for the diagnostic accuracy of serological markers for intestinal ischemia. World J Surg 2009;33(7):1374–83.
80. Padar M, Starkopf J, Starkopf L, et al. Enteral nutrition and dynamics of citrulline and intestinal fatty acid-binding protein in adult ICU patients. Clin Nutr ESPEN 2021;45:322–32.

Novel Strategies to Promote Intensive Care Unit Recovery via Personalized Exercise, Nutrition, and Anabolic Interventions

Ashley L. Artese, PhD[a], Hilary M. Winthrop, MS, RD, LDN, CNSC[b],
Megan Beyer, MS, RD, LDN[c], Krista L. Haines, DO[d],
Jeroen Molinger, MSc, PhDc[e], Amy M. Pastva, PhD[f,g],
Paul E. Wischmeyer, MD, EDIC, FASPEN, FCCM[h,*]

KEYWORDS

- Critical illness • Rehabilitation • Exercise • Nutrition • CPET testing • Testosterone
- Creatine • Cardiopulmonary exercise testing

KEY POINTS

- Survivors of critical illness experience significant morbidity, reduced physiologic reserve, and health complications that persist long into survivorship.
- Evidence is sparse regarding rehabilitation, nutrition, and anabolic agent/nutrient approaches, especially in the out-patient setting, that improve long-term outcomes and recovery.
- Promising novel strategies include multi-domain interventions, individually tailored exercise prescription, remote rehabilitation delivery, anabolic nutrients (ie, creatine and β-hydroxy-β-methylbutyrate), and anabolic agents (ie, testosterone).
- Individualized nutrition support should follow a patient well beyond the intensive care unit and include strategies to achieve adequate calories, protein, and micronutrient intake.

Continued

---

[a] Department of Exercise Science and Health Promotion, Florida Atlantic University, Boca Raton, FL, USA; [b] Duke Office of Clinical Research, Duke University School of Medicine, Durham, NC, USA; [c] Department of Anesthesiology, Duke University School of Medicine, Durham, NC, USA; [d] Department of Surgery, Division of Trauma, Critical Care, and Acute Care Surgery, Duke University Medical Center, Durham, NC 27710, USA; [e] Human Pharmacology and Physiology Lab, Department of Anesthesiology, Duke University Medical Center, Durham, NC, USA; [f] Department of Orthopaedic Surgery, Division of Physical Therapy, Duke University School of Medicine, Durham, NC, USA; [g] Center for the Study of Aging and Human Development, Duke University Medical Center, Durham, NC, USA; [h] Department of Anesthesiology and Surgery, Duke University, Durham, NC, USA
* Corresponding author. Duke University School of Medicine, DUMC, Box 3094 Mail # 41, 2301 Erwin Road, 5692 HAFS, Durham, NC 27710.
E-mail address: Paul.Wischmeyer@Duke.edu

Crit Care Clin 41 (2025) 263–281
https://doi.org/10.1016/j.ccc.2024.09.007
0749-0704/25/© 2024 Elsevier Inc. All rights reserved, including those for text and data mining, AI training, and similar technologies.

Continued

- More research is needed to further evaluate effectiveness and inform implementation of novel rehabilitation, nutrition, and anabolic nutrient/agent strategies throughout the continuum of care.

INTRODUCTION

More than 5 million patients are admitted to the intensive care unit (ICU) in the United States every year,[1] and as a result of improved treatments and care, more than 85% will survive hospitalization.[2] Despite low in-hospital mortality, ICU survivors face many challenges including significant morbidity, reduced physiologic reserve, and long-term complications that negatively impact health and quality of life.[3,4] Critical illness combined with intensive treatments and prolonged bed rest also accelerates losses in muscle mass, cardiorespiratory fitness, and physical function.[5–7] ICU-acquired weakness is experienced by approximately 40% of critical care patients,[8] with a higher incidence among those experiencing sepsis, multiple organ failure, or greater exposure to mechanical ventilation.[9] Post-ICU functional capacity is also significantly impaired, reaching 56% of predicted norms,[6] and often fails to recover overtime.[10] Impairments can continue to worsen as 54% of survivors report further decline in neuropsychological or physical function.[11] Physical, cognitive, and mental health deficits, collectively known as post-intensive care syndrome (PICS),[12] can persist years after hospitalization,[11] negatively impacting long-term recovery, rehospitalization risk,[13] and survival.[14] As a result, there has been an urgent call for an increased focus on clinical trials investigating recovery from critical illness.

One of the major pillars involved in critical illness recovery is the prevention of PICS.[12] Introduction of early mobilization and nutrition support within the first few days of ICU admission are recommended strategies for preventing and treating PICS and promoting initial recovery.[15–20] Several systematic reviews and meta-analyses support early mobilization, including walking intubated patients in ICU, to reduce the incidence of ICU-acquired weakness, shorten hospital stays, and promote short-term strength and physical function benefits.[21–24] However, results are mixed regarding the positive impacts of early rehabilitation on long-term outcomes and recovery.[22,24,25] For example, some studies have reported benefits on post-discharge physical function,[26,27] while others report no effect,[22,24] and findings related to long-term outcomes, including rehospitalization and survival, vary among studies.[26,28–31] Differing results may be confounded by differences in intervention frequency, intensity, duration, and dosage, timing, and type of outcome assessments, and heterogeneity in the control group characteristics.[23,32,33] This highlights the complexity of designing and implementing effective rehabilitation strategies to optimize long-term recovery. Nevertheless, current evidence supports the use of early ICU rehabilitation for short-term benefits but also highlights the need for high-quality research and evidence-based approaches throughout the continuum of care that focus on improving long-term outcomes.

Less is known regarding post-discharge rehabilitation, nutrition interventions, and anabolic nutrients/agents, and optimal strategies have yet to be determined. For example, results from previous studies investigating post-ICU rehabilitation programs are inconsistent, with many showing little to no effects on physical health, function, or health-related quality of life.[10,25,34,35] Despite insufficient evidence specific to rehabilitation interventions, findings from several studies support the feasibility and benefit of critical care transition and recovery programs for reducing ICU readmission and optimizing recovery.[13,36,37] However, patients face many barriers to post-ICU care including functional and cognitive impairments, limited ability to attend clinical visits, lack of knowledge regarding the importance of follow-up care, and lack of availability of coordinated post-ICU rehabilitation programs.[37] Furthermore, critical illness survivors are a heterogeneous population with varying pathophysiology, symptoms, and impairments.[38] Therefore, a one-size-fits-all approach to rehabilitation, nutrition, and anabolic nutrients/agents is not likely to be ideal for reducing ICU-related deficits and improving long-term outcomes. This warrants the need for personalized rehabilitation, nutrition, and anabolic nutrient/agent strategies that address patients' continued and changing medical needs. Furthermore, combining physical rehabilitation with personalized nutrition and anabolic strategies may further reduce ICU-related impairments and enhance recovery.[39] This review aims to discuss novel personalized multimodal rehabilitation approaches that can potentially improve patient care and promote long-term recovery. The authors also address current recommendations and new approaches to optimize patients' nutritional status and promote anabolism/muscle mass preservation and recovery throughout the critical illness care continuum.

REHABILITATION STRATEGIES
Multi-domain Rehabilitation Interventions

The implementation of multi-domain rehabilitation interventions that target several physical function domains may be an effective novel strategy to comprehensively address the numerous impairments experienced by critical illness survivors. Multi-domain exercise interventions have been found to improve strength and physical function to a greater extent than single-domain programs in frail older adults.[40,41] Although the efficacy of this type of intervention has not been fully explored within the critical care realm, the previous Physical Rehabilitation for Older Patients Hospitalized for Heart Failure (REHAB-HF) trial with older patients with heart failure,[42–44] a population with broad physical impairments as those surviving critical illness, provides a very successful model warranting further exploration. This study implemented a 12 week progressive, individualized rehabilitation program that transitioned from the hospital to an outpatient setting and targeted domains for endurance, strength, mobility, and balance. Results demonstrated high retention (82%) and session adherence (67%). The program led to significantly improved performance on the short physical performance battery and clinically important changes in 6 minute walk distance and quality of life in the intervention group.[42,43] Importantly, there was a dose-response effect such that higher session adherence associated with improved patient-centered and clinical event outcomes.[45]

Recent evidence in patients with coronavirus disease 2019 (COVID-19) offers additional insight. For example, a single-arm post-ICU study in older adults with post-COVID-19 functional impairment reported improved functional capacity, balance, and ability to perform activities of daily living following a 4 week in-hospital, exercise program with strength, cardiovascular, balance, and gait components.[46] Another single-arm 7 week multicomponent exercise study in patients with COVID-19 discharged from the hospital or ICU similarly reported increased aerobic capacity, health status, and dyspnea-related disability following the intervention.[47] A 2 year follow-up revealed that 86% of patients continued to exercise, and their health status increased.[47] Although these recent findings support the potential benefit of post-

ICU multi-domain rehabilitation approaches, neither one had a control group for comparison, thus limiting the strength of the evidence. Additional studies, including large randomized controlled trials, are needed to test the feasibility, efficacy, and implementation of multi-domain interventions in survivors of critical illness. One study of interest is an NIH-funded randomized clinical trial in patients surviving COVID-19 hospitalization (REMM-HIIT-COVID-19; clinicaltrials.gov/ct2/show/NCT04664101) that utilizes a multi-domain, progressive intervention consisting of high-intensity interval training (HIIT) guided by posthospital cardiopulmonary exercise testing (CPET) and exercises targeting strength, mobility, and balance. This study is currently underway, and in the recruitment phase, results will provide valuable insight that may be further translated to the critical care setting.

Patient-Centered Individually Personalized Rehabilitation

Many of the aforementioned multi-domain studies also utilized novel strategies for individually personalizing the intervention to match the exercise prescription to each patient's needs. Personalized and tailored interventions can be characterized by (1) rehabilitation protocols where exercise frequency, intensity, duration, and/or volume are prescribed based on each patient's individual and unique characteristics, exercise capacity, and functional needs; and (2) gradual progression that corresponds to adaptation and improvement. For example, the REMM-HIIT-COVID-19 trial (clinicaltrials.gov/ct2/show/NCT04664101) personalizes the intervention to participants by utilizing CPET testing to calculate individualized target heart rates for HIIT and prescribing strength, mobility, and balance exercises based on predetermined levels that correspond to each patient's functional assessment scores. Our team has developed a simple step-test-based CPET modality using a simple Bluetooth-based CPET mask that can be conducted at the hospital bedside or in any clinical setting without needing a large bike or CPET device (**Fig. 1**). Given the heterogeneity in critical illness survivors' characteristics, disease status, comorbidities, and

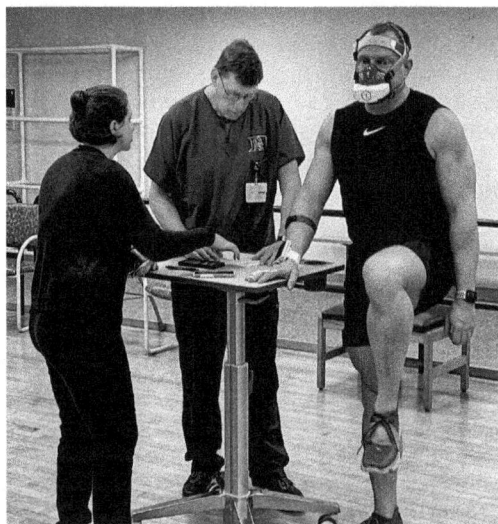

Fig. 1. Novel cardiopulmonary exercise testing (CPET) via step test that can be utilized in hospital rooms and clinic settings utilizes Bluetooth-linked CPET mask and provides VO_2-peak measures. (Mask: VO_2Master Pro, VO_2 Master Health Sensors Inc. BC, Canada).

impairments, personalized rehabilitation protocols must align the intervention with patient needs, address limitations and impairments, promote progressive improvements, and prioritize patient goals and preferences. This is supported by a recent machine learning study that defined 4 different patient groups in ICU based on clinical characteristics and demonstrated that the most effective rehabilitation strategies for increasing the likelihood of discharge to home differed between groups.[48] Furthermore, personalized exercise is perceived by patients as an essential component of successful rehabilitation programs. For example, patients participating in the REVIVE trial, which consisted of a 6 week post-ICU intervention, reported that the tailored exercise program was an important facilitator related to perceived benefit.[49] Patients participating in ICU recovery programs also highlighted the importance of programs focused on helping them set and meet their own personal care goals, which they deemed important for developing intrinsic motivation and self-efficacy.[13]

Finally, interventions that integrate personalized strategies to promote exercise adherence and address barriers to rehabilitation are needed. Few studies have focused on interventions that specifically target ICU survivors' barriers to rehabilitation, and a recent review in older adults with multi-morbidities suggested that interventions are not addressing important patient priorities and barriers to participation.[50] Therefore, current evidence supports the use and value of individually personalized rehabilitation interventions for survivors of critical illness; however, future studies are needed to expand current evidence to develop approaches that address specific facilitators and barriers to rehabilitation and explore approaches that optimize benefits based on specific patient and disease-related characteristics.

Remotely Delivered and Monitored Rehabilitation

Successfully transitioning care from the inpatient to outpatient setting poses many challenges related to resource allocation, patient communication and support, accessibility of clinics and rehabilitation services, and poor patient attendance.[37,51] Telemedicine has become more popular in recent years and has the potential to address many of these challenges. Although remotely delivered rehabilitation protocols have not been fully explored in survivors of critical illness, evidence from other patient populations demonstrates that they are feasible, cost-efficient, effective for improving symptoms and outcomes, and produce comparable results to in-person programs.[52–57] A recent review on ICU follow-up care interventions also highlighted better recruitment, delivery rates, and retention for programs that did not require in-person attendance.[58] Technology such as videoconferencing and wearable devices also enhance intervention delivery, enabling personalized high-touch instruction, goal setting, behavior change support (ie, alerts, feedback, and reminders), and continuous remote monitoring of health outcomes and exercise adherence.[59,60] The aforementioned REMM-HIIT-COVID-19 trial of post-COVID-19 rehabilitation provides all subjects with an Apple Watch and iPhone to monitor heart rate training, measure activity, and allow for personalized video coaching by a remote physical therapist or physiologist with each exercise session. Future research should identify best practices for remote rehabilitation delivery in the outpatient setting to optimize benefits and minimize barriers in critical illness survivors.

NUTRITION STRATEGIES
Protein Guidelines

Optimal protein delivery is essential for recovery from critical illness as it improves outcomes, supports immune function, and attenuates muscle mass loss.[61] For example, it has been previously suggested that there is a 1% reduction in mortality for every gram of daily ingested protein.[62] For patients in the ICU at high nutritional risk or diagnosed with severe malnutrition, enteral or parenteral nutrition (PN) should be initiated once the patient is stabilized with the goal of 1.2 to 2.0 g/kg/d.[61,63] Guidelines from the European Society for Clinical Nutrition and Metabolism state that the target of 1.3 g of protein/kg/d, with a minimum of 1.2 g/kg/d, increased in a stepwise approach following the period of critical illness.[20,64,65]

For optimal recovery, protein delivery may change over the course of the ICU stay and throughout recovery. For example, a previous study reported increased mortality for protein doses greater than 1.2 g/kg/d for ICU days 1 to 3, with lower mortality for patients provided high protein (>1.2 g/kg/d) intake after day 4. Consistently low protein throughout ICU stay (<0.8 g/kg of protein per day) showed the highest mortality.[66] The authors suggest that protein should be limited to less than 0.8 g/kg per day for the first 3 days of ICU admission and then gradually increased to 1.2 g/kg or more of protein per day by or after the sixth day.[66] In the post-ICU phase, the protein delivery goal is 1.5 to 2.0 g of protein/kg/d, and following hospital discharge, protein needs may need to be increased to 2.0 to 2.5 g/kg/d.[64,66]

Oral nutrition supplements are imperative to patients meeting protein goals in both the ICU and post-ICU setting.[64] When patients are discharged from the hospital and recovering at home, protein needs remain elevated, although there is currently no consensus on the amount of protein recommended, especially in the long-term recovery phases.[65] Increased protein consumption and exercise can stimulate muscle protein synthesis,[64] and thus, it is important for promoting recovery and mitigating further loss in muscle mass, strength, and function. There is limited research on energy and protein needs while undergoing rehabilitation, but indirect calorimetry (IC) can help provide more precise measurements.[65]

Nutrition Support Starting in the Intensive Care Unit

Early enteral and parenteral nutrition
International clinical guidelines recommend early (within 48 hours of ICU admission) initiation of enteral nutrition (EN) for improved patient outcomes, including fewer infectious complications.[19,20,67,68] In cases where enteral feeding is contraindicated, PN is recommended and can be used as early as EN with no increased risk of infection in the setting of glycemic control and eucaloric feeding.[67,69,70]

Supplemental parenteral nutrition
Although improvements have been made in the last decade or so at many centers throughout the world, nutritional adequacy has historically still been low in ICUs. One multicenter study of 2946 ICU mechanically ventilated patients showed an average intake of only 59% of prescribed calories via tube feeding for the first 12 days in the ICU.[71] Many times, the inadequacies come from interruptions in the tube feeding, such as pauses for procedures and, in some cases, being held for multiple hours each day.[72] Because of this, piqued interest in supplemental parenteral nutrition (SPN) has resulted in recent trials showing that SPN improves energy intake and reduces nosocomial infections, with no increase in hospital mortality or length of stay.[73–75] Thus, we suggest SPN should become routine worldwide for patients not at greater than 70% of nutrition goal for protein and calorie delivery at 72 hour post-ICU admission.

Oral intake
In patients who no longer require nutrition support in the form of tube feeding or PN, oral intake has also been shown to be inadequate in the critically ill. In a study

evaluating 19 patients over the course of 125 days after they were weaned from mechanical ventilation, oral intake only met 71% of predicted energy needs and 46% of predicted protein needs.[76] Average calorie delivery has been shown to be approximately 700 kcal/d post-ICU, which is far insufficient to promote recovery.[77]

Perioperative oral nutrition supplements

Given the prevalence of poor oral intake, the prescription of oral nutrition supplements (ONSs) is vital to helping patients achieve adequate calories, protein, and micronutrients to aid in recovery from their illness. A study on the use of early ONS in the postoperative period in colorectal surgery patients showed fewer infectious complications, ICU admissions, and gastrointestinal complications, along with reduced rates of pneumonia.[78] More studies are needed on using ONS in critical illness and post-ICU recovery, but it appears to be one simple solution to the problem of poor nutritional intake during recovery after the ICU.

Nutrition Care in Post-Intensive Care Unit Hospitalization

The importance of adequate nutrition does not lessen once the patient is discharged from the ICU. Instead, nutritional adequacy should follow a patient well beyond the ICU, and unfortunately, many patients continue with poor nutritional intake during their post-ICU hospitalization.

Oral intake

A cohort study published in 2018 assessed the oral intake adequacy of hospitalized patients post-critical illness during a 1 month period.[79] Out of 79 patients assessed, 62% were identified with inadequate oral intake (an average of <2/3 meal intake). This study group also showed that, in the patients with inadequate oral intake, only 32% were offered an ONS.[79] A 2019 study evaluated patients' energy and protein intake after discharge from the ICU.[80] Among 32 patients evaluated, a median intake of 1238 kcal and 60 g of protein from all sources were found, translating to 79% [41%–108%] of predicted energy needs and 73% [44%–98%] of predicted protein needs. The authors found wide ranges in nutrition intake, with median daily deficits in the post-ICU hospitalization period of −442 (−1323 to 186) kcal/d for energy and −30 (−69 to −1) g/d for protein. Another study evaluated oral intake 3 months after ICU discharge and found that reductions in appetite, oral intake, and body weight were prevalent, and ICU survivors consumed fewer calories compared to healthy controls (ICU survivors: 1876±708 vs healthy controls 2291±834 kcal; $P=.025$).[81] Therefore, future work should focus on strategies and interventions to support oral intake adequacy in hospitalized patients recovering from critical illness.

Nutrition Strategies for Posthospital Discharge

There is also an increased interest in posthospital discharge nutrition, including the use of ONSs, during recovery at home. A recent systematic review and meta-analysis of 14 studies, including 2480 participants who underwent gastrointestinal surgery, showed that patients who received ONS for at least 2 weeks after hospital discharge had improved outcomes, including reduced postoperative weight loss, increased serum albumin, and increased hemoglobin.[82] Another randomized clinical trial studying malnourished, older hospitalized patients showed that patients who received a high protein-HMB ONS during hospitalization and 90 days post-discharge had significantly lower 90-day mortality compared to placebo.[83] The number needed to treat to prevent a single death was 20.3 (95% CI 10.9–121.4) in this key trial. One study group investigated nutrition intake up to 1 year following critical illness: In 206 patients studied at 1 month, 3 month, and 12 month post-discharge, both calorie and protein intake were below target goals at all-time points (defined as 25 kcal/kg/d and 1.3 g protein/kg/d, respectively).[84] Further studies, particularly randomized controlled trials, are needed to elucidate the benefits of ONS in post-critically ill patients.

Individually Personalized Nutrition Using Indirect Calorimetry

With the use of IC, we are better able to provide patients with measured nutrition accurately. IC is a method that measures VO_2 and VCO_2, which are used to calculate resting energy expenditure (REE).[85] In the critical care setting, it can be difficult to estimate a patient's energy needs based on the degree of critical illness, thus highlighting the importance of objective assessment of REE. IC can benefit patients who are complex and have changing metabolic needs, including inflammation, increased energy needs, and insulin resistance in the critical care setting.[64,85] Utilizing results from IC testing and providing 70% of REE improved patient outcomes compared to feeding greater than 100% of REE, which was associated with longer ICU days and length of time on the ventilator.[62] Feeding less than 70% of REE was also associated with increased mortality. In addition, IC-directed nutrition recommendations have been found to provide higher amounts of protein and total calories compared to predictive energy equations, and clinical trials and multiple meta-analysis papers have shown significant reductions in mortality when IC-guided nutrition targets are utilized.[86–90] In summary, recent ICU nutrition guidelines suggest targeted energy delivery be started at approximately 10 to 15 kcal/kg or less than 70% of measured-IC REE at ICU admission whether EN/PN is used and be advanced to goal as patient stabilizes.[20,63]

There are over 200 predicative energy equations published, which have variable accuracy compared to IC, with accuracy ranging from 40% to 75%.[63,91] Patients' acute and chronic conditions can influence metabolic demands that shift throughout a patient's hospital admission.[85] There is no estimated equation that is more accurate than IC.[63] IC remains the gold standard for determining a patient's energy needs, especially in the critical care setting.[63,65] Regular IC measurements can provide a greater understanding of metabolic changes during critical illness to guide the dietitian's recommendations.[86] The International Multicentric Study Group for Indirect Calorimetry (ICALIC) developed and assessed an IC device, Q-NRG, that requires significantly less time than most other IC devices currently used, highlighting recent developments for incorporating IC into routine clinical care.[85,92] In addition, McClave and colleagues[93] reported that a 5 minute steady state reflected 24 hour total energy expenditure for mechanically ventilated patients, further supporting the use and feasibility of IC in the clinical setting. Point-of-care testing in the ICU must move toward implementing IC measures to optimize patient outcomes and personalize nutrition delivery.[86] European/American guidelines advocate IC to measure energy expenditure (EE).[20,63] In addition to IC, bedside devices are also available to measure and assess body composition to optimize individualized nutrition delivery.

A recent study that evaluated IC measurements in comparison to estimated equations in the ICU and ward setting reported a significant increase in REE compared to the mean REE within the ICU.[94] The importance and use of an activity factor in the clinical setting were not discussed but would be an area for future research. Once a patient is in a step-down level of care, feeding at 100% of their REE (or greater [up to 1.3 x REE] based on rehabilitation activities) is recommended.[64] There is little research published in the posthospital phase of care that provides recommendations for utilizing IC measurements in the outpatient setting and would provide a greater understanding to assist patients recovering from a hospitalization (see summary of personalized nutrition care pathway in **Fig. 2**).

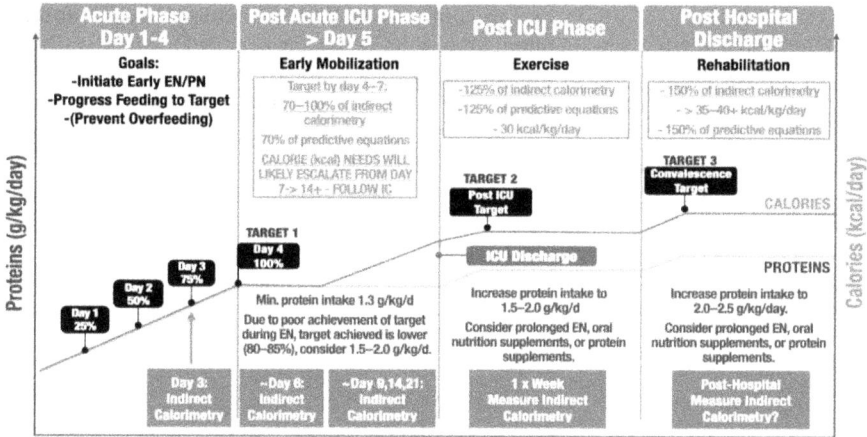

Fig. 2. Personalized IC-guided ICU nutrition algorithm. Note, suggested IC measurement days are meant as a guideline to ensure consistent IC-measurements over ICU and hospital stay. IC should optimally be performed 2 times per week in ICU or when a significant clinical change in patient status has occurred. EN, enteral nutrition; IC, indirect calorimetry; ICU, intensive care unit; PN, parenteral nutrition. (*From* Wischmeyer PE, Molinger J, Haines K. Point-counterpoint: Indirect calorimetry is essential for optimal nutrition therapy in the intensive care unit. Nutr Clin Pract. 2021;36(2):275-281. https://doi.org/10.1002/ncp.10643.)[122]

ROLE OF ANABOLIC NUTRIENTS AND ANABOLIC AGENTS

Anabolic nutrients are a mainstay for amateur and professional athletes. These are quite potentially relevant to recovering patients in ICU due to their ability to increase muscle mass, reduce muscle loss, and improve strength and function. These include creatine, β-hydroxy-β-methylbutyrate (HMB), and leucine.

Creatine

Creatine's mechanism of benefit is via increased phosphocreatine within cell, which increases ATP production essential for muscle protein synthesis. Recent reviews demonstrate that creatine supplementation shows potential benefits in a range of illness and injury states.[95] Creatine is safe for long-term use in a range of populations in multiple studies.[96] A recent meta-analysis of 33 randomized controlled trial (RCTs) in 1076 older adults with chronic disease showed creatine supplementation improves physical function via sit to stand test and also improves upper body muscle strength, handgrip strength, and lean muscle tissue.[97] Given safety and effectiveness, it seems reasonable to consider the use of creatine in recovering post-ICU patients at a dose of 5 g/d. It is also urgent that high-quality prospective RCTs utilizing creatine to improve physical function and potentially cognition in post-ICU patients are conducted.

β-hydroxy-β-methylbutyrate

HMB is a leucine metabolite that stimulates muscle protein synthesis and inhibits muscle protein breakdown via effects on the mTOR pathway; HMB also inhibits inflammation, which may lead to increased muscle catabolism. HMB is a widely studied supplement for trained/untrained athletes.[98] Many studies have looked at the effects of HMB on recovering patients post-injury and illness. One example was a study of hip fracture patients, which showed improved wound healing and a significant increase in mobile patients at the end of the study period when HMB was utilized.[99] A recent systematic review in 15 RCTs of 2137 patients by Bear and colleagues[100] reported improved muscle mass and strength in a range of clinical populations (not in ICU) at risk of muscle wasting. Two recent ICU studies reported no difference in muscle loss, as measured by ultrasound or CT,[101,102] but the possible duration of intervention was likely too short for benefit.[103,104] Finally, as muscle loss due to bed rest is a major contributor to ICU-acquired weakness and PICS, HMB has been shown to markedly reduce or almost eliminate bed rest-related muscle loss in a group of elderly subjects in a well-done study by Deutz and colleagues[105] HMB also shows great promise to improve muscle mass and reduce muscle loss in the ICU and post-ICU setting; more studies of HMB in the ICU and post-ICU setting in illness and injury are urgently needed, looking at functional outcomes such as the 6 minute walk test.

Testosterone and Anabolic Steroids

In addition to the catabolic effects of critical illness and inadequate ICU nutrition delivery, a majority (~95%) of patients in ICU demonstrate severe testosterone deficiency quite early in their ICU stay.[106] Persistent hypotestosteronemia (low-T) in acute illness is known to impair recovery/rehabilitation, and low-T at hospital admission is known to significantly increase hospital mortality and overall lifetime risk of cardiac events.[106–109] Further, in patients in ICU, low-T levels correlate with time on the ventilator, ICU LOS, disease severity, and survival.[106,109] The benefits of testosterone/oxandrolone (OX) combined with exercise on clinical outcomes and physical function has been demonstrated in a range of illnesses.[110–112] In burn injury, a range of trials show the benefits of OX,[113] and OX is a common standard of care in many burn centers worldwide.[109] Systematic reviews of OX treatment demonstrate significant benefits in burn injury, which include increased lean body mass, improved donor-site healing, reduced weight loss, and reduced LOS without increased risk of liver dysfunction, infection, or hyperglycemia.[114] Historically, concerns for testosterone replacement therapy (TRT) being associated with increased cardiovascular/stroke-related events and prostate cancer have been completely dispelled by 3 large studies.[115–117] The recent The Testosterone Replacement Therapy for Assessment of

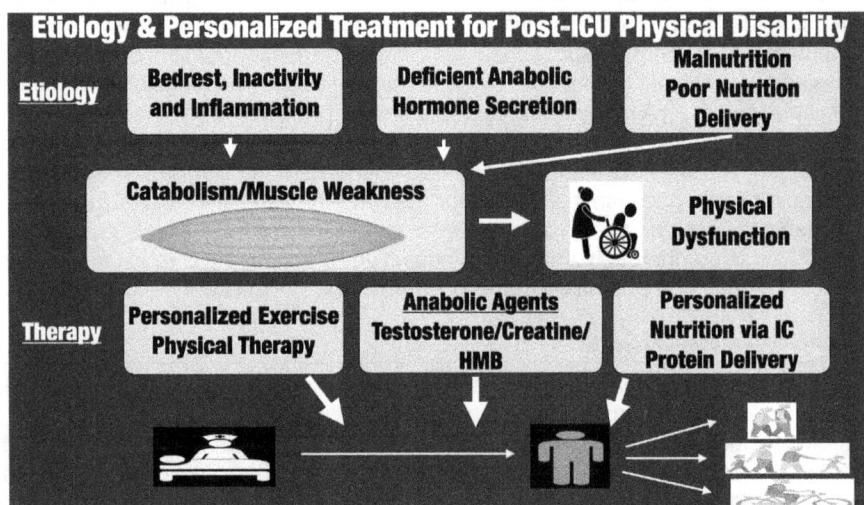

Fig. 3. Etiology and personalized treatment for post-ICU physical disability. IC, indirect calorimetry.

Long-term Vascular Events and Efficacy Response in Hypogonadal Men (TRAVERSE) trial, a large RCT published in the New England Journal of Medicine,[117] showed in men with low-T levels and preexisting or a high risk of cardiovascular disease, TRT with transdermal testosterone showed no increased risk of cardiovascular events or prostate cancer over approximately 3 years of follow-up. Further, 2 large recent studies demonstrate that subjects with low-T levels, in fact, have a significant reduction in all-cause cardiovascular events and stroke risk with TRT compared to patients with untreated low-T.[115] Low-T levels persist into the post-ICU period, with 96% of patients being T-deficient post-ICU.[118] Further, research is urgently needed on testosterone repletion to targets of 500 to 600 ng/dL in men and perhaps lower target levels in women (note there is a large National Institutes of Health (NIH) trial of TRT in women post-hip fracture ongoing[119]) as there are no current studies for interventions with testosterone agents in non-burn post-ICU settings.

SUMMARY

Countering the deleterious effects associated with critical illness and addressing patients' changing care priorities requires a multifaceted rehabilitation approach that focuses on patient-centered, personalized, multi-domain strategies that span the continuum of recovery (**Fig. 3**). Identifying novel physical rehabilitation strategies and optimizing nutritional and anabolic nutrient/agent approaches for targeting patients' energy and protein needs are the first steps to promoting meaningful recovery. More research is needed to further develop, implement, and test these strategies, especially in the out-patient setting. In addition, future work should be directed toward interventions that combine physical rehabilitation, nutrition, and anabolic nutrients/agents to minimize ICU-related deficits, optimally build and recover muscle mass, and promote recovery following critical illness.[120,121]

CLINICS CARE POINTS

- Survivors of critical illness are a heterogenous population with varying pathophysiology, symptoms, and impairments. Therefore, a one-size-fits-all approach to rehabilitation may not be ideal for reducing ICU-related deficits and improving long-term outcomes.

- Although research is limited regarding the effectiveness of post-ICU interventions, current evidence supports the implementation of multi-domain interventions that include 2 or more components to comprehensively address numerous impairments experienced by critical illness survivors.

- Current evidence suggests that rehabilitation programs should be prescribed via personalized methods where the exercise prescription is based on each patient's individual and unique characteristics, exercise capacity, and functional needs. Strategies include using baseline functional assessments to inform exercise prescription, setting personalized target exercise heart rates based on newly affordable portable CPET, and gradual progression that corresponds to adaptation and improvement.

- Although early enteral nutrition (EN) is preferred, early PN and supplemental PN should be a standard of care if patients are not at enteral or oral nutrition goals within 72 hours of ICU admission as new data and ICU nutrition guidelines show that EN and PN are equally safe and efficacious and can be used interchangeably in the ICU setting.

- Early and ongoing use of HMB (3 g/d) and creatine (5 g/d) has a strong and growing evidence base from multiple studies and meta-analysis for improving muscle mass, muscle function, and outcomes in patients with acute illness, chronic illness, and/or patients in ICU. This should be continued in the post-ICU and posthospital settings.

- Indirect calorimetry should be utilized in patients in ICU after day 3 to set accurate and personalized energy/calorie targets and needs to be repeated regularly throughout ICU stay and the post-ICU period.
- The majority of ICU and post-ICU patients are testosterone deficient. Especially in male patients (and perhaps in females as well where more data are needed), new data on the safety and benefit of intramuscular or transdermal TRT show TRT in testosterone-deficient individuals can be given safely and do not promote cardiac or prostate cancer risk but instead may reduce cardiac (ie, myocardial infarction) and stroke event rates and may be effective in improving muscle mass, muscle function, and quality of life as has been shown in burn injury settings, thus demanding further research in broad post-ICU settings.
- High protein ONSs are essential in the ICU, post-ICU, and posthospital setting and have been shown conclusively to improve clinical and functional outcomes in acutely ill patients.

DISCLOSURE

A.L. Artese, M. Beyer, and A.M. Pastva have nothing to disclose. H.M. Winthrop has served as a consultant and speaker for Baxter. K.L. Haines received grants from Fresenius Kabi, Germany, grants and personal fees from Baxter, United States, and grants from Abbott outside the submitted work. Dr P.E. Wischmeyer reported receiving grants from Abbott Ince to Duke University, serving as a consultant for Abbott Inc, honoraria for continuing medical education (CME) lectures, grants from Baxter, serving as a consultant for Baxter, honoraria for CME lectures from Fresenius serving as a consultant for Danone Nutricia, honoraria for CME lectures from Danone Nutricia, serving as a consultant for Mend Inc, and receiving honoraria for CME lectures from Mend Inc, unrestricted gift funding for research from MuscleSound and unrestricted gift funding and honoraria for CME lectures from DSM, The Netherlands, outside of the submitted work.

REFERENCES

1. Society of Critical Care Medicine. Critical care statistics. 2024. Available at: https://www.sccm.org/Communications/Critical-Care-Statistics. Accessed May 20, 2024.
2. Zimmerman JE, Kramer AA, Knaus WA. Changes in hospital mortality for United States intensive care unit admissions from 1988 to 2012. Crit Care 2013; 17(2):R81.
3. Hiser SL, Fatima A, Ali M, et al. Post-intensive care syndrome (PICS): recent updates. J Intensive Care 2023;11(1):23.
4. Schwitzer E, Jensen KS, Brinkman L, et al. Survival ≠ Recovery: a narrative review of post-intensive care syndrome. Chest Crit Care 2023;1(1):100003.
5. Parry SM, Puthucheary ZA. The impact of extended bed rest on the musculoskeletal system in the critical care environment. Extrem Physiol Med 2015; 4(1):1–8.
6. Benington S, McWilliams D, Eddleston J, et al. Exercise testing in survivors of intensive care-is there a role for cardiopulmonary exercise testing? J Crit Care 2012;27(1):89–94.
7. Denehy L, Lanphere J, Needham DM. Ten reasons why ICU patients should be mobilized early. Intensive Care Med 2017;43(1):86–90.
8. Appleton RTD, Kinsella J, Quasim T. The incidence of intensive care unit-acquired weakness syndromes: a systematic review. J Intensive Care Soc 2015;16(2): 126–36.

9. Fan E, Cheek F, Chlan L, et al. An official American Thoracic Cociety clinical practice guideline: the diagnosis of intensive care unit-acquired weakness in adults. Am J Respir Crit Care Med 2014;190(12):1437–46.

10. Denehy L, Skinner EH, Edbrooke L, et al. Exercise rehabilitation for patients with critical illness: a randomized controlled trial with 12 months of follow-up. Crit Care 2013;17:R156.

11. Maley JH, Brewster I, Mayoral I, et al. Resilience in survivors of critical illness in the context of the survivors' experience and recovery. Ann Am Thorac Soc 2016; 13(8):1351–60.

12. Inoue S, Nakanishi N, Amaya F, et al. Post-intensive care syndrome: recent advances and future directions. Acute Med Surg 2024;11:e929. https://doi.org/10.1002/ams2.929.

13. McPeake J, Boehm LM, Hibbert E, et al. Key components of ICU recovery programs: what did patients report provided benefit? Crit Care Explor 2020;2(4): E0088.

14. Yanagi N, Kamiya K, Hamazaki N, et al. Post-intensive care syndrome as a predictor of mortality in patients with critical illness: a cohort study. PLoS One 2021; 16(3):e0244564.

15. Devlin JW, Skrobik Y, Gélinas C, et al. Clinical practice guidelines for the prevention and management of pain, agitation/sedation, delirium, immobility, and sleep disruption in adult patients in the ICU. Crit Care Med 2018;46. https://doi.org/10.1097/CCM.0000000000003299.

16. National Institute for Health and Care Excellence (NICE). 2018 Surveillance of Rehabilitation after Critical Illness in Adults (NICE Guideline CG83).; 2018. nice.org.uk.

17. National Insititute for Health and Care Excellence. Rehabilitation after critical illness in adults [QS158]. Nice. 2009. Available at: https://www.ncbi.nlm.nih.gov/books/NBK550275/.

18. Tian F, Heighes PT, Allingstrup MJ, et al. Early enteral nutrition provided within 24 hours of ICU admission: a meta-analysis of randomized controlled trials. Crit Care Med 2018;46(7):1049–56.

19. Reintam Blaser A, Starkopf J, Alhazzani W, et al. Early enteral nutrition in critically ill patients: ESICM clinical practice guidelines. Intensive Care Med 2017; 43(3):380–98.

20. Singer P, Blaser AR, Berger MM, et al. ESPEN guideline on clinical nutrition in the intensive care unit. Clin Nutr 2019;38(1):48–79.

21. Menges D, Seiler B, Tomonaga Y, et al. Systematic early versus late mobilization or standard early mobilization in mechanically ventilated adult ICU patients: systematic review and meta-analysis. Crit Care 2021;25:1–24.

22. Fuke R, Hifumi T, Kondo Y, et al. Early rehabilitation to prevent postintensive care syndrome in patients with critical illness: a systematic review and meta-analysis. BMJ Open 2018;8(5):e019998.

23. Zhang L, Hu W, Cai Z, et al. Early mobilization of critically ill patients in the intensive care unit: a systematic review and meta-analysis. PLoS One 2019;14(10):1–16.

24. Okada Y, Unoki T, Matsuishi Y, et al. Early versus delayed mobilization for in-hospital mortality and health-related quality of life among critically ill patients: a systematic review and meta-analysis. J Intensive Care 2019;7:57.

25. Held N, Moss M. Optimizing post-intensive care unit rehabilitation. Turkish Thorac J 2019;20(2):147–52.

26. Paton M, Chan S, Tipping CJ, et al. The effect of mobilization at 6 months after critical illness — meta-analysis. NEJM Evid 2023;2(2).

27. Patel BK, Wolfe KS, Patel SB, et al. Effect of early mobilisation on long-term cognitive impairment in critical illness in the USA: a randomised controlled trial. Lancet Respir Med 2023;11(6):563–72.

28. Murooka Y, Sasabuchi Y, Takazawa T, et al. Long-term prognosis following early rehabilitation in the ICU: a retrospective cohort study. Crit Care Med 2023;51(8): 1054–63.

29. Waldauf P, Jiroutková K, Krajčová A, et al. Effects of rehabilitation interventions on clinical outcomes in critically ill patients: systematic review and meta-analysis of randomized controlled trials. Crit Care Med 2020;48(7):1055–65.

30. Morris PE, Griffin L, Berry M, et al. Receiving early mobility during an ICU admission is a predictor of improved outcomes in acute respiratory failure. Am J Med Sci 2011;341(5):373–7.

31. Watanabe S, Liu K, Morita Y, et al. Effects of mobilization among critically ill patients in the intensive care unit: a single-center retrospective study. Prog Rehabil Med. 2022;7:20220013.

32. de Queiroz RS, Saquetto MB, Martinez BP, et al. Evaluation of the description of active mobilisation protocols for mechanically ventilated patients in the intensive care unit: a systematic review of randomized controlled trials. Hear Lung 2018; 47(3):253–60.

33. O'Grady HK, Reid JC, Farley C, et al. Comparator groups in ICU-based studies of physical rehabilitation: a scoping review of 125 studies. Crit Care Explor 2023; 5(5):E0917.

34. Walsh TS, Salisbury LG, Merriweather JL, et al. Increased hospital-based physical rehabilitation and information provision after intensive care unit discharge: the RECOVER randomized clinical trial. JAMA Intern Med 2015;175(6):901–10.

35. Cuthbertson BH, Rattray J, Campbell MK, et al. The PRaCTICaL study of nurse led, intensive care follow-up programmes for improving long term outcomes fromcritical illness: a pragmatic randomised controlled trial. BMJ 2009;339.

36. Niven DJ, Bastos JF, Stelfox HT. Critical care transition programs and the risk of readmission or death after discharge from an ICU: a systematic review and meta-analysis. Crit Care Med 2014;42(1):179–87.

37. Sevin CM, Bloom SL, Jackson JC, et al. Comprehensive care of ICU survivors: development and implementation of an ICU recovery center. J Crit Care 2018; 46:141–8.

38. Liu P, Li S, Zheng T, et al. Subphenotyping heterogeneous patients with chronic critical illness to guide individualised fluid balance treatment using machine learning: a retrospective cohort study. eClinicalMedicine 2023;59:101970.

39. Heyland DK, Stapleton RD, Mourtzakis M, et al. Combining nutrition and exercise to optimize survival and recovery from critical illness: conceptual and methodological issues. Clin Nutr 2016;35(5):1196–206.

40. Nash KCM. The effects of exercise on strength and physical performance in frail older people: a systematic review. Rev Clin Gerontol 2012;22(4):274–85.

41. Theou O, Stathokostas L, Roland KP, et al. The effectiveness of exercise interventions for the management of frailty: a systematic review. J Aging Res 2011;2011(1):569194.

42. Kitzman DW, Whellan DJ, Duncan P, et al. Physical rehabilitation for older patients hospitalized for heart failure. N Engl J Med 2021;385(3):203–16.

43. Reeves GR, Whellan DJ, Duncan P, et al. Rehabilitation therapy in older acute heart failure patients (REHAB-HF) trial: design and rationale. Am Heart J 2017; 185:130–9.

44. Pastva AM, Duncan PW, Reeves GR, et al. Strategies for supporting intervention fidelity in the rehabilitation therapy in older acute heart failure patients (REHAB-HF) trial. Contemp Clin Trials 2018;64:118–27.

45. Nelson MB, Gilbert ON, Duncan PW, et al. Intervention adherence in REHAB-HF:Predictors and relationship with physical function, quality of life, and clinical events. J Am Heart Assoc 2022;11:e024246.

46. Cuenca-Zaldivar JN, Monroy Acevedo Á, Fernández-Carnero J, et al. Effects of a multicomponent exercise program on improving frailty in post-COVID-19 older adults after intensive care units: a single-group retrospective cohort study. Biology 2022;11(7):1084.

47. Martínez Rolando L, Villafañe JH, Cercadillo García S, et al. Sánchez Romero EA. Multicomponent exercise program to improve the immediate sequelae of COVID-19: a prospective study with a brief report of 2-year follow-up. Int J Environ Res Public Health 2022;19(19):12396.

48. Fuest KE, Ulm B, Daum N, et al. Clustering of critically ill patients using an individualized learning approach enables dose optimization of mobilization in the ICU. Crit Care 2023;27(1).

49. Ferguson K, Bradley JM, McAuley DF, et al. Patients' perceptions of an exercise program delivered following discharge from hospital after critical illness (the Revive Trial). J Intensive Care Med 2019;34(11–12):978–84.

50. Forsyth F, Soh CL, Elks N, et al. Exercise modalities in multi-component interventions for older adults with multi-morbidity: a systematic review and narrative synthesis. J Frailty Aging 2024;1–8. https://doi.org/10.14283/jfa.2024.28.

51. Bloom SL, Stollings JL, Kirkpatrick O, et al. Randomized clinical trial of an ICU recovery pilot program for survivors of critical illness. Crit Care Med 2019; 47(10):1337–45.

52. Pehlivan E, Palalı İ, Atan SG, et al. The effectiveness of POST-DISCHARGE tele-rehabilitation practices in COVID-19 patients: tele-COVID study-randomized controlled trial. Ann Thorac Meedicine 2022;17:110–7.

53. Brown RCC, Coombes JS, Jungbluth Rodriguez K, et al. Effectiveness of exercise via telehealth for chronic disease: a systematic review and meta-analysis of exercise interventions delivered via videoconferencing. Br J Sports Med 2022; 56:1042–52.

54. Hwang R, Bruning J, Morris NR, et al. Home-based telerehabilitation is not inferior to a centre-based program in patients with chronic heart failure: a randomised trial. J Physiother 2017;63(2):101–7.

55. Pescaru CC, Crisan AF, Marc M, et al. A systematic review of telemedicine-driven pulmonary rehabilitation after the acute phase of COVID-19. J Clin Med 2023;12(14):4854.

56. Muñoz-Tomás MT, Burillo-Lafuente M, Vicente-Parra A, et al. Telerehabilitation as a therapeutic exercise tool versus face-to-face physiotherapy: a systematic review. Int J Environ Res Public Health 2023;20(5). https://doi.org/10.3390/ijerph20054358.

57. Mayer KP, Parry SM, Kalema AG, et al. Safety and feasibility of an interdisciplinary treatment approach to optimize recovery from critical coronavirus disease 2019. Crit Care Explor 2021;3(8):e0516.

58. Dimopoulos S, Leggett NE, Deane AM, et al. Models of intensive care unit follow-up care and feasibility of intervention delivery: a systematic review. Aust Crit Care 2024;37(3):508–16.

59. Artese AL, Rawat R, Sung AD. The use of commercial wrist-worn technology to track physiological outcomes in behavioral interventions. Curr Opin Clin Nutr Metab Care 2023;26(6):534–40.
60. Artese AL, Winthrop HM, Bohannon L, et al. A pilot study to assess the feasibility of a remotely monitored high-intensity interval training program prior to allogeneic hematopoietic stem cell transplantation. PLoS One 2023;18(11):e0293171.
61. Wischmeyer PE, Bear DE, Berger MM, et al. Personalized nutrition therapy in critical care: 10 expert recommendations. Crit Care 2023;27:261.
62. Zusman O, Theilla M, Cohen J, et al. Resting energy expenditure, calorie and protein consumption in critically ill patients: a retrospective cohort study. Crit Care 2016;20:367.
63. McClave SA, Taylor BE, Martindale RG, et al. Guidelines for the provision and assessment of nutrition support therapy in the adult critically ill patient: Society of Critical Care Medicine (SCCM) and American Society for Parenteral and Enteral Nutrition (A.S.P.E.N.). J Parenter Enter Nutr 2016;40(2):159–211.
64. Van Zanten ARH, De Waele E, Wischmeyer PE. Nutrition therapy and critical illness: practical guidance for the icu, post-icu, and long-term convalescence phases. Crit Care 2019;23:368.
65. Weijs PJM, Looijaard WGPM, Dekker IM, et al. Lessons from the ICU: Post-intensive care syndrome. In: Imaging. Cham, Switzerland: Springer Nature Switzerland AG; 2019. p. 109–24.
66. Koekkoek WAC, van Setten CH, Olthof LE, et al. Timing of PROTein INtake and clinical outcomes of adult critically ill patients on prolonged mechanical VENTilation: the PROTINVENT retrospective study. Clin Nutr 2019;38(2):883–90.
67. Reignier J, Boisramé-Helms J, Brisard L, et al. Enteral versus parenteral early nutrition in ventilated adults with shock: a randomised, controlled, multicentre, open-label, parallel-group study (NUTRIREA-2). Lancet 2018;391(10116):133–43.
68. Compher C, Bingham AL, McCall M, et al. Guidelines for the provision of nutrition support therapy in the adult critically ill patient: the American Society for Parenteral and Enteral Nutrition. J Parenter Enter Nutr 2022;46(1):12–41.
69. Harvey SE, Parrott F, Harrison DA, et al. Trial of the route of early nutritional support in critically ill adults. N Engl J Med 2014;371(18):1673–84.
70. Elke G, van Zanten ARH, Lemieux M, et al. Enteral versus parenteral nutrition in critically ill patients: an updated systematic review and meta-analysis of randomized controlled trials. Crit Care 2016;20:1–14.
71. Cahill NE, Dhaliwal R, Day AG, et al. Nutrition therapy in the critical care setting: what is "best achievable" practice? An international multicenter observational study. Crit Care Med 2010;38(2):395–401.
72. Kozeniecki M, McAndrew N, Patel JJ. Process-related barriers to optimizing enteral nutrition in a tertiary medical intensive care unit. Nutr Clin Pract 2016;31(1):80–5.
73. Heidegger CP, Berger MM, Graf S, et al. Optimization of energy provision with supplemental parenteral nutrition in critically ill patients: a randomized controlled trial. Lancet 2013;381(9864):385–93.
74. Russell MK, Wischmeyer PE. Supplemental parenteral nutrition: review of the literature and current nutrition guidelines. Nutr Clin Pract 2018;33(3):359–69.
75. Ridley EJ, Davies AR, Parke R, et al. Supplemental parenteral nutrition versus usual care in critically ill adults: a pilot randomized controlled study. Crit Care 2018;22(12):1–11.

76. Moisey LL, Pikul J, Keller H, et al. Adequacy of protein and energy intake in critically all adults following liberation from mechanical ventilation is dependent on route of nutrition delivery. Nutr Clin Pract 2021;36(1):201–11.
77. Peterson SJ, Tsai AA, Scala CM, et al. Adequacy of oral intake in critically ill patients 1 week after extubation. J Am Diet Assoc 2010;110(3):427–33.
78. Williams DGA, Ohnuma T, Krishnamoorthy V, et al. Impact of early postoperative oral nutritional supplement utilization on clinical outcomes in colorectal surgery. Perioper Med 2020;9(29). https://doi.org/10.1186/s13741-020-00160-6.
79. Jarden RJ, Sutton-Smith L, Boulton C. Oral intake evaluation in patients following critical illness: an ICU cohort study. Nurs Crit Care 2018;23(4):179–85.
80. Ridley EJ, Parke RL, Davies AR, et al. What happens to nutrition intake in the post–intensive care unit hospitalization period? An observational cohort study in critically ill adults. J Parenter Enter Nutr 2019;43(1):88–95.
81. Chapple LS, Weinel LM, Abdelhamid YA, et al. Observed appetite and nutrient intake three months after ICU discharge. Clin Nutr 2019;38(3):1215–20.
82. Rowley A, Adiamah A, Kushairi A, et al. The effect of post-discharge oral nutritional supplements on outcomes after gastrointestinal surgery: a systematic review and meta-analysis. Clin Nutr 2023;42(7):1189–201.
83. Deutz NE, Matheson EM, Matarese LE, et al. Readmission and mortality in malnourished, older, hospitalized adults treated with a specialized oral nutritional supplement: a randomized clinical trial. Clin Nutr 2016;35(1):18–26.
84. Rousseau AF, Lucania S, Fadeur M, et al. Adequacy of nutritional intakes during the year after critical illness: an observational study in a post-ICU follow-Up clinic. Nutrients 2022;14(18):3797.
85. Oshima T, Berger MM, De Waele E, et al. Indirect calorimetry in nutritional therapy. A position paper by the ICALIC study group. Clin Nutr 2017;36(3):651–62.
86. Rattanachaiwong S, Singer P. Indirect calorimetry as point of care testing. Clin Nutr 2019;38(6):2531–44.
87. Singer P, Anbar R, Cohen J, et al. The tight calorie control study (TICACOS): a prospective, randomized, controlled pilot study of nutritional support in critically ill patients. Intensive Care Med 2011;37(4):601–9.
88. Pertzov B, Bar-Yoseph H, Menndel Y, et al. The effect of indirect calorimetry guided isocaloric nutrition on mortality in critically ill patients—a systematic review and meta-analysis. Eur J Clin Nutr 2022;76:5–15.
89. Duan JY, Zheng WH, Zhou H, et al. Energy delivery guided by indirect calorimetry in critically ill patients: a systematic review and meta-analysis. Crit Care 2021;25:88.
90. Moonen HPFX, Beckers KJH, van Zanten ARH. Energy expenditure and indirect calorimetry in critical illness and convalescence: current evidence and practical considerations. J Intensive Care 2021;9:8.
91. De Waele E, van Zanten ARH. Routine use of indirect calorimetry in critically ill patients: pros and cons. Crit Care 2022;26:123.
92. Oshima T, Dupertuis YM, Delsoglio M, et al. In vitro validation of indirect calorimetry device developed for the ICALIC project against mass spectrometry. Clin Nutr ESPEN 2019;32(2019):50–5.
93. McClave SA, Spain DA, Skolnick JL, et al. Achievement of steady state optimizes results when performing indirect calorimetry. J Parenter Enter Nutr 2003;27(1):16–20.
94. Moonen HPFX, Hermans AJH, Bos AE, et al. Resting energy expenditure measured by indirect calorimetry in mechanically ventilated patients during ICU

stay and post-ICU hospitalization: a prospective observational study. J Crit Care 2023;78:154361.

95. Harmon KK, Stout JR, Fukuda DH, et al. The application of creatine supplementation in medical rehabilitation. Nutrients 2021;13(6):1825.

96. Kreider RB. Effects of creatine supplementation on performance and training adaptations. Mol Cell Biochem 2003;244(1–2):89–94.

97. Davies TW, Watson N, Pilkington JJ, et al. Creatine supplementation for optimization of physical function in the patient at risk of functional disability: a systematic review and meta-analysis. J Parenter Enter Nutr 2024;48(4):389–405.

98. Wilson JM, Fitschen PJ, Campbell B, et al. International society of sports nutrition position stand: beta-hydroxy-beta-methylbutyrate (HMB). J Int Soc Sports Nutr 2013;10:6.

99. Ekinci O, Yanık S, Bebitoğlu BT, et al. Effect of calcium β-Hydroxy-β-Methylbutyrate (CaHMB), vitamin D, and protein supplementation. Nutr Clin Pract 2016; 31(6):829–35.

100. Bear DE, Langan A, Dimidi E, et al. β-Hydroxy-β-methylbutyrate and its impact on skeletal muscle mass and physical function in clinical practice: a systematic review and meta-analysis. Am J Clin Nutr 2019;109(4):1119–32.

101. Nakamura K, Kihata A, Naraba H, et al. β-Hydroxy-β-methylbutyrate, arginine, and glutamine complex on muscle volume loss in critically ill patients: a randomized control trial. J Parenter Enter Nutr 2020;44(2):205–12.

102. Viana MV, Becce F, Pantet O, et al. Impact of β–hydroxy-β–methylbutyrate (HMB) on muscle loss and protein metabolism in critically ill patients: a RCT. Clin Nutr 2021;40(8):4878–87.

103. Bear DE, Puthucheary ZA. Designing nutrition-based interventional trials for the future: addressing the known knowns. Crit Care 2019;23:53.

104. Bear DE, Wandrag L, Merriweather JL, et al. The role of nutritional support in the physical and functional recovery of critically ill patients: a narrative review. Crit Care 2017;21:226.

105. Deutz NEP, Pereira SL, Hays NP, et al. Effect of β-hydroxy-β-methylbutyrate (HMB) on lean body mass during 10 days of bed rest in older adults. Clin Nutr 2013;32(5):704–12.

106. Almoosa KF, Gupta A, Pedroza C, et al. Low testosterone levels are frequent in patients with acute respiratory failure and are associated with poor outcomes. Endocr Pract 2014;20(10):1057–63.

107. Iglesias P, Prado F, Macías MC, et al. Hypogonadism in aged hospitalized male patients: prevalence and clinical outcome. J Endocrinol Invest 2014;37(2): 135–41.

108. Mulhall JP, Trost LW, Brannigan RE, et al. Evaluation and management of testosterone deficiency: AUA Guideline. J Urol 2018;200(2):423–32.

109. Wischmeyer PE, Suman OE, Kozar R, et al. Role of anabolic testosterone agents and structured exercise to promote recovery in ICU survivors. Curr Opin Crit Care 2020;26(5):508–15.

110. Toma M, McAlister FA, Coglianese EE, et al. Testosterone supplementation in heart failure: a meta-analysis. Circ Hear Fail 2012;5(3):315–21.

111. Sardar P, Jha A, Roy D, et al. Therapeutic effects of nandrolone and testosterone in adult male HIV patients with AIDS wasting syndrome (AWS): a randomized, double-blind, placebo-controlled trial. HIV Clin Trials 2010;11(4):220–9.

112. Schols AM, Soeters PB, Mostert R, et al. Physiologic effects of nutritional support and anabolic steroids in patients with chronic obstructive pulmonary disease. A

placebo-controlled randomized trial. Am J Respir Crit Care Med 1995;152(4 Pt 1): 1268–74.

113. Stanojcic M, Finnerty CC, Jeschke MG. Anabolic and anticatabolic agents in critical care. Curr Opin Crit Care 2016;22(4):325–31.

114. Li H, Guo Y, Yang Z, et al. The efficacy and safety of oxandrolone treatment for patients with severe burns: a systematic review and meta-analysis. Burns 2016; 42(4):717–27.

115. Cheetham TC, An JJ, Jacobsen SJ, et al. Association of testosterone replacement with cardiovascular outcomes among men with androgen deficiency. JAMA Intern Med 2017;177(4):491–9.

116. Anderson JL, May HT, Lappé DL, et al. Impact of testosterone replacement therapy on myocardial infarction, stroke, and death in men with low testosterone concentrations in an integrated health care system. Am J Cardiol 2016;117(5):794–9.

117. Lincoff AM, Bhasin S, Flevaris P, et al. Cardiovascular safety of testosterone-replacement therapy. N Engl J Med 2023;389(2):107–17.

118. Nierman DM, Mechanick JI. Hypotestosteronemia in chronically critically ill men. Crit Care Med 1999;27(11):2418–21.

119. Binder EF, Christensen JC, Stevens-lapsley J, et al. A multi-center trial of exercise and testosterone therapy in women after hip fracture: design, methods and impact of the COVID-19 pandemic. Contemp Clin Trials 2021;104:106356.

120. Nakano H, Naraba H, Hashimoto H, et al. Novel protocol combining physical and nutrition therapies, Intensive Goal-directed REhabilitation with Electrical muscle stimulation and Nutrition (IGREEN) care bundle. Crit Care 2021;25:415.

121. Nakanishi N, Oto J, Tsutsumi R, et al. Upper limb muscle atrophy associated with in-hospital mortality and physical function impairments in mechanically ventilated critically ill adults: a two-center prospective observational study. J Intensive Care 2020;8:87.

122. Wischmeyer PE, Molinger J, Haines K. Point-counterpoint: indirect calorimetry is essential for optimal nutrition therapy in the intensive care unit. Nutr Clin Pract 2021;36(2):275–81.

Body Composition Assessment in Critically Ill Adults – Where are We now?

Kate J. Lambell, BHSc, MNutrDiet, PhD[a,b,*], Michael T. Paris, PhD[c],
Maria Cristina Gonzalez, PhD, MD[d], Carla M. Prado, PhD, RD[e]

KEYWORDS

- Skeletal muscle mass • Body composition • Critical illness • Intensive care unit
- Computed tomography • Ultrasound

KEY POINTS

- Muscle mass depletion is associated with a range of negative clinical and functional outcomes and is a key characteristic in a number of conditions, including sarcopenia, malnutrition, and cachexia.
- Assessing muscle health may help identify patients at-risk for prolonged recovery and to evaluate interventions aimed at attenuating muscle loss to optimize function and recovery.
- Computed tomography, ultrasound, bioelectrical impedance analysis, and anthropometric methods have been used to assess muscle health during critical illness, with varying levels of validity and utility in this population.

INTRODUCTION

Skeletal muscle mass forms the largest portion of lean mass in the body. It serves as the body's structural support and facilitates movement. Furthermore, and importantly, skeletal muscle acts as a metabolically active tissue with immunologic properties, providing a critical reserve for amino acids to aid with cell repair when needed.[1] The amount of skeletal muscle mass an individual has is influenced by a number of factors, with increasing age, lack of physical activity, inadequate nutrition intake (particularly low protein), and the presence of chronic and acute diseases all contributing to reduced muscle mass.[2]

---

[a] Alfred Health, Melbourne, Australia; [b] Australian and New Zealand Intensive Care Research Centre, Monash University, Melbourne, Australia; [c] School of Kinesiology and Health Science, York University, Toronto, Canada; [d] Postgraduate Program in Nutrition and Food, Federal University of Pelotas, Brazil; [e] Department of Agricultural, Food and Nutritional Science, University of Alberta, Canada
* Corresponding author. Department of Nutrition and Dietetics, Alfred Health, 55 Commercial Road, Melbourne, Victoria 3004, Australia.
E-mail address: k.lambell@alfred.org.au

Crit Care Clin 41 (2025) 283–297
https://doi.org/10.1016/j.ccc.2024.09.006
0749-0704/25/Crown Copyright © 2024 Published by Elsevier Inc. All rights reserved, including those for text and data mining, AI training, and similar technologies.

Muscle mass depletion is associated with a range of negative clinical and functional outcomes and conditions.[3] As such, muscle mass assessment is included as a key criterion for the diagnosis of sarcopenia,[4] cachexia,[5] and malnutrition.[6] Specifically in critical illness, low muscle mass at admission to the intensive care unit (ICU) has been associated with in-hospital and 6-month mortality, ICU and ventilator days, and reduced likelihood of being discharged home.[7–11] Furthermore, it is well-characterized that critically ill patients experience rapid and catastrophic losses of skeletal muscle mass, at ∼2% per day over the first week,[12] which continues over the first 2 to 3 weeks,[13] and then may be maintained post-ICU (with a lack of recovery to baseline mass).[14] Skeletal muscle loss is the key contributor to muscle weakness and functional deficits,[15–17] which may continue long after ICU discharge.[18,19] The reasons for such severe losses are likely multifactorial, including immobility, inflammation, catabolism, and anabolic resistance that occur during early critical illness.[19,20]

Similarly, in parallel to the emerging importance of muscle mass, there is also evidence suggesting that skeletal muscle composition may be important for recovery from critical illness. Muscle composition can be worsened by the infiltration of adipose and/or fibrous tissue into skeletal muscle,[21] and low muscle density at ICU admission using computed tomography (CT) has been associated with mortality at ICU discharge and at 6 to 12 months.[22–24] Unlike muscle mass, there have been differing reports of changes in muscle composition during critical illness, with some studies reporting no change over time,[16,25–27] whereas others reporting negative changes over time[15,17,24,27] and associated weakness.[15]

As survival of critical illness has improved over the last decade, the focus is now on the quality of survival.[28] There is an urgent need to identify high-risk populations for prolonged recovery and to develop and test interventions (eg, nutrition and/or physical therapy) to optimize function and quality of life, including the attenuation of the negative changes to muscle health throughout the trajectory of illness. As recommended in clinical guidelines, nutrition-trained clinicians should incorporate muscle assessment into a broader nutrition assessment to individualize, guide, and evaluate nutrition interventions.[6,29] This review provides an overview of the body composition methods available for use in critically ill patients, with a focus on the evidence relating to the validity and use of methods for muscle assessment, identifying patients with lower-than-normal muscularity, and future directions.

BODY COMPOSITION MODALITIES

There are a number of modalities available for body composition analysis, each measuring different body compartments.[30] To help clarify what component is being measured by a particular body composition technique, frameworks have been developed to describe the relationships between major body compartments. **Fig. 1** outlines a framework commonly used in modern-day clinical environments including the whole-body, molecular, and tissue-organ levels and commonly used body composition assessment methods.[31,32]

The remaining part of this section provides an overview of body composition modalities available for use in critically ill patients: CT image analysis, ultrasonography, bioelectrical impedance analysis (BIA), and anthropometry. Advantages and disadvantages of each method are summarized in **Fig. 2**. It is important to note that while dual-energy x-ray absorptiometry and magnetic resonance imaging (MRI) are considered reference methods for body composition analysis due to measurement precision and reliability, the techniques have limited applicability for the use for critically ill

A. Whole body	B. Molecular			C. Tissue-Organ
Body weight Body shape	Fat mass	Fat mass	Fat mass	Adipose tissue
	Bone Minerals		Bone mineral content	Bones
	Total body water			Organs and blood
	Protein	Fat-free mass	Lean soft tissue	Skeletal muscle
	Carbohydrates			
	Soft tissue minerals			

Model:	2-compartment	3-compartment	Skeletal muscle
Modality commonly used:	Bioimpedance technology, arm and calf circumference	DXA, Bioimpedance technology[a]	CT, MRI, Ultrasound

Muscle composition: CT, MRI, ultrasound

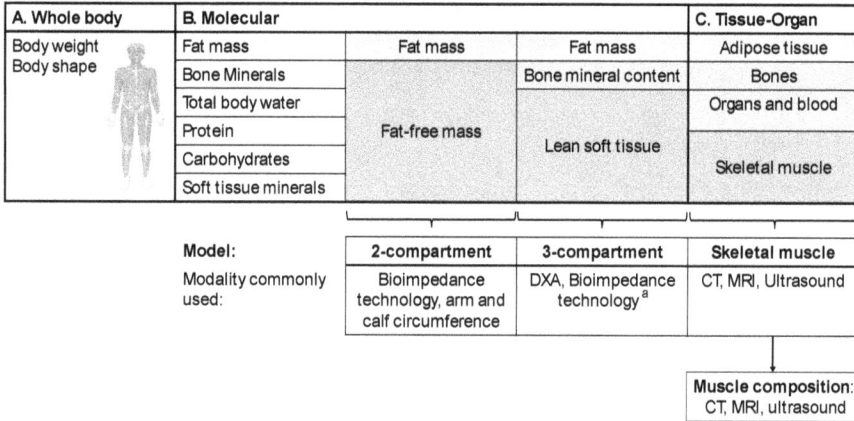

Fig. 1. Body composition framework depicting levels and compartments measured by commonly used body composition modalities. [a]Modern bioimpedance equations can estimate appendicular lean soft tissue. CT, Computed Tomography; DXA, dual-energy x-ray absorptiometry; MRI, magnetic resonance imaging. (*Adapted from* Refs.[31,32])

patients due to cost, time, logistical, and safety issues with patient transportation to specialized machinery and will not be discussed.

Computed Tomography Image Analysis

CT scans, traditionally used for diagnostic purposes in clinical populations, are considered a reference method for assessing body composition.[33] CT scans deliver high-resolution, precise images, which can be used for the secondary purpose of body composition analysis.[31] Skeletal muscle mass and radiodensity (indicative of myosteatosis), as well as adipose tissue depots, can be quantified using these images.[31]

The analysis of CT images involves a single cross-sectional area (CSA), which is used to estimate whole-body composition. The third lumbar vertebra (L3) is traditionally used as the best correlate of whole-body skeletal muscle and adipose tissues.[34] Additional landmarks have also been proposed; for example, skeletal muscle cross-sectional assessment at L1 is reliable (96% acceptable quality evaluations) when L3 is not available.[35,36] Notably, total muscle CSA is recommended versus the analysis of individual muscle groups,[37,38] such as psoas, for example.

CT scanning is a promising modality to assess abnormal body composition in critically ill patients.[39] To date, the majority of studies in ICU have utilized CT scans that are available as a part of routine clinical practice (due to the high cost and radiation exposure). Most studies have retrospectively included patients who had a scan at the L3 area performed on or around ICU admission and investigated associations with CT-measured muscle mass and/or radiodensity and outcomes, reporting strong correlations with clinical and discharge outcomes[7–11,22,23,40] as outlined earlier.

There are a number of small studies that have used CT image analysis to describe changes in muscularity in the abdominal region by including patients who had 2 or more CT scans as a part of clinical practice.[24,26,27,41–43] Reported changes in CT-derived muscle mass and radiodensity are highly variable, and comparing the results across studies is limited by the different muscle variables reported, heterogenous study populations, and variable and often undefined time between CT scans. Although clinical practice differs worldwide, unless there is a significant shift in practice, it is

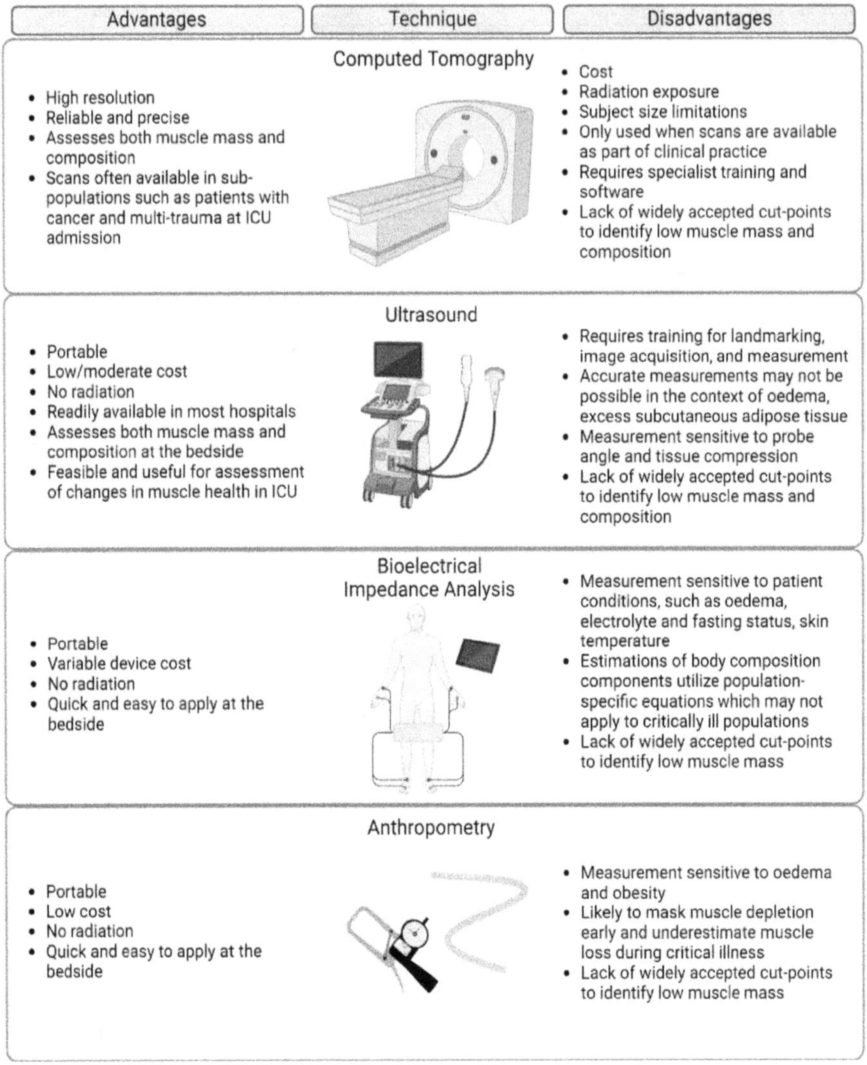

Advantages	Technique	Disadvantages
• High resolution • Reliable and precise • Assesses both muscle mass and composition • Scans often available in sub-populations such as patients with cancer and multi-trauma at ICU admission	**Computed Tomography**	• Cost • Radiation exposure • Subject size limitations • Only used when scans are available as part of clinical practice • Requires specialist training and software • Lack of widely accepted cut-points to identify low muscle mass and composition
• Portable • Low/moderate cost • No radiation • Readily available in most hospitals • Assesses both muscle mass and composition at the bedside • Feasible and useful for assessment of changes in muscle health in ICU	**Ultrasound**	• Requires training for landmarking, image acquisition, and measurement • Accurate measurements may not be possible in the context of oedema, excess subcutaneous adipose tissue • Measurement sensitive to probe angle and tissue compression • Lack of widely accepted cut-points to identify low muscle mass and composition
• Portable • Variable device cost • No radiation • Quick and easy to apply at the bedside	**Bioelectrical Impedance Analysis**	• Measurement sensitive to patient conditions, such as oedema, electrolyte and fasting status, skin temperature • Estimations of body composition components utilize population-specific equations which may not apply to critically ill populations • Lack of widely accepted cut-points to identify low muscle mass
• Portable • Low cost • No radiation • Quick and easy to apply at the bedside	**Anthropometry**	• Measurement sensitive to oedema and obesity • Likely to mask muscle depletion early and underestimate muscle loss during critical illness • Lack of widely accepted cut-points to identify low muscle mass

Fig. 2. Advantages and disadvantages of body composition modalities in critical care. *Adapted from* Ref.[29]

unlikely that CT scans can be available for routine monitoring of changes in muscularity in critically ill patients, as many do not undergo multiple scanning procedures.

In addition to the routine availability of CT scans for analysis, there are also a number of limitations for its use in critically ill patients. Patient dimensions (such as weight and height) may exceed equipment's capacity. Challenges also include transporting medically unstable patients out of the ICU for scanning, inconsistent image acquisition protocols, issues with image cropping and artifacts, and limited validation for populations with obesity.[29,44,45] Furthermore, validation studies are needed to ensure the accuracy of these measures in the ICU population and to define specific cutoffs for low muscularity and radiodensity.[39] Finally, as with many body composition techniques, edema can affect assessments; such data/information must be interpreted with caution.[46]

The use of CT scans in critical illness is a field that continues to rapidly evolve, marked by innovations such as semi-automated or fully-automated software.[37,47] These evolving tools not only promise to enhance analytical efficiency but may also enable researchers and health care professionals to seamlessly incorporate CT assessments to enhance patient care and treatment outcomes. For patient subgroups who routinely have CT scans at or during ICU admission at the L3 level (eg, patients with traumatic injuries, abdominal surgery), this advancement will be particularly valuable in offering clinicians timely information. This information can in turn be used to identify patients at high nutritional risk and help to target and evaluate nutrition support, with the potential for further enhancement of precision and effectiveness of nutritional interventions.[48]

Ultrasound

Ultrasound has emerged as a useful tool for bedside assessment of muscle health in the ICU due to its increasingly routine availability and capacity to prospectively quantify changes in muscle size and composition noninvasively.[49] Using high-frequency sound waves (2–20 MHz), ultrasound devices generate 2-dimensional, high contrast images of the underlying musculature at specific anatomic landmarks, permitting precise quantification of muscle health.[39] Most commonly, muscle CSA and thickness (centimeter) are extracted from these images as surrogates of muscle mass, as displayed in **Fig. 3**. Across a wide variety of limb and trunk anatomic landmarks, ultrasound-derived muscle CSA and thickness are strongly correlated with reference measures of muscle mass (eg, MRI muscle volume) in healthy adults across the life span,[50–52] highlighting the strong criterion validity of ultrasound as a tool to measure muscle size. However, far less is known about the criterion validity of single-site anatomic landmarks in critically ill patients, which may be further challenged by additional clinical considerations (eg, fluid imbalances).

Among a few studies, ultrasound-derived measures of quadriceps muscle thickness or CSA have shown moderate to strong correlations with L3 muscle CSA from CT scans in critically ill patients.[53–55] In a study of 50 patients at ICU admission, there were stronger associations with CT L3 CSA when including the anterior upper arm muscle thickness alongside the quadriceps, further reinforcing the strong criterion validity of this tool.[54] However, these evaluations are confounded due to different muscle groups being compared. In a more direct comparison, CT and ultrasound measures of muscle thickness at the same anatomic landmark of the quadriceps showed very strong agreement,[56,57] similar to those observed in noncritically ill populations.[58] In addition to single-timepoint validity, the ability to monitor muscle atrophy is a strong focal point of ultrasound in the ICU and has been more widely explored.[12,59] A recent systematic review investigating the rate of muscle atrophy and methods used to measure muscle mass during critical illness included 52 studies and reported that ultrasound was used in 85% of the studies.[12] Importantly, in a scoping review of muscle ultrasound use in critically ill patients, the feasibility (defined as capturing >70% of attempted measurements) and reproducibility of ultrasound-measured muscle health was reviewed, with all studies reporting feasibility of the method and intraobserver and interobserver reliabilities ranging from good to excellent, confirming ultrasound as a viable tool in this setting.[59]

Skeletal muscle composition is another commonly assessed feature of muscle health in critically ill patients, often evaluated as mean echo intensity of ultrasound images. Muscle echo intensity is the average pixel brightness from a region of interest within the muscle on ultrasound images (scaled from 0 to 255).[60] Previous literature in healthy adults has shown that increased muscle echo intensity is correlated with

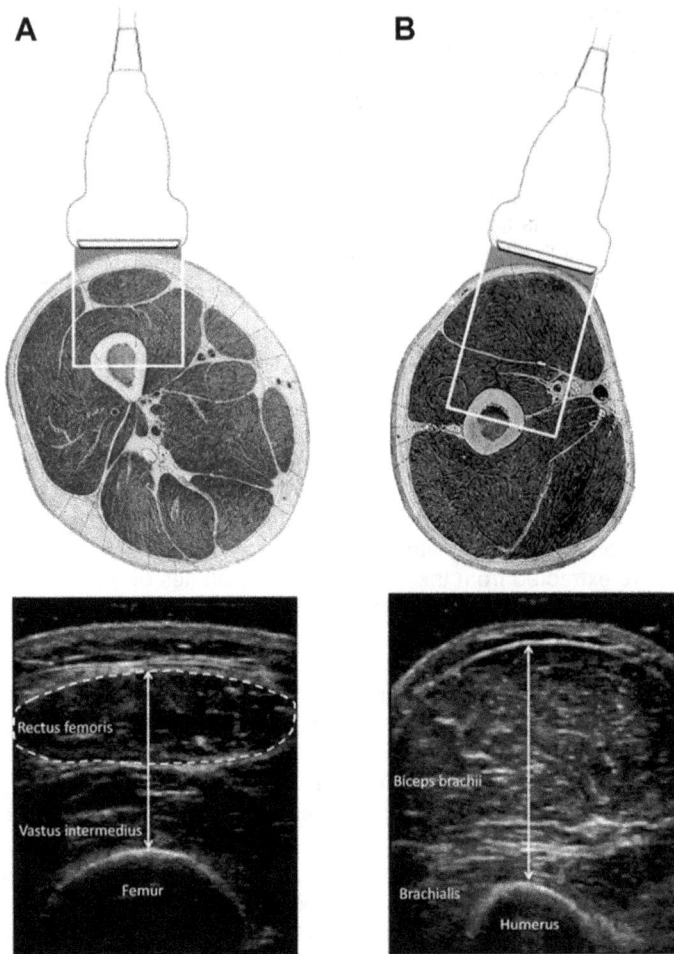

Fig. 3. MRIs demonstrating location of ultrasound probe on quadriceps (*A*) and anterior mid-upper arm (*B*), and corresponding ultrasound images with readily measured muscle groups and measurements (rectus femoris cross-sectional area and quadriceps and mid-upper arm muscle thickness). MRI images from Gray, H (1918). Anatomy of the Human Body. 20th ed. Philadelphia, Lea and Febiger.

a higher degree of intramuscular adipose tissue (ie, adipose tissue surrounding individual muscle fibers but not lipids stored intramyocellularly) across diverse anatomic landmarks.[61] However, many factors confound muscle echo intensity, which may become exacerbated in critically ill patients, including hydration status and fibrotic infiltration.[60] Thus, muscle echo intensity as a sole indicator of intramuscular adipose tissue is unwarranted, hence our reference to overall muscle composition. Nonetheless, echo intensity in critically ill patients has shown to increase over an acute length of stay compared with admission and has been associated with myonecrosis,[21] poor muscle function,[17] and ICU-acquired weakness.[15] Unlike thickness or CSA, no cutpoints have been established for muscle echo intensity, as the brightness of the muscle image is highly dependent on the ultrasound equipment, limiting comparisons across different setups.

Although ultrasound has emerged as a clinically applicable tool to quantify features of skeletal muscle health at the bedside, several significant barriers remain (in addition to those discussed earlier, reviewed extensively by Lima and colleagues[59]) and require clarification to determine how best to capture these indices and subsequently utilize these features to improve patient outcomes.

Bioelectrical Impedance Analysis

BIA is one of the most used bedside body composition assessment techniques in hospitals.[62] BIA measures the tissue conductivity, or impedance (Z), in response to the passage of an electric current of one or several frequencies. Impedance comprises 2 components: resistance (R), inversely related to the amount of water and electrolytes in tissues, and reactance (Xc), directly associated with the quantity of cells and their membrane integrity.[63,64] BIA methodology is based on assumptions such as fixed fat-free mass hydration, body geometry, and stable extracellular water/intracellular water ratio (ECW/ICW). Body composition is estimated using prediction equations/algorithms derived from the reference body composition methods or biophysical modeling (bioelectrical impedance spectroscopy).[45,65] These predictive equations include data from BIA (Z, R, and Xc) from one or multiple frequencies, and other variables, for example, height, weight, sex, and age. They are specific to the population and the device used. However, some BIA devices do not disclose these equations, which may impair the accuracy of results if applied to a different population.[66] Fat mass and various muscle-related compartments, such as fat-free mass, appendicular lean soft tissue, or skeletal muscle mass, can be estimated using BIA, according to the reference method used to generate the prediction equation. Phase angle (PhA) is another parameter obtained directly from the raw BIA parameters Xc and R. It is defined as the phase shift caused by the cell membranes, acting as capacitors when the electric current flows into the cells. PhA is correlated with the quality and the quantity of soft tissues. It is also directly associated with cell mass and membrane integrity and inversely associated with the ECW/ICW ratio. Thus, PhA is considered an emergent marker of the quantity and the quality of muscle mass and a prognostic tool in several clinical conditions.[67]

Few studies have validated the muscle mass compartments estimated by BIA with CT measurements in ICU patients.[68–71] Overall, they demonstrated a good correlation and agreement in identifying patients with low muscularity, except in one study in ICU patients with COVID-19.[71] However, differences in absolute values between CT measurements and BIA estimations were found. PhA also showed a good correlation with CT-derived skeletal muscle area and density,[70] but these results were not confirmed by Osuna-Padilla and colleagues.[71] Two meta-analyses investigated PhA prognostic value in critically ill patients.[67,72] The results showed that PhA may be considered an important prognostic factor in this population, as it was associated with higher mortality and ICU length of stay. PhA also showed a prognostic value for 60-day mortality, postextubation dysphagia, prolonged LOS, and disease severity in critically ill patients with COVID-19.[73–77]

Advantages of BIA include safety, noninvasiveness, radiation-free, relatively affordable, portability, and availability at the bedside. However, some factors affect body compartment estimations from BIA in critical illness. Most of the BIA equations use weight and height for the body composition estimations, which are not measured accurately in these patients. BIA estimations rely on the assumption of fixed tissue hydration, which might not be valid in critically ill patients. For this reason, BIA is not validated in patients with large and rapid hydration changes and in the presence of ascites, pleural effusion, or urine retention, situations commonly found in ICU patients.[64,78] Most of the equations were developed for healthy subjects with a normal BMI range, limiting even more its use in subjects with obesity.[45]

The aforementioned limitations and the absence of well-established cut-off points limit the applicability of BIA-derived body compartment estimates and PhA in ICU patients.[64] Changes in fluid balance commonly found in ICU patients also hinder its use to monitor changes in muscle mass.[79] Nonetheless, longitudinal changes in PhA may reflect more favorable or unfavorable outcomes.[80] PhA can also be used as a sensitive marker of global health after interventional studies.[81] While BIA has limited utility in estimating body composition in ICU patients, PhA is emerging as a valuable parameter for use as a prognostic tool and for monitoring the patient's progress and response to interventions.

Anthropometric Measures (Arm and Calf Circumference)

Anthropometric measurements, such as arm and calf circumferences, can be used as a surrogate measure of muscle mass in the absence of more technical approaches described earlier.[82] Although these measures are inexpensive, quick, portable, and noninvasive, they are not as accurate as the more technical approaches, are influenced by edema and obesity, and generally are not sensitive enough to detect short-term changes in muscle mass,[82] as described in more detail later.

In critical illness, there is limited data comparing anthropometric measurements to a reference method for muscle assessment. In a study of 41 patients at ICU admission, arm anthropometry was compared with CT-derived muscle CSA.[69] There were moderate-poor correlations between methods, with mid-arm muscle circumference more strongly correlated with CT muscle area than mid-upper arm circumference ($r = 0.665$, $P<.001$ vs $r = 0.342$, $P=.029$).[69] Additionally, both methods had a poor ability to classify participants with low CT muscle area, with 4 (31%) being correctly classified using mid-upper arm circumference and 5 (38%) using mid-arm muscle circumference.[69]

Arm anthropometry and calf circumference have been used in a number of small studies evaluating the relationship between baseline measurements and clinical outcomes, with inconsistent findings.[83–86] Other studies have measured longitudinal changes in arm anthropometry during ICU admission alongside other body composition methods. Campbell and colleagues investigated 9 patients with multiorgan failure and measured ultrasound-derived muscle thickness and mid-upper arm circumference every 1 to 4 days in early critical illness.[87] Despite ultrasound imaging showing a significant decrease in muscle thickness over time, arm circumference measurements showed an inconsistent pattern of change.[87] These findings are consistent with a more recent study ($n = 34$), where changes in ultrasound-derived rectus femoris CSA, mid-upper arm circumference, and calf circumference were measured at baseline and 7 days after.[88] Compared with baseline, the median percentage change was 16% (6.6–28.9), 5.5% (0–7.9), and 3.7% (0–5.9), respectively.[88] These findings indicate that anthropometric methods, at least in early critical illness, are likely influenced by edema and possibly other factors such as positioning and landmarking, and may overestimate muscle mass early and underestimate muscle loss over time. Considering the low cost and ease of use of anthropometric measurements, the validation of these methods to provide proxy assessments of muscle mass and/or strength later in critical illness (ie, ICU discharge) and in the post-ICU phase is warranted.

IDENTIFYING CRITICALLY ILL PATIENTS WITH LOW MUSCLE MASS

Broadly, at present, there are currently no universally accepted cut-points to define low muscle mass using any of the body composition modalities for critically ill patients.

To date, several cut-points using CT and ultrasound have been derived to identify critically ill patients with low muscle mass, mostly at ICU admission. While several different approaches have been used, most studies have been primarily focused on regression modeling or receiver operator characteristic (ROC) analysis for predicting clinical outcomes such as mortality, ICU and hospital length of stay, weaning from a ventilator, and ICU-acquired weakness.[7,9–11,59] While these analyses are useful at a group level to show associations, they are only applicable to the populations with the same characteristics: ethnicity, admission diagnosis, disease severity, age, gender, device and method of muscle assessment, muscle variable measured, and outcome.

Identification of patients experiencing significant muscle atrophy throughout their ICU stay is important for targeted therapies to mitigate muscle depletion. Similar to cut-points developed for identifying low muscle mass at admission, using ultrasound ROC analysis has been applied to determine what relative change in muscle size, for a given length of time (eg, 7 days), is associated with poor outcomes. Importantly, because a relative change from baseline is compared, there is perhaps less variability for the reported cut-points, as differences in imaging protocols (eg, anatomic landmark) would be minimized between studies. For example, many studies have reported that 7 days following ICU admission, a reduction in rectus femoris CSA between 18% and 20% is associated with worse outcomes, which represents a narrower range than the use of an absolute value for a cut-point. However, thus far, all cut-points have been derived within a cohort they are being applied to, future work should look toward validating either previously established cut-points[59] or those derived from normative data.[50]

FUTURE DIRECTIONS

Challenges surrounding the quantification of muscle health in the ICU setting underline a significant gap in the application of these methods into clinical practice and standardization in research. A promising future direction would be a Delphi consensus involving a diverse group of global experts to establish a unified definition and measurement protocol for low muscle mass in critically ill patients. This effort should aim to standardize the diagnostic tools and techniques, perhaps focusing on innovative imaging technologies and biochemical markers that can provide reliable data even in challenging ICU settings. Upcoming work on (general) body composition methodological standards, as well as cut-points for low muscle mass based on reference populations may further inform such effort. Such a consensus could pave the way for more standardized research studies, enhance interdisciplinary communication, and ultimately lead to improved clinical guidelines that are essential for optimizing patient care and outcomes in critical illnesses.

SUMMARY

Poor muscle health at admission to ICU and muscle atrophy during critical illness influences recovery from critical illness. Methods for muscle assessment in critically ill patients include CT image analysis, ultrasound, BIA, and anthropometry. While all modalities have merit, none can be currently recommended for routine use to identify critically ill patients with lower-than-normal muscularity. Muscle ultrasound shows the greatest promise for bedside assessment of muscle health during critical illness, although more work is required to develop standardized protocols for muscle assessment to ensure consistency and application in use both in clinical practice and research.

CLINICS CARE POINTS

- Assessment of muscle health may help identify patients at-risk for prolonged recovery and to evaluate interventions aimed at attenuating muscle loss to optimize function and recovery.
- Computed tomography, ultrasound, bioelectrical impedance analysis, and anthropometric methods have been used to assess muscle health during critical illness, and all have varying levels of validity in this population.
- Further research is needed to standardize measurement protocols and develop and review cut-points that can be used in critically ill patients to progress muscle health assessment into clinical practice.

ACKNOWLEDGMENTS

The authors would like to thank Julia Montenegro for her assistance with graphic designing of figures (using BioRender.com).

DISCLOSURE

K.J. Lambell and M. Paris have nothing to disclose. M.C. Gonzalez has received honoraria and/or paid consultancy from Abbott Nutrition, Nutricia Danone, and Nestlé Brazil. C.M. Prado has received honoraria and/or paid consultancy from Abbott Nutrition, Nutricia Danone, Nestlé Health Science, Pfizer and AMRA medical.

REFERENCES

1. Pedersen BK, Febbraio MA. Muscles, exercise and obesity: skeletal muscle as a secretory organ. Nat Rev Endocrinol 2012;8(8):457–65.
2. Baumgartner RN, Waters DL, Gallagher D, et al. Predictors of skeletal muscle mass in elderly men and women. Mech Ageing Dev 1999;107(2):123–36.
3. Prado CM, Landi F, Chew STH, et al. Advances in muscle health and nutrition: a toolkit for healthcare professionals. Clin Nutr 2022;41(10):2244–63.
4. Zanker J, Sim M, Anderson K, et al. Consensus guidelines for sarcopenia prevention, diagnosis and management in Australia and New Zealand. J Cachexia Sarcopenia Muscle 2023;14(1):142–56.
5. Fearon K, Strasser F, Anker SD, et al. Definition and classification of cancer cachexia: an international consensus. Lancet Oncol 2011;12(5):489–95.
6. Cederholm T, Jensen GL, Correia M, et al. GLIM criteria for the diagnosis of malnutrition - a consensus report from the global clinical nutrition community. Clin Nutr 2019;38(1):1–9.
7. Weijs PJ, Looijaard WG, Dekker IM, et al. Low skeletal muscle area is a risk factor for mortality in mechanically ventilated critically ill patients. Crit Care 2014;18(2):R12.
8. Moisey LL, Mourtzakis M, Cotton BA, et al. Skeletal muscle predicts ventilator-free days, ICU-free days, and mortality in elderly ICU patients. Crit Care 2013;17(5):R206.
9. Jaitovich A, Dumas CL, Itty R, et al. ICU admission body composition: skeletal muscle, bone, and fat effects on mortality and disability at hospital discharge-a prospective, cohort study. Crit Care 2020;24(1):566.
10. Ng CC, Lee ZY, Chan WY, et al. Low muscularity as assessed by abdominal computed tomography on intensive care unit admission is associated with

mortality in a critically ill asian population. JPEN - J Parenter Enter Nutr 2020; 44(3):425–33.

11. Fuchs G, Thevathasan T, Chretien YR, et al. Lumbar skeletal muscle index derived from routine computed tomography exams predict adverse post-extubation outcomes in critically ill patients. J Crit Care 2018;44:117–23.

12. Fazzini B, Markl T, Costas C, et al. The rate and assessment of muscle wasting during critical illness: a systematic review and meta-analysis. Crit Care 2023; 27(1):2.

13. Gruther W, Benesch T, Zorn C, et al. Muscle wasting in intensive care patients: ultrasound observation of the M. quadriceps femoris muscle layer. J Rehabil Med 2008;40(3):185–9.

14. Chapple LAS, Deane AM, Williams LT, et al. Longitudinal changes in anthropo-metrics and impact on self-reported physical function after traumatic brain injury. Critical Care and Resuscitation 2017;19(1):29–36.

15. Mayer KP, Thompson Bastin ML, Montgomery-Yates AA, et al. Acute skeletal muscle wasting and dysfunction predict physical disability at hospital discharge in patients with critical illness. Crit Care 2020;24(1):637.

16. Hayes K, Holland AE, Pellegrino VA, et al. Acute skeletal muscle wasting and relation to physical function in patients requiring extracorporeal membrane oxygenation (ECMO). J Crit Care 2018;48:1–8.

17. Parry SM, El-Ansary D, Cartwright MS, et al. Ultrasonography in the intensive care setting can be used to detect changes in the quality and quantity of muscle and is related to muscle strength and function. J Crit Care 2015;30(5):1151 e1159–e1114.

18. Dos Santos C, Hussain SN, Mathur S, et al. Mechanisms of chronic muscle wasting and dysfunction after an intensive care unit stay. a pilot study. Am J Re-spir Crit Care Med 2016;194(7):821–30.

19. Batt J, Herridge MS, Dos Santos CC. From skeletal muscle weakness to func-tional outcomes following critical illness: a translational biology perspective. Tho-rax 2019;74(11):1091–8.

20. Chapple LS, Kouw IWK, Summers MJ, et al. Muscle protein synthesis after pro-tein administration in critical illness. Am J Respir Crit Care Med 2022;206(6): 740–9.

21. Puthucheary ZA, Phadke R, Rawal J, et al. Qualitative ultrasound in acute critical illness muscle wasting. Crit Care Med 2015;43(8):1603–11.

22. Looijaard WG, Dekker IM, Stapel SN, et al. Skeletal muscle quality as assessed by CT-derived skeletal muscle density is associated with 6-month mortality in me-chanically ventilated critically ill patients. Crit Care 2016;20(1):386.

23. Loosen SH, Schulze-Hagen M, Pungel T, et al. Skeletal muscle composition pre-dicts outcome in critically ill patients. Crit Care Explor 2020;2(8):e0171.

24. Bear DE, MacGowan L, Elstad M, et al. Relationship between skeletal muscle area and density and clinical outcome in adults receiving venovenous extracor-poreal membrane oxygenation. Crit Care Med 2021;49(4):e350–9.

25. Casaer MP, Langouche L, Coudyzer W, et al. Impact of early parenteral nutrition on muscle and adipose tissue compartments during critical illness. Crit Care Med 2013;41(10):2298–309.

26. Dusseaux MM, Antoun S, Grigioni S, et al. Skeletal muscle mass and adipose tis-sue alteration in critically ill patients. PLoS One 2019;14(6):e0216991.

27. Yeh DD, Ortiz-Reyes LA, Quraishi SA, et al. Early nutritional inadequacy is asso-ciated with psoas muscle deterioration and worse clinical outcomes in critically ill surgical patients. J Crit Care 2018;45:7–13.

28. Iwashyna TJ. Survivorship will be the defining challenge of critical care in the 21st century. Ann Intern Med 2010;153(3):204–5.
29. Wischmeyer PE, Bear DE, Berger MM, et al. Personalized nutrition therapy in critical care: 10 expert recommendations. Crit Care 2023;27(1):261.
30. Heymsfield SBL TG, Wang Z, Going SB. Human body composition. Second Edition edition. United States of America: Human Kinetics; 2005.
31. Prado CM, Heymsfield SB. Lean tissue imaging: a new era for nutritional assessment and intervention. JPEN - J Parenter Enter Nutr 2014;38(8):940–53.
32. Lambell K.J., Skeletal muscle mass in critically ill adults: assessment, changes and association with nutrition delivery, 2021, La Trobe University Research Repository, La Trobe University. Available at: https://opal.latrobe.edu.au/articles/thesis/Skeletal_Muscle_Mass_in_Critically_ill_Adults_Assessment_Changes_and_Association_with_Nutrition_Delivery/16865023.
33. Earthman CP. Body composition tools for assessment of adult malnutrition at the bedside: a tutorial on research considerations and clinical applications. JPEN - J Parenter Enter Nutr 2015;39(7):787–822.
34. Shen W, Punyanitya M, Wang Z, et al. Total body skeletal muscle and adipose tissue volumes: estimation from a single abdominal cross-sectional image. J Appl Physiol (1985) 2004;97(6):2333–8.
35. Recio-Boiles A, Galeas JN, Goldwasser B, et al. Enhancing evaluation of sarcopenia in patients with non-small cell lung cancer (NSCLC) by assessing skeletal muscle index (SMI) at the first lumbar (L1) level on routine chest computed tomography (CT). Support Care Cancer 2018;26(7):2353–9.
36. Derstine BA, Holcombe SA, Ross BE, et al. Skeletal muscle cutoff values for sarcopenia diagnosis using T10 to L5 measurements in a healthy US population. Sci Rep 2018;8(1):11369.
37. Baracos VE. Psoas as a sentinel muscle for sarcopenia: a flawed premise. J Cachexia Sarcopenia Muscle 2017;8(4):527–8.
38. Abbass T, Tsz Ho YT, Horgan PG, et al. The relationship between computed tomography derived skeletal muscle index, psoas muscle index and clinical outcomes in patients with operable colorectal cancer. Clin Nutr ESPEN 2020;39:104–13.
39. Paris M, Mourtzakis M. Assessment of skeletal muscle mass in critically ill patients: considerations for the utility of computed tomography imaging and ultrasonography. Curr Opin Clin Nutr Metab Care 2016;19(2):125–30.
40. Toledo DO, Carvalho AM, Oliveira A, et al. The use of computed tomography images as a prognostic marker in critically ill cancer patients. Clin Nutr ESPEN 2018;25:114–20.
41. Lambell KJ, Goh GS, Tierney AC, et al. Marked losses of computed tomography-derived skeletal muscle area and density over the first month of a critical illness are not associated with energy and protein delivery. Nutrition 2021;82:111061.
42. Brewster DJ, Strauss BJ, Crozier TM. Measuring visceral fat, subcutaneous fat and skeletal muscle area changes by computed tomography in acute pancreatitis: a retrospective, single-centre study. Crit Care Resusc 2014;16(1):42–7.
43. Braunschweig CA, Sheean PM, Peterson SJ, et al. Exploitation of diagnostic computed tomography scans to assess the impact of nutrition support on body composition changes in respiratory failure patients. JPEN - J Parenter Enter Nutr 2014;38(7):880–5.
44. Prado CM, Cushen SJ, Orsso CE, et al. Sarcopenia and cachexia in the era of obesity: clinical and nutritional impact. Proc Nutr Soc 2016;75(2):188–98.

45. Price KL, Earthman CP. Update on body composition tools in clinical settings: computed tomography, ultrasound, and bioimpedance applications for assessment and monitoring. Eur J Clin Nutr 2019;73(2):187–93.

46. Baggerman MR, van Dijk DPJ, Winkens B, et al. Edema in critically ill patients leads to overestimation of skeletal muscle mass measurements using computed tomography scans. Nutrition 2021;89:111238.

47. Prado CM, Ford KL, Gonzalez MC, et al. Nascent to novel methods to evaluate malnutrition and frailty in the surgical patient. JPEN - J Parenter Enter Nutr 2023;47:S54–68 (Suppl 1.

48. Looijaard W, Molinger J, Weijs PJM. Measuring and monitoring lean body mass in critical illness. Curr Opin Crit Care 2018;24(4):241–7.

49. Mourtzakis M, Parry S, Connolly B, et al. Skeletal muscle ultrasound in critical care: a tool in need of translation. Ann Am Thorac Soc 2017;14(10):1495–503.

50. Paris MT, Lafleur B, Dubin JA, et al. Development of a bedside viable ultrasound protocol to quantify appendicular lean tissue mass. J Cachexia Sarcopenia Muscle 2017;8(5):713–26.

51. Takai Y, Ohta M, Akagi R, et al. Validity of ultrasound muscle thickness measurements for predicting leg skeletal muscle mass in healthy Japanese middle-aged and older individuals. J Physiol Anthropol 2013;32:12.

52. Sanada K, Kearns CF, Midorikawa T, et al. Prediction and validation of total and regional skeletal muscle mass by ultrasound in Japanese adults. Eur J Appl Physiol 2006;96(1):24–31.

53. Paris MT, Mourtzakis M, Day A, et al. Validation of bedside ultrasound of muscle layer thickness of the quadriceps in the critically ill patient (VALIDUM Study). JPEN - J Parenter Enter Nutr 2017;41(2):171–80.

54. Lambell KJ, Tierney AC, Wang JC, et al. Comparison of ultrasound-derived muscle thickness with computed tomography muscle cross-sectional area on admission to the intensive care unit: a pilot cross-sectional study. JPEN - J Parenter Enter Nutr 2021;45(1):136–45.

55. Fetterplace K, Corlette L, Abdelhamid YA, et al. Assessment of muscle mass using ultrasound with minimal versus maximal pressure compared with computed tomography in critically ill adult patients. Aust Crit Care 2020;34(4):303–10.

56. Peres LM, Luis-Silva F, Menegueti MG, et al. Validation study of ultrasonography versus computed tomography for measuring muscle mass loss in critically ill patients: CT mUS study. Crit Care 2023;27(1):310.

57. Tourel C, Burnol L, Lanoisele J, et al. Reliability of standardized ultrasound measurements of quadriceps muscle thickness in neurological critically ill patients: a comparison to computed tomography measures. J Rehabil Med 2020;52(3): jrm00032.

58. Sipila S, Suominen H. Muscle ultrasonography and computed tomography in elderly trained and untrained women. Muscle Nerve 1993;16(3):294–300.

59. Lima J, Foletto E, Cardoso RCB, et al. Ultrasound for measurement of skeletal muscle mass quantity and muscle composition/architecture in critically ill patients: a scoping review on studies' aims, methods, and findings. Clin Nutr 2024;43(1):95–110.

60. Paris MT, Bell KE, Avrutin E, et al. Ultrasound image resolution influences analysis of skeletal muscle composition. Clin Physiol Funct Imag 2020;40(4):277–83.

61. Young HJ, Jenkins NT, Zhao Q, et al. Measurement of intramuscular fat by muscle echo intensity. Muscle Nerve 2015;52(6):963–71.

62. Smith LO, Olieman JF, Berk KA, et al. Clinical applications of body composition and functional status tools for nutrition assessment of hospitalized adults: a systematic review. JPEN - J Parenter Enter Nutr 2023;47(1):11–29.

63. Lukaski HC, Kyle UG, Kondrup J. Assessment of adult malnutrition and prognosis with bioelectrical impedance analysis: phase angle and impedance ratio. Curr Opin Clin Nutr Metab Care 2017;20(5):330–9.

64. Moonen H, Van Zanten ARH. Bioelectric impedance analysis for body composition measurement and other potential clinical applications in critical illness. Curr Opin Crit Care 2021;27(4):344–53.

65. Gonzalez MC. Using bioelectrical impedance analysis for body composition assessment: sorting out some misunderstandings. JPEN - J Parenter Enter Nutr 2019;43(8):954–5.

66. Gonzalez MC, Barbosa-Silva TG, Heymsfield SB. Bioelectrical impedance analysis in the assessment of sarcopenia. Curr Opin Clin Nutr Metab Care 2018;21(5):366–74.

67. Lima J, Eckert I, Gonzalez MC, et al. Prognostic value of phase angle and bioelectrical impedance vector in critically ill patients: a systematic review and meta-analysis of observational studies. Clin Nutr 2022;41(12):2801–16.

68. Kim D, Sun JS, Lee YH, et al. Comparative assessment of skeletal muscle mass using computerized tomography and bioelectrical impedance analysis in critically ill patients. Clin Nutr 2019;38(6):2747–55.

69. Lambell KJ, Earthman CP, Tierney AC, et al. How does muscularity assessed by bedside methods compare to computed tomography muscle area at intensive care unit admission? A pilot prospective cross-sectional study. J Hum Nutr Diet 2021;34(2):345–55.

70. Looijaard W, Stapel SN, Dekker IM, et al. Identifying critically ill patients with low muscle mass: agreement between bioelectrical impedance analysis and computed tomography. Clin Nutr 2020;39(6):1809–17.

71. Osuna-Padilla IA, Rodriguez-Moguel NC, Rodriguez-Llamazares S, et al. Low muscle mass in COVID-19 critically-ill patients: prognostic significance and surrogate markers for assessment. Clin Nutr 2022;41(12):2910–7.

72. Zheng WH, Zhao YH, Yao Y, et al. Prognostic role of bioelectrical impedance phase angle for critically ill patients: a systemic review and meta-analysis. Front Med 2022;9:1059747.

73. Lakenman PLM, van Marwijk I, van der Hoven B, et al. Association between fat-free mass and survival in critically ill patients with COVID-19: a prospective cohort study. JPEN - J Parenter Enter Nutr 2024;48(2):192–8.

74. Moonen H, van Zanten FJL, Driessen L, et al. Association of bioelectric impedance analysis body composition and disease severity in COVID-19 hospital ward and ICU patients: the BIAC-19 study. Clin Nutr 2021;40(4):2328–36.

75. Osuna-Padilla IA, Rodriguez-Moguel NC, Rodriguez-Llamazares S, et al. Low phase angle is associated with 60-day mortality in critically ill patients with COVID-19. JPEN - J Parenter Enter Nutr 2022;46(4):828–35.

76. Reyes-Torres CA, Flores-Lopez A, Osuna-Padilla IA, et al. Phase angle and overhydration are associated with post-extubating dysphagia in patients with COVID-19 discharged from the ICU. Nutr Clin Pract 2022;37(1):110–6.

77. Simon-Frapolli VJ, Vegas-Aguilar IM, Fernandez-Jimenez R, et al. Phase angle and rectus femoris cross-sectional area as predictors of severe malnutrition and their relationship with complications in outpatients with post-critical SARS-CoV2 disease. Front Nutr 2023;10:1218266.

78. Dong V, Karvellas CJ. Using technology to assess nutritional status and optimize nutrition therapy in critically ill patients. Curr Opin Clin Nutr Metab Care 2021; 24(2):189–94.
79. Nakanishi N, Tsutsumi R, Okayama Y, et al. Monitoring of muscle mass in critically ill patients: comparison of ultrasound and two bioelectrical impedance analysis devices. J Intensive Care 2019;7:61.
80. Ellegard LH, Petersen P, Ohrn L, et al. Longitudinal changes in phase angle by bioimpedance in intensive care patients differ between survivors and non-survivors. Clin Nutr ESPEN 2018;24:170–2.
81. Viana MV, Becce F, Pantet O, et al. Impact of beta-hydroxy-beta-methylbutyrate (HMB) on muscle loss and protein metabolism in critically ill patients: a RCT. Clin Nutr 2021;40(8):4878–87.
82. Barazzoni R, Jensen GL, Correia M, et al. Guidance for assessment of the muscle mass phenotypic criterion for the Global Leadership Initiative on Malnutrition (GLIM) diagnosis of malnutrition. Clin Nutr 2022;41(6):1425–33.
83. Santer D, Schneider N, de Carvalho YSS, et al. The association between reduced calf and mid-arm circumferences and ICU mortality in critically ill COVID-19 patients. Clin Nutr ESPEN 2023;54:45–51.
84. Simpson F, Doig GS, Early PNTIG. Physical assessment and anthropometric measures for use in clinical research conducted in critically ill patient populations: an analytic observational study. JPEN - J Parenter Enter Nutr 2015;39(3): 313–21.
85. Ravasco P, Camilo ME, Gouveia-Oliveira A, et al. A critical approach to nutritional assessment in critically ill patients. Clin Nutr 2002;21(1):73–7.
86. Bernardes S, Stello BB, Milanez DSJ, et al. Absence of association between low calf circumference, adjusted or not for adiposity, and ICU mortality in critically ill adults: a secondary analysis of a cohort study. JPEN - J Parenter Enter Nutr 2024; 48(3):291–9.
87. Campbell IT, Watt T, Withers D, et al. Muscle thickness, measured with ultrasound, may be an indicator of lean tissue wasting in multiple organ failure in the presence of edema. Am J Clin Nutr 1995;62(3):533–9.
88. Kangalgil M, Ulusoy H, Turan S, et al. Association between skeletal muscle changes, anthropometric measurements, and clinical outcomes in critically ill trauma and surgical patients: a prospective observational study. Nutr Clin Pract 2022;37(6):1326–35.

Skeletal Muscle
A Critical Organ for Survival and Recovery in Critical Illness

Check for updates

Matthew J. Lees, PhD[a], Carla M. Prado, PhD[b],
Paul E. Wischmeyer, MD[c], Stuart M. Phillips, PhD[a],*

KEYWORDS

- Skeletal muscle • Intensive care unit • Atrophy • Bed rest • Amino acids
- Immobilization

KEY POINTS

- The intensive care unit (ICU) represents one of the most challenging environments in which to preserve skeletal muscle mass and function.
- Parameters of skeletal muscle health on admission (eg, muscle mass and composition/quality) are predictors of clinically important outcomes and survival; the sarcopenia of aging compounds these risks.
- Patients in critical care exhibit a blunting of skeletal muscle protein synthesis and elevated breakdown, despite comparable protein digestion and amino acid availability to healthy individuals.
- Patients can lose ~2% of skeletal muscle mass per day in the first week of admission to the ICU and are at risk for intensive care unit-acquired weakness.
- Early mobilization/stimulation of muscle (by physical therapy, ambulation and/or neuromuscular electrical stimulation) alongside the adequate provision of protein/amino acids, preferably with higher leucine content, can improve physical function, maintain muscle mass, and increase survival.

INTRODUCTION

Skeletal muscle constitutes around 40% of total body weight and contains approximately 50 - 75% of all body proteins.[1] It is one of the most dynamic and plastic tissues in the human body and is an indispensable organ involved in a broad array of mechanical and metabolic processes.[1,2] Through the conversion of chemical to

[a] Exercise Metabolism Research Group, Department of Kinesiology, McMaster University, Hamilton, Ontario, Canada; [b] Human Nutrition Research Unit, Department of Agricultural, Food and Nutritional Science, University of Alberta, Edmonton, Alberta, Canada; [c] Department of Anesthesiology and Surgery, Duke University, Durham, NC, USA
* Corresponding author. McMaster University, 1280 Main Street West, Hamilton, Ontario L8S 4K1, Canada.
E-mail address: phillis@mcmaster.ca

Crit Care Clin 41 (2025) 299–312
https://doi.org/10.1016/j.ccc.2024.08.011
0749-0704/25/© 2024 Elsevier Inc. All rights reserved, including those for text and data mining, AI training, and similar technologies.
criticalcare.theclinics.com

mechanical energy, skeletal muscle contractile activity enables locomotion, maintains posture, and facilitates respiration.[2] In terms of metabolism, skeletal muscle serves as a principal reservoir for amino acids needed by other vital tissues to maintain organ-specific protein synthesis in the absence of amino acid absorption from the gut, which are mobilized during trauma and infection.[1,3] Furthermore, muscle mass is intimately related to the immune system in a bidirectional relationship. While the immune system plays a crucial role in maintaining muscle health, muscles produce and release myokines responsible for proliferation, activation, and distribution of immune cells. Consequently, low muscle mass has been associated with compromised immunity and an increased risk of infection.[4] The breakdown of skeletal muscle in the fasted state maintains plasma amino acid concentrations, provided sufficient muscle mass is available, which contributes to the maintenance of blood glucose levels during periods of starvation.[3] Reduced muscle mass, therefore, could impede the ability to respond to stress and chronic illness.[1] Moreover, altered skeletal muscle metabolism is implicated in the genesis of many common pathologies and chronic diseases.[3]

Critical care represents one of the most challenging environments for the maintenance of skeletal muscle health. It is common for patients admitted to the intensive care unit (ICU) to experience a rapid loss of muscle cross-sectional area (CSA) and strength due to prolonged bed rest (ie, muscle disuse) and other major risk factors[5] such as multiple organ failure, systemic inflammatory response syndrome (SIRS), hyperglycemia, prolonged mechanical ventilation (more than one week), and the use of drugs such as corticosteroids[6] and neuromuscular blocking agents[5] that contribute to accelerated catabolism. Furthermore, suboptimal energy intake further exacerbates the imbalance between muscle protein synthesis and breakdown. The loss of muscle mass and strength in critical care contributes to long-term ICU-acquired weakness (ICUAW),[7] which is an independent predictor of survival following critical illness.[7,8] Older ICU patients, particularly those affected by sarcopenia and anabolic resistance, have a compounded risk for ICUAW in critical care.[9,10] The interplay between these assorted factors is shown in **Fig. 1**.

The purpose of this review is to discuss the importance of skeletal muscle for survival and recovery in critical care and the challenges posed by this environment. The additive impact of aging and its associated risk factors for muscle health in the ICU will also be examined. Finally, we consider strategies that support the preservation, restoration, and recovery of skeletal muscle during and after periods of critical care.

DISCUSSION
An Overview of Muscle Protein Turnover

Skeletal muscle mass is regulated by the intricate balance between muscle protein synthesis (MPS) and breakdown (MPB). The algebraic difference between MPS and MPB, termed net balance, dictates whether proteins within muscle are accrued (ie, anabolism/hypertrophy) or degraded and lost from skeletal muscle tissue (ie, catabolism/atrophy).[2,10] These opposing, interrelated kinetic processes are continuous and normally exist in dynamic equilibrium.[11] They determine the overall rate of muscle protein turnover, a process encompassing the efficient repair and renewal of damaged or misfolded proteins,[12] and the principal determinant of skeletal muscle mass.[2]

Changes in skeletal muscle mass occur when net protein balance favors MPS (leading to protein accretion) or MPB (leading to protein loss).[2,13] Some of the major influences on skeletal muscle proteostasis are dietary protein intake, physical (in)activity

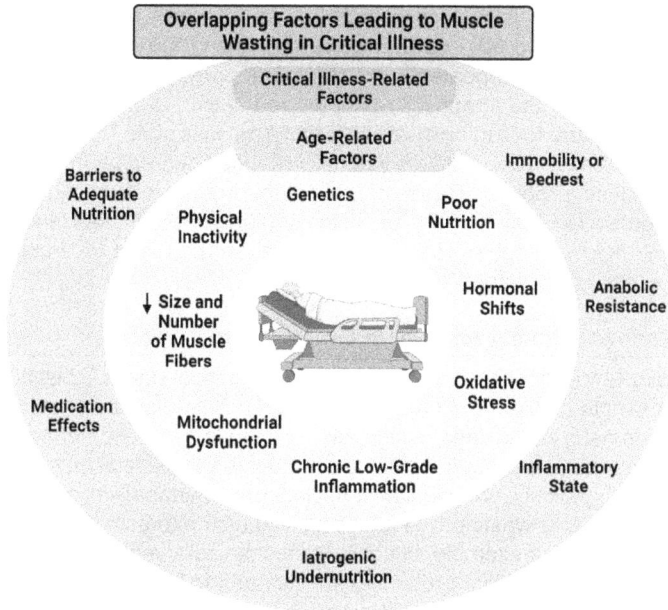

Fig. 1. A schematic representation of factors driving skeletal muscle loss during an indeterminate period in critical care and how these factors can be compounded with aging.

and aging.[11,14] Ingestion of a mixed meal induces a rise in plasma amino acids (AAs) and insulin that stimulates MPS whilst suppressing MPB, leading to net protein accretion or hypertrophy.[12] Over a 24 hour timeframe, these transient periods of anabolism are interspersed with periods of postabsorptive catabolism (in a 'fasted-loss/fed-gain' cycle), wherein muscle protein is broken down, and the resultant AAs are deaminated and either oxidized, used to supply the free AA pool or directed toward other metabolic pathways.[2,11,12] In healthy adults not engaged in a regular program of resistance training, the consumption of adequate dietary protein (specifically the essential amino acids [EAAs] and leucine[13,15]) ensures MPS and MPB are in equilibrium and skeletal muscle mass remains relatively constant.[2,13]

Uncomplicated Disuse Atrophy and Muscle Protein Turnover

As discussed above, skeletal muscle is a highly plastic tissue that can alter its phenotype in response to the loading demands placed upon it.[12] Physical exercise, particularly resistance exercise (RE), represents a powerful anabolic stimulus that complements the effects of protein ingestion.[16,17] Through the loading it imparts on the contractile apparatus, RE sensitizes the muscle protein translational machinery to the presence of AAs for at least 24 - 48 hours and potentiates the effect of hyperaminoacidemia alone on MPS.[12,16,18] It induces acute mechanical, metabolic, and neuronal perturbations that underpin physiologic adaptation[19] and drive changes in intracellular gene and protein expression that ultimately lead to long-term structural remodeling.[2,20]

In contrast to the anabolic stimulus provided by physical exercise, the loss of mechanical input brings about a pro-catabolic environment and consequent unloading-induced atrophy of skeletal muscle.[21,22] The primary driving process underlying the loss of muscle protein over time in human uncomplicated ('simple') disuse-induced atrophy is a decline in MPS, as opposed to elevated MPB.[21–26] Indeed, declines of up to 50 - 60% in both fasting and fed MPS during unloading have been demonstrated repeatedly.[22,27–32] The atrophy of 'simple disuse' is not a systemic condition (ie, the atrophy is restricted to the limb(s) exposed to the disuse), however, and is characterized by the absence of a disease state.[22,24,29] Local unloading, a short-term illness, and voluntary inactivity-induced decreases in physical activity can result in disuse atrophy.[22] Disuse of this nature promotes 'anabolic resistance' of the MPS response to EAAs.[29,32] The provision of high doses of EAAs (and particularly leucine) may help attenuate short-term disuse atrophy and overcome disuse-associated anabolic resistance.[33]

Skeletal Muscle and Protein Turnover in Critical Illness

The disuse atrophy experienced under conditions of critical illness is distinct from that observed in simple disuse. It is characterized by muscle disuse in conjunction with elevated inflammatory cytokines,[34] increased systemic catabolic hormones, with or without undernutrition, leading to enhanced proteolysis of skeletal muscle tissue.[22,35] Proinflammatory cytokines can regulate muscle protein metabolism, playing a key role in the onset of muscle wasting by increasing ubiquitin expression and proteasome enzymatic activity.[34] For example, critically ill mechanically ventilated patients exhibit comparable fasted myofibrillar protein synthesis rates to healthy controls, as well as normal protein digestion kinetics and amino acid availability following a duodenal protein bolus (20 g administered over 60 minutes).[36] Despite this, these patients demonstrate a blunted ability to use ingested protein for MPS. Undoubtedly, the disuse-induced combination of reductions in MPS and increases in MPB combine to result in the rapid loss of muscle mass observed in critical illness. The modified schematic from an earlier review by Morton and colleagues[37] depicts whole-body and muscle protein kinetics in the fasted and postprandial state and the impact of aging and critical illness on these responses (**Fig. 2**).

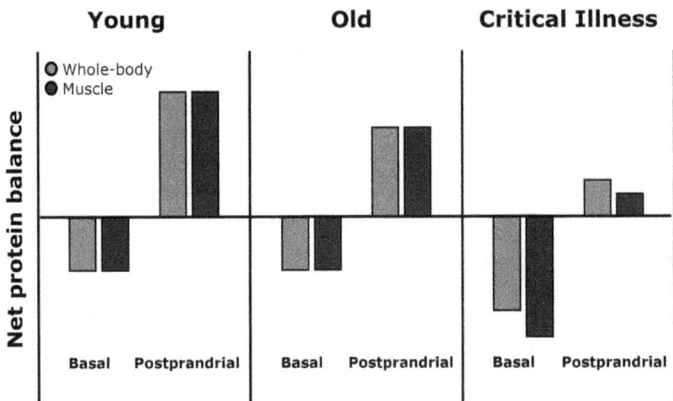

Fig. 2. Schematic depicting net whole-body and muscle protein balance in the fasted and postprandial state. Basal whole-body protein turnover does not differ between young and older individuals but is substantially reduced in critical illness, predominantly due to skeletal muscle. The anabolic resistance that is a common feature of aging is exacerbated during critical illness due to the severity of disuse. (*From* Morton RW, Traylor DA, Weijs PJM, Phillips SM. Defining anabolic resistance: implications for delivery of clinical care nutrition. Curr Opin Crit Care. Apr 2018;24(2):124-130. https://doi.org/10.1097/MCC. 0000000000000488.)

Critically ill patients can lose more than 15% of their muscle mass in one week, and ICUAW can manifest in ~50% of patients during this time.[38] The early and rapid nature of this type of atrophy[39] can have long-term detrimental effects on health. Recent meta-analytic evidence suggests that, on average, critically ill patients lose nearly 2% of skeletal muscle per day during the first week of ICU admission.[38] Puthucheary and colleagues[39] reported a reduction in ultrasonography-derived rectus femoris CSA of 10.3% after one week, with a corresponding decrease in histology-derived muscle fiber CSA of 17.5% and a decrease in the ratio of protein to DNA of 29.5%. The decrease in rectus femoris CSA was exacerbated in patients who experienced multi-organ failure as opposed to single-organ failure. The daily loss of CSA in both type I and type II fibers has been shown to be ~7% and ~14%, respectively, in critically ill patients. These rapid changes have been shown to preferentially affect the lower limbs, particularly the vastus lateralis, evidenced by reduced muscle thickness and muscle pennation angle five days following admission.[40] Alterations of this magnitude are unlikely to be due solely to reductions in MPS or increases in MPB but rather a simultaneous reduction in the former and increase in the latter. The skeletal muscle wasting that occurs during critical illness is implicated in the concomitant loss of muscle strength, which is another important risk factor for survival.[8]

Alongside these rapid early losses in skeletal muscle tissue, an altered metabolic profile of skeletal muscle is observed,[41] as evidenced by decreased mitochondrial biogenesis, dysregulated lipid oxidation, intramuscular inflammation, and reduced intramuscular ATP content. In patients with protracted (50 ± 21 days in ICU) critical illness and ICUAW, skeletal muscle demonstrates a reduction in its capacity for aerobic ATP synthesis per mg of muscle wet weight of ~50%.[42] Furthermore, critically ill patients exhibit a state of hypermetabolism, as shown by severe glycogen depletion in skeletal muscle.[43] This depletion is of a greater degree than that observed in competitive athletes and is suggestive of heightened catabolism to support higher energy needs.[43]

The early and rapid muscle atrophy experienced in critical care can have long-term implications for health, quality of life, and mortality (see below). Patients who experience muscle wasting have a greater risk of ICUAW,[44] increased length of ICU stay, and the loss of muscle mass within the first week of admission is associated with increased 60-day mortality.[45] For example, Dinglas and colleagues[46] showed that more than one-third of acute respiratory distress syndrome patients had muscle weakness and that greater strength at discharge and throughout follow-up was associated with improved 5-year survival.

Aging Exacerbates the Catabolic Stress of Critical Illness

Aging compounds the catabolic stressors of critical illness, as an older patient (>60 years of age) may present with sarcopenia and anabolic resistance.[9,47] Sarcopenia, the age-associated loss of muscle mass, strength and function, principally affects older adults and is often accompanied by a blunted MPS response to the normally robust anabolic stimuli of amino acids and resistance exercise (so-called age-related 'anabolic resistance').[48] For instance, older people typically require ~1.5 to 2 times the amount of high-quality protein required to maximally stimulate MPS versus their younger counterparts.[22,49] In this sense, an older patient can already be assumed to be losing muscle mass, have a blunted muscle protein synthetic response to feeding, and be at increased risk of frailty on discharge from the ICU.[10] The muscle loss from sarcopenia is slower and likely due to a convergence of factors resulting from poor diet quality, decreased physical activity levels, as well as chronic imbalances between anabolic and catabolic hormones.[22] Nevertheless, the presence of sarcopenia increases the risk of mortality in critical illness[50] and represents a compounding variable in a critical care setting.

Skeletal Muscle Parameters at Intensive Care Unit Admission Predict Survival

Baseline (ie, prior to ICU admission) skeletal muscle mass and composition/quality are associated with important clinical outcomes and mortality in an ICU setting. Although a higher body mass index (BMI) has been associated with lower mortality in ICU patients,[51,52] when muscle area is accounted for, BMI appears to have no impact on mortality.[53] In fact, larger erector spinae muscle area derived from computed tomography (CT) scans on ICU admission were associated with decreased odds of 6-month mortality and disability at discharge.[54] The concept of high BMI masking low muscle mass has been discussed elsewhere.[55] This observation was also true for bone density, whereas subcutaneous adipose tissue was not associated with mortality.[54] Importantly, erector spinae muscle area remained a significant predictor of 6-month mortality and survival even after adjusting for other covariates such as preadmission comorbidities, albumin, preadmission functional independence, severity scores, age, and exercise capacity.[54]

In addition to muscle mass (ie, quantity), its composition is also an important prognostic factor, for example the presence and extent of myosteatosis (the ectopic fat infiltration of muscle tissue).[56–58] Patients with adequate muscle quantity or mass may nevertheless exhibit disadvantageous muscle composition. Abnormalities in several parameters of body composition such as higher muscle echo intensity and lower phase angle are associated with higher mortality in critically ill patients.[59] Loosen and colleagues[56] reported that critically ill patients with a skeletal muscle index or mean skeletal muscle attenuation below defined cutoff values (74.9 mm^2/cm or 29 Hounsfield units, respectively) showed a significantly reduced overall survival. In critically ill patients with SARS-CoV-2 pneumonia, Sabatino and colleagues[57] found that muscle mass and myosteatosis determined from chest CT scans of paravertebral skeletal muscle were associated with higher mortality. Similarly, Looijaard and colleagues[60] observed that low skeletal muscle quality defined from CT-derived skeletal muscle density was independently associated with higher 6-month mortality in mechanically-ventilated ICU patients. Collectively, these findings demonstrate the prognostic value of skeletal muscle health (ie, mass and composition parameters) in critical care settings, particularly in the 24 hours following admission.

Strategies to Mitigate Intensive Care Unit-Induced Muscle Mass and Strength Losses

Given the importance of skeletal muscle mass at ICU admission and the challenges posed by atrophic muscle losses during critical care, strategies that promote the growth, maintenance, and recovery of skeletal muscle in critical care settings could be of great therapeutic value.[9] The leveraging of innovative technologies and targeted/personalized nutrition and exercise interventions holds promise for increasing ICU survivorship into the future.[61] The modified schematic from Morton and colleagues[37] provides an overview of recommendations for preserving muscle mass in healthy and critically ill patients (**Fig. 3**).

Protein
Nutrition is essential for muscle health, and both the quantity and quality of nutrients are important. Although a comprehensive review of all nutritional interventions for muscle health in critically ill patients is beyond the scope of this paper, we will focus specifically on protein. When energy intake is optimized, adequate and prompt provision of protein

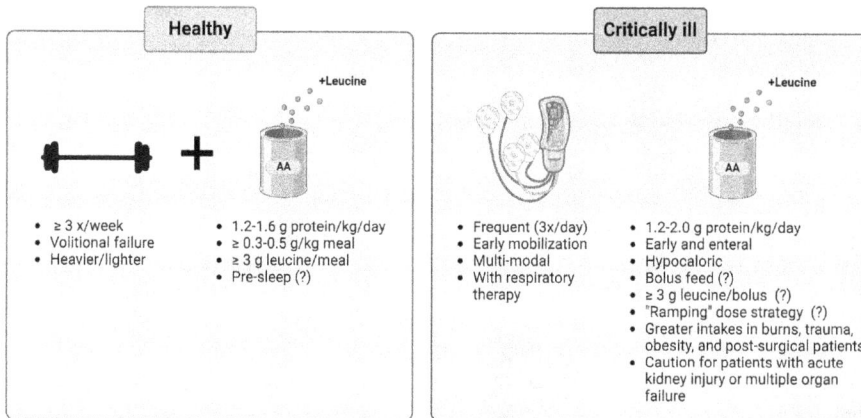

Fig. 3. Recommendations for preserving muscle mass in healthy and critically ill individuals. AA, amino acids; NMES, neuromuscular electrical stimulation (an example of a potential therapy to induce muscle contraction).

has been recognized as a cornerstone in the treatment of the critically ill.[62,63] This notion is of particular importance given the blunted anabolic response to protein provision in this population.[36] Current evidence appears to support the provision of dietary protein, and particularly leucine, in excess of the recommended daily allowance (RDA) of 0.8 g/kg/day to help prevent and treat muscle loss during critical illness.[64–66] As of 2022, the American Society of Parenteral and Enteral Nutrition (ASPEN) recommends a protein dose of 1.2 to 2.0 g/kg/day and for higher amounts to be provided to patients with burns, obesity, or trauma.[67] In critically ill patients with low skeletal muscle area and density on admission, Looijaard and colleagues[68] observed that early high protein intake (≥1.2 g/kg/day) was associated with lower mortality, whereas this was not the case for patients with normal skeletal muscle area. Although this was a retrospective study, the findings nevertheless point toward a personalized approach to protein nutrition in a critical care setting. For enteral infusion, free amino acids may augment the effects of intact protein as recent work has shown this approach to be advantageous for plasma amino acid availability in critically ill patients.[69] For older adults, the consumption of higher leucine-containing proteins or amino acid mixtures through enteral and/or parenteral means is a strategy that holds promise.[10]

Although greater protein intakes might be warranted for patients with burns, trauma, obesity, or those recovering from surgery, the provision of considerably higher (≥2.2 g/kg/day) protein intakes may be contraindicated in critically ill patients with acute kidney injury and multiple organ failure at baseline.[70] Further, some observational data suggest that "ramping" up protein delivery at ICU admission may improve outcome and survival. These data showed early high protein (>0.8 g/kg/day) over the first 1 - 3 days in the ICU was associated with higher mortality; subsequently higher protein delivery (>1.2 g/kg/day) beyond day 4 was associated with improved survival.[71] These findings further reinforce the need for a personalized nutrition approach that takes the nutritional and metabolic status of the patient into account. Early and continuous nutrition intervention is essential for optimal muscle health and should be provided well beyond ICU-discharge for optimal recovery.[72,73] Interestingly, the concept of adjusting protein based on lean mass has been introduced as a superior approach to individualized protein requirements.[74] Since the lean mass compartment determined protein needs, the wide variability in lean mass per kg of body weight could result in underfeeding or overfeeding in some patients. This concept has started to be tested and explored in different populations and should be further investigated in the ICU environment.[74–76]

Skeletal muscle loading

Physical activity, and in particular resistance exercise, is known as a potent anabolic stimulus at any age.[2,10] Physical therapy (PT) can improve quality of life and physical function, increase ventilator-free days, and reduce the length of stay in the hospital and ICU.[77,78] When initiated early (eg, within one week of ICU admission and four days of invasive mechanical ventilation),[79] the mobilization of critically ill patients appears to decrease the incidence of ICUAW.[80] Another important feature of skeletal muscle loading is its ability to sensitize muscle to the aminoacidemia induced by protein feeding. Such sensitization, even if small, would be important for highly immobile ICU patients, given the anabolic blunting that is known to occur.[36] Evidence from mechanically ventilated patients has shown that early mobilization (two daily 15-min sessions of cycle ergometry) coupled with high protein intake (median = 1.48 g/kg/day) results in improved physical component scores at three and six months compared with routine physiotherapy and lower protein intake (median = 1.19 g/kg/day).[81] This approach also brought about improved survival compared with the control group.

Loading exercise is difficult to conduct in the ICU environment for a variety of reasons[82]; however, some activities can be performed, such as sitting up at the bedside, walking, cycling (in and/or out of bed), resistive work using bands, and neuromuscular electrical stimulation (NMES).[10] Understandably, there are groups of ICU patients for which ambulation and PT will be difficult, if not impossible, such as trauma, brain injury, and burns patients. However, even relatively modest skeletal muscle contractions in these patients, for example, those brought about using NMES, can increase MPS and have beneficial outcomes for muscle health. Indeed, NMES has been identified as a safe alternative to active exercise for critically ill patients who cannot perform voluntary muscle contractions, ideally within the first two days of ICU admission.[83]

Older patients require special attention, as they are less likely to recover from periods of disuse due to age-related anabolic resistance.[22] Smeuninx and colleagues[84] recently reported that a single bout of unilateral resistance exercise performed the evening prior to five days of bed rest attenuated the decline in myofibrillar protein synthesis and muscle atrophy, using a model that mimicked a traditional inpatient hospital stay. While this model did not replicate the more extreme conditions of critical care, the optimal strategy to recover from such catabolic stress is physical activity, especially resistance exercise, and the provision of adequate protein nutrition.

SUMMARY

Skeletal muscle is a critical tissue for survival and recovery in the ICU environment. On admission, baseline skeletal muscle mass and composition/quality are predictive of clinically important outcomes and survival. The ICU setting represents one of the most challenging for skeletal muscle, particularly if mechanical ventilation is required and/or the patient is older (>60 years). Research suggests that the early provision of high amounts of dietary protein, provided there is no evidence of acute kidney injury or multiple organ failure, alongside early mobilization using a variety of methods, can support skeletal muscle health and other clinically important outcomes and reduce mortality. Importantly, these findings emphasize the importance of a personalized/targeted approach based on the functional capacity and nutritional risk of the patient.

CLINICS CARE POINTS

- Skeletal muscle mass is regulated by the opposing processes of muscle protein synthesis and breakdown.
- The critical care setting represents one of the most challenging environments for skeletal muscle health.
- Patients in the ICU, particularly those undergoing invasive mechanical ventilation, exhibit an anabolic blunting of muscle protein synthesis.
- In the first week of admission, patients can lose ~2% of muscle mass per day, and around ~50% will manifest ICUAW.
- Skeletal muscle parameters, including mass and composition/quality, on admission predict ventilator-free days, ICU-free days, and mortality in younger and older patients.
- The goals of treatment should be the early provision of high-quality protein through the optimal means available (oral, enteral, or parenteral) as well as mobilization through PT, ambulation, or neuromuscular electrical stimulation.
- Higher protein doses (2.2 g/kg/day) appear to be contraindicated in critically ill patients, particularly in those with acute kidney injury and multiple organ failure at baseline.
- An individualized/targeted approach that considers physical and nutritional requirements should be pursued.

ACKNOWLEDGMENTS

The authors thank Montserrat Montes-Ibarra and Leticia Ramos Da Silva for their contributions in the design and development of the figures.

DISCLOSURES

S.M. Phillips has received grant funding from the Canadian Institutes of Health Research, Canada, the Natural Sciences and Engineering Research Council of Canada, Canada, the US National Institutes for Health, Roquette Freres, France, Nestle Health Science, Friesland Campina, The Netherlands, The US National Dairy Council, Dairy Farmers of Canada and Myos. S.M. Phillips has received travel expenses and honoraria for speaking from Nestle Health Science. S.M. Phillips holds patents licensed to Exerkine Inc. but reports no financial gains. S.M. Phillips and C.M. Prado are supported by a Tier 1 Canada Research Chair award. M.J. Lees is supported by a Canadian Institutes of Health Research (CIHR) Postdoctoral Fellowship award (Funding Reference Number 187773). C.M. Prado has received honoraria and/or paid consultancy from Abbott Nutrition, Nutricia, Nestle Health Science, Pfizer, Amra Medical, Novo Nordisk and funding from Almased for unrelated research. Dr P.E. Wischmeyer reports receiving investigator-initiated grant funding related to this work from National Institutes of Health, United States, Department of Defense, United States, Abbott, Baxter, United States, and Fresenius. Dr P.E. Wischmeyer has served as a consultant to Abbott, Fresenius, Baxter, Cardinal Health, Mend Inc and Nutricia, for research related to this work. Dr P.E. Wischmeyer has received unrestricted gift donation for nutrition research from Musclesound and DSM. Dr P.E. Wischmeyer has received honoraria or travel expenses for CME lectures on improving nutrition care from Abbott, Baxter, Fresenius, Danone-Nutricia, and DSM.

REFERENCES

1. Frontera WR, Ochala J. Skeletal muscle: a brief review of structure and function. Calcif Tissue Int 2015;96(3):183–95.
2. McKendry J, Stokes T, McLeod JC, et al. Resistance exercise, aging, disuse, and muscle protein metabolism. Compr Physiol 2021;11(3):2249–78.
3. Wolfe RR. The underappreciated role of muscle in health and disease. Am J Clin Nutr 2006;84(3):475–82.
4. Nelke C, Dziewas R, Minnerup J, et al. Skeletal muscle as potential central link between sarcopenia and immune senescence. EBioMedicine 2019;49:381–8.
5. de Jonghe B, Lacherade JC, Sharshar T, et al. Intensive care unit-acquired weakness: risk factors and prevention. Crit Care Med 2009;37(10 Suppl):S309–15.
6. Yang T, Li Z, Jiang L, et al. Corticosteroid use and intensive care unit-acquired weakness: a systematic review and meta-analysis. Crit Care 2018;22(1):187.
7. Jolley SE, Bunnell AE, Hough CL. ICU-acquired weakness. Chest 2016;150(5): 1129–40.
8. Puthucheary Z, Montgomery H, Moxham J, et al. Structure to function: muscle failure in critically ill patients. J Physiol 2010;588(Pt 23):4641–8.
9. McKendry J, Thomas ACQ, Phillips SM. Muscle mass loss in the older critically ill population: potential therapeutic strategies. Nutr Clin Pract 2020;35(4):607–16.
10. Phillips SM, Dickerson RN, Moore FA, et al. Protein Turnover and metabolism in the elderly intensive care unit patient. Nutr Clin Pract 2017;32(1_suppl):112S–20S.
11. Atherton PJ, Smith K. Muscle protein synthesis in response to nutrition and exercise. J Physiol 2012;590(5):1049–57.
12. Joanisse S, McKendry J, Lim C, et al. Understanding the effects of nutrition and post-exercise nutrition on skeletal muscle protein turnover: insights from stable isotope studies. Clinical Nutrition Open Science 2021;36:56–77.
13. Phillips SM. A brief review of critical processes in exercise-induced muscular hypertrophy. Sports Med 2014;44(Suppl 1):S71–7.
14. Deane CS, Ely IA, Wilkinson DJ, et al. Dietary protein, exercise, ageing and physical inactivity: interactive influences on skeletal muscle proteostasis. Proc Nutr Soc 2021;80(2):106–17.
15. Churchward-Venne TA, Breen L, Di Donato DM, et al. Leucine supplementation of a low-protein mixed macronutrient beverage enhances myofibrillar protein synthesis in young men: a double-blind, randomized trial. Am J Clin Nutr 2014; 99(2):276–86.
16. Biolo G, Tipton KD, Klein S, et al. An abundant supply of amino acids enhances the metabolic effect of exercise on muscle protein. Am J Physiol 1997;273(1 Pt 1): E122–9.
17. Reidy PT, Rasmussen BB. Role of ingested amino acids and protein in the promotion of resistance exercise-induced muscle protein anabolism. J Nutr 2016; 146(2):155–83.
18. Burd NA, West DW, Moore DR, et al. Enhanced amino acid sensitivity of myofibrillar protein synthesis persists for up to 24 h after resistance exercise in young men. J Nutr 2011;141(4):568–73.
19. Fluck M. Functional, structural and molecular plasticity of mammalian skeletal muscle in response to exercise stimuli. J Exp Biol 2006;209(Pt 12):2239–48.
20. Perry CG, Lally J, Holloway GP, et al. Repeated transient mRNA bursts precede increases in transcriptional and mitochondrial proteins during training in human skeletal muscle. J Physiol 2010;588(Pt 23):4795–810.

21. Phillips SM, Glover EI, Rennie MJ. Alterations of protein turnover underlying disuse atrophy in human skeletal muscle. J Appl Physiol 2009;107(3):645–54.
22. Nunes EA, Stokes T, McKendry J, et al. Disuse-induced skeletal muscle atrophy in disease and nondisease states in humans: mechanisms, prevention, and recovery strategies. Am J Physiol Cell Physiol 2022;322(6):C1068–84.
23. Phillips SM, McGlory C. CrossTalk proposal: the dominant mechanism causing disuse muscle atrophy is decreased protein synthesis. J Physiol 2014;592(24): 5341–3.
24. Rudrappa SS, Wilkinson DJ, Greenhaff PL, et al. Human skeletal muscle disuse atrophy: effects on muscle protein synthesis, breakdown, and insulin resistance-a qualitative review. Front Physiol 2016;7:361.
25. Brook MS, Stokes T, Gorissen SHM, et al. Declines in muscle protein synthesis account for short-term muscle disuse atrophy in humans in the absence of increased muscle protein breakdown. J Cachexia Sarcopenia Muscle 2022; 13(4):2005–16.
26. Atherton PJ, Greenhaff PL, Phillips SM, et al. Control of skeletal muscle atrophy in response to disuse: clinical/preclinical contentions and fallacies of evidence. Am J Physiol Endocrinol Metab 2016;311(3):E594–604.
27. Gibson JN, Halliday D, Morrison WL, et al. Decrease in human quadriceps muscle protein turnover consequent upon leg immobilization. Clin Sci (Lond) 1987; 72(4):503–9.
28. Gibson JN, Smith K, Rennie MJ. Prevention of disuse muscle atrophy by means of electrical stimulation: maintenance of protein synthesis. Lancet 1988;2(8614): 767–70.
29. Glover EI, Phillips SM, Oates BR, et al. Immobilization induces anabolic resistance in human myofibrillar protein synthesis with low and high dose amino acid infusion. J Physiol 2008;586(24):6049–61.
30. Ferrando AA, Lane HW, Stuart CA, et al. Prolonged bed rest decreases skeletal muscle and whole body protein synthesis. Am J Physiol 1996;270(4 Pt 1):E627–33.
31. Wall BT, Snijders T, Senden JM, et al. Disuse impairs the muscle protein synthetic response to protein ingestion in healthy men. J Clin Endocrinol Metab 2013; 98(12):4872–81.
32. Wall BT, Dirks ML, Snijders T, et al. Short-term muscle disuse lowers myofibrillar protein synthesis rates and induces anabolic resistance to protein ingestion. Am J Physiol Endocrinol Metab 2016;310(2):E137–47.
33. Holloway TM, McGlory C, McKellar S, et al. A novel amino acid composition ameliorates short-term muscle disuse atrophy in healthy young men. Front Nutr 2019; 6:105.
34. Costamagna D, Costelli P, Sampaolesi M, et al. Role of Inflammation in muscle homeostasis and myogenesis. Mediators Inflamm 2015;2015:805172.
35. Sartori R, Romanello V, Sandri M. Mechanisms of muscle atrophy and hypertrophy: implications in health and disease. Nat Commun 2021;12(1):330.
36. Chapple LS, Kouw IWK, Summers MJ, et al. Muscle protein synthesis after protein administration in critical illness. Am J Respir Crit Care Med 2022;206(6): 740–9.
37. Morton RW, Traylor DA, Weijs PJM, et al. Defining anabolic resistance: implications for delivery of clinical care nutrition. Curr Opin Crit Care 2018;24(2):124–30.
38. Fazzini B, Markl T, Costas C, et al. The rate and assessment of muscle wasting during critical illness: a systematic review and meta-analysis. Crit Care 2023; 27(1):2.

39. Puthucheary ZA, Rawal J, McPhail M, et al. Acute skeletal muscle wasting in critical illness. JAMA 2013;310(15):1591–600.

40. Turton P, Hay R, Taylor J, et al. Human limb skeletal muscle wasting and architectural remodeling during five to ten days intubation and ventilation in critical care - an observational study using ultrasound. BMC Anesthesiol 2016;16(1):119.

41. Puthucheary ZA, Astin R, McPhail MJW, et al. Metabolic phenotype of skeletal muscle in early critical illness. Thorax 2018;73(10):926–35.

42. Jiroutkova K, Krajcova A, Ziak J, et al. Mitochondrial function in skeletal muscle of patients with protracted critical illness and ICU-acquired weakness. Crit Care 2015;19:448.

43. Millan IS, Hill J, Wischmeyer P. Measurement of skeletal muscle glycogen status in critically ill patients: a new approach in critical care monitoring. Crit Care 2015; 19(Suppl 1):P400.

44. Mayer KP, Thompson Bastin ML, Montgomery-Yates AA, et al. Acute skeletal muscle wasting and dysfunction predict physical disability at hospital discharge in patients with critical illness. Crit Care 2020;24(1):637.

45. Hrdy O, Vrbica K, Kovar M, et al. Incidence of muscle wasting in the critically ill: a prospective observational cohort study. Sci Rep 2023;13(1):742.

46. Dinglas VD, Aronson Friedman L, Colantuoni E, et al. Muscle weakness and 5-year survival in acute respiratory distress syndrome survivors. Crit Care Med 2017;45(3):446–53.

47. Churchward-Venne TA, Breen L, Phillips SM. Alterations in human muscle protein metabolism with aging: protein and exercise as countermeasures to offset sarcopenia. Biofactors 2014;40(2):199–205.

48. Paulussen KJM, McKenna CF, Beals JW, et al. Anabolic resistance of muscle protein turnover comes in various shapes and sizes. Front Nutr 2021;8:615849.

49. Moore DR, Churchward-Venne TA, Witard O, et al. Protein ingestion to stimulate myofibrillar protein synthesis requires greater relative protein intakes in healthy older versus younger men. J Gerontol A Biol Sci Med Sci 2015;70(1):57–62.

50. Zhang XM, Chen D, Xie XH, et al. Sarcopenia as a predictor of mortality among the critically ill in an intensive care unit: a systematic review and meta-analysis. BMC Geriatr 2021;21(1):339.

51. Pickkers P, de Keizer N, Dusseljee J, et al. Body mass index is associated with hospital mortality in critically ill patients: an observational cohort study. Crit Care Med 2013;41(8):1878–83.

52. Li S, Zhang W, Fu Z, et al. Impact of obesity on all-cause and cause-specific mortality among critically ill men and women: a cohort study on the eICU database. Front Nutr 2023;10:1143404.

53. Weijs PJ, Looijaard WG, Dekker IM, et al. Low skeletal muscle area is a risk factor for mortality in mechanically ventilated critically ill patients. Crit Care 2014; 18(2):R12.

54. Jaitovich A, Khan M, Itty R, et al. ICU admission muscle and fat mass, survival, and disability at discharge: a prospective cohort study. Chest 2019;155(2): 322–30.

55. Prado CM, Gonzalez MC, Heymsfield SB. Body composition phenotypes and obesity paradox. Curr Opin Clin Nutr Metab Care 2015;18(6):535–51.

56. Loosen SH, Schulze-Hagen M, Pungel T, et al. Skeletal muscle composition predicts outcome in critically ill patients. Crit Care Explor 2020;2(8):e0171.

57. Sabatino A, Pacchiarini MC, Regolisti G, et al. The impact of muscle mass and myosteatosis on mortality in critically ill patients with Sars-Cov2-related pneumonia. Clin Nutr ESPEN 2023;58:409–15.

58. Giani M, Rezoagli E, Grassi A, et al. Low skeletal muscle index and myosteatosis as predictors of mortality in critically ill surgical patients. Nutrition 2022;101: 111687.
59. Montes-Ibarra M, Orsso CE, Limon-Miro AT, et al. Prevalence and clinical implications of abnormal body composition phenotypes in patients with COVID-19: a systematic review. Am J Clin Nutr 2023;117(6):1288–305.
60. Looijaard WG, Dekker IM, Stapel SN, et al. Skeletal muscle quality as assessed by CT-derived skeletal muscle density is associated with 6-month mortality in mechanically ventilated critically ill patients. Crit Care 2016;20(1):386.
61. Wischmeyer PE, Puthucheary Z, San Millán I, et al. Muscle mass and physical recovery in ICU: innovations for targeting of nutrition and exercise. Curr Opin Crit Care 2017;23(4):269–78.
62. Bendavid I, Zusman O, Kagan I, et al. Early administration of protein in critically ill patients: a retrospective cohort study. Nutrients 2019;11(1):106.
63. Wischmeyer PE, Bear DE, Berger MM, et al. Personalized nutrition therapy in critical care: 10 expert recommendations. Crit Care 2023;27(1):261.
64. Phillips SM, Paddon-Jones D, Layman DK. Optimizing adult protein intake during catabolic health conditions. Adv Nutr 2020;11(4):S1058–69.
65. Bauer J, Biolo G, Cederholm T, et al. Evidence-based recommendations for optimal dietary protein intake in older people: a position paper from the PROT-AGE Study Group. J Am Med Dir Assoc 2013;14(8):542–59.
66. McClave SA, Taylor BE, Martindale RG, et al. Guidelines for the provision and assessment of nutrition support therapy in the adult critically ill patient: society of Critical Care Medicine (SCCM) and American Society for Parenteral and Enteral Nutrition (A.S.P.E.N.). JPEN J Parenter Enteral Nutr 2016;40(2):159–211.
67. Compher C, Bingham AL, McCall M, et al. Guidelines for the provision of nutrition support therapy in the adult critically ill patient: the American society for parenteral and enteral nutrition. JPEN J Parenter Enteral Nutr 2022;46(1):12–41.
68. Looijaard WGPM, Dekker IM, Beishuizen A, et al. Early high protein intake and mortality in critically ill ICU patients with low skeletal muscle area and -density. Clin Nutr 2020;39(7):2192–201.
69. van Gassel RJ, Weijzen ME, Kouw IW, et al. Administration of free amino acids improves exogenous amino acid availability when compared with intact protein in critically ill patients: a randomized controlled study. J Nutr 2024;154(2):554–64.
70. Heyland DK, Patel J, Compher C, et al. The effect of higher protein dosing in critically ill patients with high nutritional risk (EFFORT Protein): an international, multi-centre, pragmatic, registry-based randomised trial. Lancet 2023;401(10376): 568–76.
71. Koekkoek W, van Setten CHC, Olthof LE, et al. Timing of PROTein INtake and clinical outcomes of adult critically ill patients on prolonged mechanical VENTilation: the PROTINVENT retrospective study. Clin Nutr 2019;38(2):883–90.
72. Prado CM, Anker SD, Coats AJS, et al. Nutrition in the spotlight in cachexia, sarcopenia and muscle: avoiding the wildfire. J Cachexia Sarcopenia Muscle 2021; 12(1):3–8.
73. Wischmeyer PE. Are we creating survivors…or victims in critical care? Delivering targeted nutrition to improve outcomes. Curr Opin Crit Care 2016;22(4):279–84.
74. Weijs PJ, Sauerwein HP, Kondrup J. Protein recommendations in the ICU: g protein/kg body weight - which body weight for underweight and obese patients? Clin Nutr 2012;31(5):774–5.

75. Geisler C, Prado CM, Müller MJ. Inadequacy of body weight-based recommendations for individual protein intake-lessons from body composition analysis. Nutrients 2016;9(1):23.

76. Prado CM, Cushen SJ, Orsso CE, et al. Sarcopenia and cachexia in the era of obesity: clinical and nutritional impact. Proc Nutr Soc 2016;75(2):188–98.

77. Connolly B, Salisbury L, O'Neill B, et al. Exercise rehabilitation following intensive care unit discharge for recovery from critical illness. Cochrane Database Syst Rev 2015;2015(6):CD008632.

78. Kayambu G, Boots R, Paratz J. Physical therapy for the critically ill in the ICU: a systematic review and meta-analysis. Crit Care Med 2013;41(6):1543–54.

79. Kho ME, Molloy AJ, Clarke FJ, et al. Multicentre pilot randomised clinical trial of early in-bed cycle ergometry with ventilated patients. BMJ Open Respir Res 2019;6(1): e000383.

80. Zhang L, Hu W, Cai Z, et al. Early mobilization of critically ill patients in the intensive care unit: a systematic review and meta-analysis. PLoS One 2019;14(10): e0223185.

81. de Azevedo JRA, Lima HCM, Frota P, et al. High-protein intake and early exercise in adult intensive care patients: a prospective, randomized controlled trial to evaluate the impact on functional outcomes. BMC Anesthesiol 2021;21(1):283.

82. Dubb R, Nydahl P, Hermes C, et al. Barriers and strategies for early mobilization of patients in intensive care units. Ann Am Thorac Soc 2016;13(5):724–30.

83. Sepúlveda-Jofré P, Guerra-Vega P, Fu C, et al. Skeletal muscle atrophy in critical ill patients and the use of electrical stimulation as a treatment strategy: recommendations for clinical practice. Trends in Anaesthesia and Critical Care 2021; 40:14–22.

84. Smeuninx B, Elhassan YS, Sapey E, et al. A single bout of prior resistance exercise attenuates muscle atrophy and declines in myofibrillar protein synthesis during bed-rest in older men. J Physiol 2023. https://doi.org/10.1113/JP285130.

Patients' Experience of Nutrition Therapy During Critical Illness and Recovery

A Narrative Review

Georgia Hardy, BSc, MNutrDiet[a,b], Andrea P. Marshall, RN, PhD[c,d],
Dashiell Gantner, MBBS, PhD[a,e], Emma J. Ridley, PhD[a,b],*

KEYWORDS

- Nutrition • Critical illness • Patient experience • Oral nutrition • Enteral nutrition
- Nasogastric tube

KEY POINTS

- Nutrition interventions and symptoms can have strong emotional and psychological implications for patients.
- Hospital food service systems affect patients' nutritional intake and experience of nutrition throughout hospitalization.
- The patient experience of nutrition can be impacted by family involvement, clinician knowledge and communication, and the hospital environment.
- Including the patient experience is crucial to inform clinical practice, research, and hospital food services.
- Further investigation of the patient experience of nutrition in the critically ill may help optimize the delivery of this essential intervention.

INTRODUCTION

Medical nutrition therapy (MNT) is considered a mainstay of supportive treatment for the critically ill.[1,2] This may encompass oral, enteral, and parenteral nutrition support.

a Australian and New Zealand Intensive Care Research Centre, School of Public Health and Preventive Medicine, Monash University, Melbourne, Australia; b Nutrition and Dietetics Department, Alfred Health, Melbourne, Australia; c Intensive Care Unit, Gold Coast Health, Gold Coast University Hospital, Queensland, Australia; d School of Nursing and Midwifery, Griffith University, Gold Coast, Queensland, Australia; e Intensive Care Unit, Alfred Health, Melbourne, Australia
* Corresponding author. Australian and New Zealand Intensive Care Research Centre, School of Public Health and Preventive Medicine, Monash University, Level 3, 553 St Kilda Road, Melbourne, Victoria 3004, Australia.
E-mail address: emma.ridley@monash.edu
Twitter: @georgia_hardy (G.H.); @AndreaM_au (A.P.M.); @ICUnutrition (E.J.R.)

Crit Care Clin 41 (2025) 313–325
https://doi.org/10.1016/j.ccc.2024.09.004
criticalcare.theclinics.com
0749-0704/25/© 2024 Elsevier Inc. All rights are reserved, including those for text and data mining, AI training, and similar technologies.

MNT has been associated with benefits during critical illness such as supporting the immune system, promoting gut integrity, and aiding wound healing.[1,2] While many studies have investigated the route, amount, and timing of nutrition, patients' experience of nutrition during critical illness and recovery remains largely uninvestigated.

Clinical practice guidelines recommend that intubated patients commence MNT via enteral nutrition (EN) within 24 to 48 hours of intensive care unit (ICU) admission.[1,2] During this early phase, patients' awareness of medical interventions may be limited due to sedation, brain injury, or delirium, with decisions regarding nutrition directed by clinicians. As patients' conditions stabilize, their awareness of interventions will increase, and their experience of MNT becomes highly relevant to ongoing care.

In the ICU, following the cessation of invasive mechanical ventilation, oral intake may commence. In the absence of ongoing brain illness or sedation, patients may be able to engage in decision-making about MNT by communicating individual preferences and challenges with nutrition; however, this has not been described in the literature. Following extubation, nutrition intake from oral diet alone has been described as well below clinician recommendations.[3-5] Barriers affecting oral intake in the ICU include symptoms which affect oral intake such as poor appetite, altered consciousness, nausea and many others (termed nutrition-impacting symptoms), issues with food service, and clinician-related factors. These experiences also affect patients who do not require intubation and can eat and drink throughout their ICU admission.

Following transfer to the ward, ongoing MNT (including EN or oral nutrition support) is often indicated as intake from oral diet frequently continues to be inadequate, with studies reporting 37% to 54% of energy targets and 48% to 65% of protein targets achieved.[6,7] Providing adequate nutrition for recovery can be challenging and must be balanced with patients' preferences. A lack of understanding by ward clinicians regarding nutritional needs in this patient group may contribute to this challenge.[8]

Following hospital discharge to a rehabilitation setting or home, nutrition-impacting symptoms may last for months, affecting nutritional intake.[9,10] However, little is known about the nutrition experiences of patients following discharge from acute-care hospital settings. After hospital discharge, patients may need to integrate MNT (most commonly oral nutrition support) into everyday life. Therefore, understanding patients' individual preferences and situations is imperative. It is also important to consider that eating and drinking is much more than simply consuming nutrients for the body, and can have complex cultural, emotional, and social implications.[11]

In this narrative review, key aspects of the patient experience, and clinician and hospital-related factors influencing nutrition are summarized. Factors that both directly and indirectly impact the patient's experience of nutrition will be discussed (**Fig. 1**).

DISCUSSION
Patient Experiences of Enteral Nutrition Therapy

Nasogastric feeding tubes
For mechanically ventilated patients, the predominant form of nutrition is EN delivered via a nasogastric tube (NGT), of which there are 2 main types. Larger polyvinyl-chloride tubes are termed "wide-bore" tubes and are relatively rigid. "Fine-bore" tubes are smaller, more pliable, and usually made of polyurethane. In the early stages of critical illness, when the risk of gastric and enteric dysfunction is high, wide-bore NGTs are commonly used for gastric drainage and checking of gastric residual volumes while also being used to administer EN.[12] Changing to a fine-bore tube may occur,

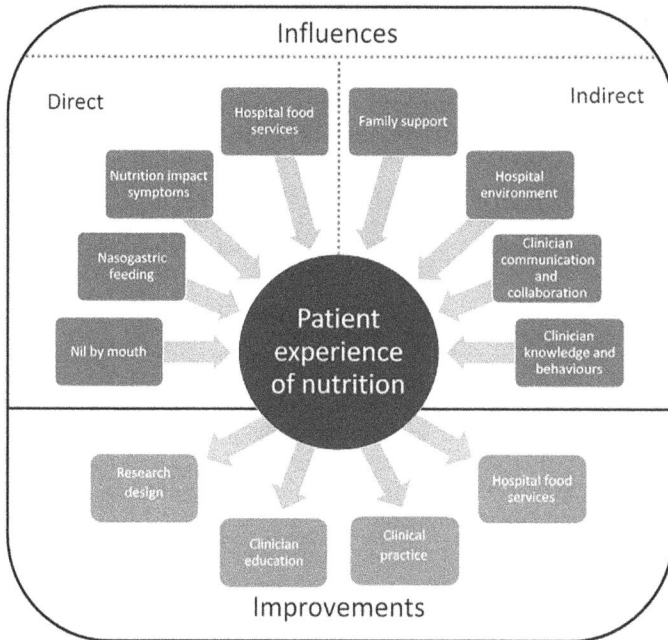

Fig. 1. Influences on the patient experience of nutrition and areas that can be improved with increased understanding of the patient experience.

although when or if this happens varies widely. International critical care nutrition guidelines currently do not make recommendations regarding NGT type or size[1,2]; however, it is plausible that the type of NGT could impact the patient experience. Furthermore, patients may have pre-existing preferences regarding tube feeding before becoming ill.

The patients' experience regarding NGTs is poorly described in patients with critical illness, although there are some reports of discomfort and distress. In a study investigating the experiences of intubated patients within the ICU, NGT insertion was described by one patient as the hardest procedure to endure.[13] Having an NGT has also been briefly described as being unpleasant or repulsive.[14] In a study outside the ICU context, the experiences of patients with malignant small bowel obstruction were explored. In this study, wide-bore NGTs were used for gastric decompression, one patient described the discomfort of the tube: "I hated that up my nose because it was so uncomfortable. It hurt me…it was horrible and uncomfortable in my throat."[15] There is some evidence that NGTs may impact swallowing function in healthy volunteers, though no clear differences between fine-bore and wide-bore tubes have been reported.[16,17] Several authors describe fine-bore tubes as more comfortable for patients[18–20]; however, no data are provided to substantiate these claims. Given a large number of critically ill patients experience NGT use, and it is at times an essential route for nutrition, this is an important gap in the literature and an area of patient experience that should be explored.

Receiving enteral feeds

Divergent experiences of receiving EN in ICU have been reported by Persenius and colleagues.[14] The patients who described positive experiences with EN appeared unphased and reassured. This is evidenced by the quote "I don't really know much about it, what has come through the tube, but it seems to have worked quite well in my opinion."[14] A sense of convenience and safety at having their nutrition supplied without having to eat and drink was also described.

Conversely, other patients expressed frustration and a sense of helplessness with symptoms related to EN. One patient stated "I think the food you are given through the tube upsets the bowels. That you feel so distended and bloated, I feel it now and it hurts a lot. Nothing seems to help... It's very frustrating."[14] This lived experience of powerlessness was described as changing to relief and hope when gastrointestinal symptoms resolved. This highlights the potential emotional overlay to physical experiences for patients.

Patient Experiences of Oral Nutrition and Impacting Factors

Fasting
The experience of fasting for procedures is common in critically ill patients.[21,22] This experience has been explored in hospital patients, with thirst and xerostomia described as the most difficult aspects, accompanied by a sense of helplessness. Conversely, for patients who were fasting due to gastrointestinal symptoms, fasting was experienced with a sense of relief.[23]

Nil by mouth
Not being allowed to consume food or fluids orally due to dysphagia, mechanical ventilation via a tracheostomy, and illness or injury despite being alert is a challenging experience for patients. Despite receiving EN to meet their nutritional needs, patients have described not being allowed to eat and drink as difficult and contributing to a sense of abnormality.[24] However, it is again often a sensation of thirst that is most distressing,[14] as expressed in the quote, "For a lot of the time I didn't really think about eating, but drinking was very important, much more so than eating. I really wanted to drink but just had no appetite. I wasn't craving food, I wasn't the least bit hungry."[24]

Starting oral diet
Patients describe commencing oral intake as a meaningful symbol of recovery.[24] It can help to bring a sense of normality and routine to an otherwise abnormal environment: "In [the] ICU there is not really any routine or pattern, it's just 12 hours of blur. Whereas, with eating, it breaks this up and makes it more like your normal day. The routine helped as I had a set pattern and knew what to expect. It also really helped me in getting ready to be transferred to the ward."[24] Linking eating and drinking to the next step in recovery gives a sense of hope and optimism.

In contrast, a sense of fear when commencing oral intake when a tracheostomy is in place has been described. This is epitomized by the quote "It had been a long time without taking anything by mouth, also there was fear that it may go down the wrong way. There was concern that if it went down into the lungs it would put the whole process back. This made me feel very apprehensive."[24] Difficulties with swallowing and not meeting goals related to eating have also been linked with feelings of failure.[14,24] Patients also described frustration at restrictions on allowed foods and drinks and needing to slow their eating speed.[24]

Nutrition impacting symptoms
The patients' experience of nutrition may also be shaped by a range of symptoms, most commonly poor appetite.[3,5,10,25] This may be related to changes in appetite hormones, which take several weeks to normalize.[26] Other reported symptoms both in ICU and following transfer to the ward include early satiety, taste changes, nausea and vomiting, dislike of the hospital food, difficulty chewing and swallowing, and

changed levels of consciousness.[3,5,9,10] Given the range of symptoms patients may experience, it is unsurprising that oral intake at this point is consistently reported to be below nutritional needs.[3–5] Ongoing MNT can help patients meet their macro and micronutrient needs during this time[6]; however, the patient's preferred options regarding the mode of MNT are unclear.

Oral intake may also be hindered by difficulty self-feeding due to weakness, injuries, or changes in cognition; feeding assistance is an intervention valued by patients.[27] However, patients may be reluctant to ask for this, as described in this quote "I didn't want to ask them because I knew they were busy and yet they would put my breakfast in front of me and I couldn't take it and I couldn't take my drugs, whatever."[28] This suggests there should be a low threshold to offer patients feeding assistance in the post-ICU period. Whilst this task is usually designated to nurses, it can be difficult to find the time within busy clinical workloads.[29] Nutrition assistants or allied health assistants may be well placed to provide feeding assistance if available; alternatively, trained volunteers have also been shown to provide effective feeding assistance.[30] Family members may also be able to help provide feeding assistance when they are present at meal times.[27,29]

Unsurprisingly, these symptoms influence the patient's experience of nutrition and contribute to the difficulty of consuming enough nutrients from diet alone to support recovery without MNT. These challenges have been described as removing the pleasure from eating and drinking, as exemplified by a quote collected by Merriweather and colleagues: "'I'm eating because I have to. . . I'm eating because it is necessary to live, to eat. You've got to get your dietary stuff, your nutrition, all the stuff you need to get by in life but it's a struggle now."[10] Potential strategies to positively influence the patient's experience of nutrition are outlined in **Table 1**.

Weight and body composition changes

Patients undergo weight and body composition changes throughout their illness, their experience of which could impact patients' feelings about their bodies and self-esteem. This may then affect patient decisions regarding nutrition interventions. Muscle loss is rapid in ICU with patients losing 2% of skeletal muscle per day in the first week of admission[31] and weight and muscle loss continues during the post-ICU hospitalization period.[7,32] Persenius and colleagues[14] found patients experience maintaining weight positively, whereas weight loss was viewed negatively. This may be related to clinicians' focus on weight maintenance and education regarding the harm of unintentional weight and lean tissue loss. However, Johansson and colleagues[33] describe a difference in responses depending on whether the individual was satisfied with their pre-admission weight.

Post-hospital discharge

Limited studies have reported on the nutritional experiences of patients who were critically ill following discharge from acute hospital settings. The prevalence of nutrition-impacting symptoms may decrease in patients following transfer to sub-acute care, with improvements in patients' levels of alertness being a primary improvement and the number of patients requiring enteral nutrition support decreasing.[9] Appetite generally improves with time,[34] with patients at 3 months post ICU discharge having similar self-rated appetite scores compared to healthy volunteers.[35] However, for other patients, poor appetite can persist for months following hospital discharge.[10,36] In a cohort of patients who were critically ill with coronavirus disease 2019 (COVID-19), other nutrition-impacting symptoms that were still present at the time of a post-ICU follow-up clinic included breathlessness, fatigue, taste changes, and dysphagia.[36]

Table 1
Practical bedside interventions that may improve the patient experience of nutrition

Issue	Potential Interventions
Discomfort associated with the feeding tube	• Ensure feeding tubes do not create pressure on the nostril or mucosa • Regularly check for signs of pressure injury • Consider change to a smaller more flexible tube before extubation
Gastrointestinal symptoms attributed to enteral feeds	• Identify and address the root cause of symptoms (ie, medication, anxiety, constipation, slow gastric emptying, administration of cold feed, rapid administration of feed) • Trial a feed with a different composition that is, add or remove fiber, try a more or less dilute feed
Taste changes	• Encourage patients to try different foods that they may not have previously liked • Encourage the use of condiments which counteract the taste change
Poor appetite or early satiety	• Encourage the intake of protein and energy-rich food first • Encourage small frequent intake
Nausea and vomiting	• Administer antiemetics half an hour before meals
Difficulty self-feeding	• Identify patients who require feeding assistance (such as a colored meal tray) • Have designated personnel to provide feeding assistance • Encourage family to provide feeding assistance (where safe and appropriate)
Dislike of eating in a clinical environment	• If clinically appropriate, facilitate the patient to get out of bed and into a chair or wheel the bed to a window • Provide headphones to help block out unit noise
Social isolation at mealtimes	• Encourage visitors at mealtimes • Use volunteers to provide conversation • Facilitate hands-free phone or video calls during meals
Dislike of hospital food or issues with the timing of hospital meals	• Encourage visitors to bring food • Facilitate visits to the cafeteria • Have a stock of snacks available on the ward

Patients may be prescribed nutrition supplement drinks to help meet nutritional needs at home; however, poor compliance has been described.[8] The reasons behind this and the experience of eating and continuing nutrition support following hospital discharge remain areas for further study.

Following discharge home, some patients regain lost weight, whilst others may continue to lose weight,[35] which may change the nutritional advice sought. Changes relating to decreased function of the body as a result of weight loss and decreased lean tissue stores have been described by patients as affecting their mood, with one patient stating "… it's the sheer frustration as well, the sheer frustration of not being able to do what you want to do and obviously the tiredness is a contributory factor to that."[10] Evidence suggests that regained weight may be a higher percentage of adipose tissue compared to lean tissue, with over 70% of regained weight being fat mass.[37] Consistent with this finding, ICU survivors had an average of 6.8 kg more fat mass and 0.96 kg less lean mass compared to matched controls. In a COVID-19 population, reasons for dietitian referral from a post-ICU follow-up clinic included helping with weight restoration in 43% of patients, but conversely helping with weight loss in 16%.[36] The effect of the complex emotions and societal pressures relating to weight change and body image and how these experiences affect compliance with nutrition recommendations is an area deserving of investigation.

Hospital-Related Factors

The environment
The ICU environment itself can affect some patients' desire to eat. This is exemplified by this quote from research undertaken by Segaran: "Seeing people ill around me really influenced my ability to eat. The lights, the noise, and the people around. It's so horrible to have to eat in the same bed as you've been in all day and even been to the toilet in."[24] Another element of the ICU environment that affects patients' mealtime experiences is the absence of social interaction that is part of a normal meal.[24] This experience may affect how much is eaten and is an area where families may be a key resource to provide a more normalized and social aspect to hospital meals.[24]

Similarly, ward patients have described the clinical aspects of the environment as negatively affecting the mealtime experience.[38] Eating in social isolation was also described as negatively affecting intake, with one patient stating "I think being alone you don't eat as well as if you've got somebody with you."[10] However, some patients prefer to eat alone due to self-consciousness about symptoms at mealtimes, and sharing rooms with patients who may be vomiting, coughing, burping, or yelling is described as affecting appetite and intake.[38] One solution that has been proposed is to provide a communal dining space on the ward.[10] This would allow patients who would like a less clinical and more social environment to enhance their mealtime experience, whilst allowing more privacy for patients in shared rooms who would prefer to eat alone due to their symptoms.

Food service
In ICU, reported food service-related issues include dislike of the hospital meals and difficulty with food packaging.[3,5,9] Altered levels of consciousness are a common barrier to oral intake in ICU.[9] This was also a primary factor in a study of patients' ability to self-report barriers to oral intake, even though these patients were eating and drinking.[3] Given patients are required to select food options from hospital menus, any barrier to the ability to perform this will lead to default meals being served. More in-depth evaluation of food-service issues in the ICU is warranted. Filling out menus for patients who are unable to is a task family members could assist with. Qualitative evidence tells us that critically ill patients value family bringing in preferred food.[10,24,27]

On the post-ICU ward, meal timing, which is system-centric, has been highlighted as a significant problem. Typically, hospital meals are served relatively early and have a set structure. This was strongly highlighted by Merriweather and colleagues[8,10] with quotes relating to both the time and meal patterns in hospital being foreign and out of the patients' control: "You know this sort of breakfast, lunch, supper, I mean that's just not for me you know, I sort of ate when I felt like it."[8]

Changing to a "room service" style hospital meal ordering system, involving patients ordering from a menu at any time within a set period (ie, 6 AM to 7 PM) may help to overcome this issue. Meals are prepared on demand and delivered within 45 minutes and this has been shown to improve energy and protein intake, decrease plate waste, improve patient satisfaction, and lower costs.[39,40]

Other options have been proposed, including having a variety of snacks available on the unit to enable food intake outside of meal times and facilitating food purchasing from the food outlets in the hospital.[10] This can help accommodate different timings and food preferences. Similarly, a randomized trial in post-ICU patients found that receiving assistance from a rehabilitation assistant to get food from the hospital canteen was valued.[27]

Failures in food service delivery have also been reported to negatively affect patients' nutrition experiences. This relates to oral nutrition supplement drinks and snacks not being delivered from the kitchen.[8] This highlights the importance of auditing hospital meal trays and implies an unmet need in hospitals to help troubleshoot issues and assist with the practical tasks related to nutrition that can make an important difference in the patient's experience. The benefits of similar interventions have been reported. In a population of trauma patients with hip fractures, dietitian assistants helped check patient food preferences and food selection, encouraged intake, and provided meal set-up and feeding assistance. This not only improved nutritional intake but reduced mortality.[41]

Clinician Factors

Education and knowledge

Nutrition has been identified as a shortcoming in medical education across the continuum of training.[42] In a study regarding patients with traumatic brain injuries,[43] doctors described their understanding of the evidence regarding nutrition as either lacking or a belief that studies show no difference in important outcomes. Knowledge was described as being largely influenced by the modeling of senior medical staff, as opposed to being based on published literature or formal teaching.

Huang and colleagues[44] reported that ICU nurses indicated that insufficient education on nutrition was one of the top 3 factors affecting the delivery of EN, and showed that nurses with more frequent education regarding EN reported fewer perceived barriers to enteral feeding.

It should be acknowledged that large randomized control trials investigating nutrition interventions in critically ill patients have failed to show benefits,[45–47] leading to an assumption that nutrition is not important; however, this is not necessarily the case. Methodological issues including the use of primary outcomes such as mortality as opposed to functional or health-related quality of life measures and limited timeframes of nutrition interventions (often 1 week or less) are potential explanations for these results.[48]

A lack of knowledge is hypothesized to underlie the premature removal of feeding tubes,[8] a key barrier to adequate nutrition in critically ill patients following extubation. In post-operative patients, the early removal of NGTs is recommended in enhanced recovery after surgery protocols[49,50]; however, these protocols were not designed for, or tested in critically ill populations. Merriweather and colleagues[10] described close to 70% of feeding tubes being removed within 48 hours of transfer from the ICU to the ward, despite no formal assessment of nutrition intake having taken place. Documented rationale for decisions to remove feeding tubes in patients with poor oral intake included encouraging oral intake[8] or improving appetite.[27] However, oral intake was minimal following NGT removal.[8] Preliminary evidence published as an abstract showed that in ICU, patients receiving oral diet alone, or oral diet plus EN did not have significantly different oral intakes or self-rated appetite scores.[51] This is also supported by observational research showing patients with combined oral and EN have significantly better nutritional adequacy compared to oral diet alone.[3,4,6] This suggests that ceasing EN is not the answer to improving oral intake or helping patients meet their nutritional needs. However, patient wishes and any NGT-related discomfort also need to be considered.

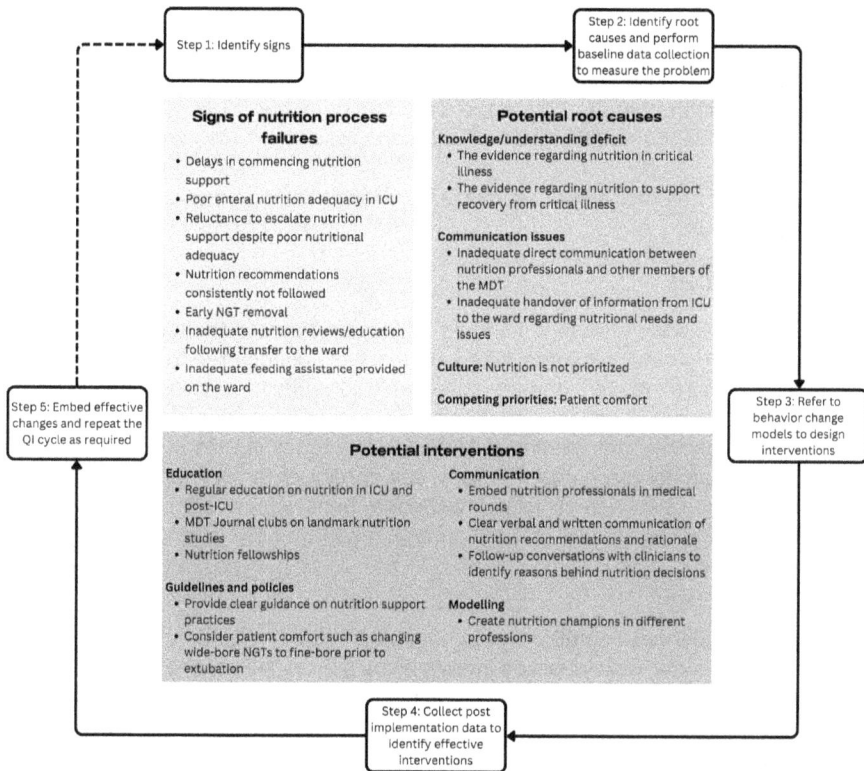

Step 1: Identify signs

Step 2: Identify root causes and perform baseline data collection to measure the problem

Signs of nutrition process failures
- Delays in commencing nutrition support
- Poor enteral nutrition adequacy in ICU
- Reluctance to escalate nutrition support despite poor nutritional adequacy
- Nutrition recommendations consistently not followed
- Early NGT removal
- Inadequate nutrition reviews/education following transfer to the ward
- Inadequate feeding assistance provided on the ward

Potential root causes
Knowledge/understanding deficit
- The evidence regarding nutrition in critical illness
- The evidence regarding nutrition to support recovery from critical illness

Communication issues
- Inadequate direct communication between nutrition professionals and other members of the MDT
- Inadequate handover of information from ICU to the ward regarding nutritional needs and issues

Culture: Nutrition is not prioritized

Competing priorities: Patient comfort

Step 5: Embed effective changes and repeat the QI cycle as required

Step 3: Refer to behavior change models to design interventions

Potential interventions

Education
- Regular education on nutrition in ICU and post-ICU
- MDT Journal clubs on landmark nutrition studies
- Nutrition fellowships

Guidelines and policies
- Provide clear guidance on nutrition support practices
- Consider patient comfort such as changing wide-bore NGTs to fine-bore prior to extubation

Communication
- Embed nutrition professionals in medical rounds
- Clear verbal and written communication of nutrition recommendations and rationale
- Follow-up conversations with clinicians to identify reasons behind nutrition decisions

Modelling
- Create nutrition champions in different professions

Step 4: Collect post implementation data to identify effective interventions

Fig. 2. Ways to improve medical nutrition therapy at a local level. Nutrition process issues can be addressed using quality improvement cycles to optimize multidisciplinary team work.

Insufficient knowledge of factors affecting patients following ICU discharge on the ward may also be an important element. In a study, ward nurses expressed frustration at the high level of care patients require due to ICU-acquired weakness which can affect a patient's ability to self-feed, with patients' dependence seen as demanding.[8] This lack of understanding by ward staff may also extend to dietitians and dietetic support staff. It has been suggested that ward dietitians underestimate the needs of post-ICU patients, as evidenced by limited nutrition reviews, and an unmet need for nutrition education following discharge home.[8]

Communication and collaboration
Nutrition care is acknowledged as a responsibility that intersects with multiple disciplines.[29,43] Despite this, a lack of coordinated and collaborative care has been reported.[10,29] One issue is a lack of integration of the dietitian or other nutrition expert into medical rounds,[43] as well as issues with communication between staff.[10] This may lead to patients experiencing unclear or conflicting messaging regarding their nutrition.

Transfer from ICU to the ward is a key time when communication and handover regarding a patient's nutrition occurs between staff. Patients have described breakdowns in communication as greatly affecting their experience. In a study, a patient was quoted as saying"So when I was discharged from intensive care, the idea was that I would be eating food. I would start off with soup, ice cream, that sort of thing, to get myself back into the habit of eating again. When I got down to the general ward, there had been no communication from intensive care to the general ward what I should be doing. They could not actually supply the right food for me. So, my wife and son had to bring food in for me to eat."[28] Limited documented handover regarding nutrition information from the ICU to the ward has been described and is postulated to negatively influence nutritional care[8] and can create confusion and frustration for patients.

Fig. 2 outlines potential ways to address knowledge and communication issues at a local hospital level.

FUTURE DIRECTIONS

The patient experience of nutrition should be included across the research process, from design to outcome measures; however, this has not occurred to date. Rectifying this will help ensure interventions are acceptable to patients, and identify if changes are required to improve patient compliance. Evidence gaps identified in this review include patient experiences relating to MNT; feeding tubes, routes of MNT, and nutrition following hospital discharge. Similarly, the impact of family-based interventions and the interaction between clinician knowledge, behaviors, and attitudes regarding nutrition on patient experience of nutrition requires further investigation.

SUMMARY

The patient experience of nutrition throughout the trajectory of critical illness is diverse and can be emotional. Individualized interventions are required along the care journey to address difficulties and enhance the patient experience. Improving clinician knowledge and collaboration and redesigning hospital food services and environments are all potential ways to improve patient care. Resources which may improve nutrition experience and intake in patients include family support, and assistant roles focused on providing additional nutrition-related care such as feeding assistance. Gaining a better understanding of patient experiences is key to unlocking improvements in clinical care, research design, and hospital food service systems.

CLINICS CARE POINTS

- Consideration should be given to the physical as well as emotional and psychological effects of MNT interventions and restrictions.
- Poor appetite is a common and persistent symptom across the recovery trajectory. Strategies to improve intake may be helpful but it takes time for this to resolve.
- Families should be empowered to assist with nutrition where appropriate such as bringing in preferred foods and providing feeding assistance and social interaction at meals.
- Hospital food service systems should be designed to serve various patient preferences, including flexible meal times (such as a room-service style ordering system), readily available snacks, and culturally appropriate options.
- Education to staff regarding the complex nutritional needs of critically ill patients should be embedded into hospital orientation for ICU, wards, and rehabilitation units.
- The decision to remove NGTs should be made in partnership with the multidisciplinary team and the patient.
- Collaborative multidisciplinary work is required to ensure appropriate handover and consistent messaging to patients about nutritional plans and the importance of nutrition.

DISCLOSURES

This work was supported by an Australian Government Research Training Program (RTP) scholarship (G.H.). The Australian Government had no role in the writing of this article.

REFERENCES

1. Singer P, Blaser AR, Berger MM, et al. ESPEN guideline on clinical nutrition in the intensive care unit. Clin Nutr 2019;38(1):48–79.
2. Taylor BE, McClave SA, Martindale RG, et al. Guidelines for the provision and assessment of nutrition support therapy in the adult critically ill patient: society of critical care medicine (SCCM) and American Society for Parenteral and Enteral Nutrition (A.S.P.E.N.). Crit Care Med 2016;44(2):390–438.
3. Moisey LL, Pikul J, Keller H, et al. Adequacy of protein and energy intake in critically ill adults following liberation from mechanical ventilation is dependent on route of nutrition delivery. Nutr Clin Pract 2021;36(1):201–12.
4. Rougier L, Preiser JC, Fadeur M, et al. Nutrition during critical care: an audit on actual energy and protein intakes. JPEN - J Parenter Enter Nutr 2021;45(5):951–60.
5. Peterson SJ, Tsai AA, Scala CM, et al. Adequacy of oral intake in critically ill patients 1 week after extubation. J Am Diet Assoc 2010;110(3):427–33.
6. Ridley EJ, Parke RL, Davies AR, et al. What happens to nutrition intake in the post-intensive care unit hospitalization period? an observational cohort study in critically ill adults. JPEN - J Parenter Enter Nutr 2019;43(1):88–95.
7. Wittholz K, Fetterplace K, Clode M, et al. Measuring nutrition-related outcomes in a cohort of multi-trauma patients following intensive care unit discharge. J Hum Nutr Diet 2020;33(3):414–22.
8. Merriweather J, Smith P, Walsh T. Nutritional rehabilitation after ICU - does it happen: a qualitative interview and observational study. J Clin Nurs 2014;23(5–6):654–62.
9. Amon JN, Tatucu-Babet OA, Hodgson CL, et al. Nutrition care processes from intensive care unit admission to inpatient rehabilitation: a retrospective observational study. Nutrition 2023;113:112061.
10. Merriweather JL, Salisbury LG, Walsh TS, et al. Nutritional care after critical illness: a qualitative study of patients' experiences. J Hum Nutr Diet 2016;29(2):127–36.
11. Brown L, Edwards J, Hartwell H. Eating and emotion: focusing on the lunchtime meal. Br Food J 2013;115(2):196–208.
12. Ohbe H, Matsui H, Fushimi K, et al. Small-bore feeding tube versus large-bore sump tube for early enteral nutrition in mechanically ventilated patients: a nationwide inpatient database study. Clin Nutr 2021;40(6):4113–9.
13. Pakmehr M, Rahnama M, Firouzkouhi M, et al. Lived experience of intubated patients: a phenomenological study. Indian J Public Health Res Dev 2017;8(1):296–301.
14. Persenius MW, Hall-Lord ML, Wilde-Larsson B. Grasping the nutritional situation: a grounded theory study of patients' experiences in intensive care. Nurs Crit Care 2009;14(4):166–74.
15. Singh Curry R, Evans E, Raftery A-M, et al. Percutaneous venting gastrostomy/gastrojejunostomy for malignant bowel obstruction: a qualitative study. BMJ Support Palliat Care 2019;9(4):381–8.
16. Pryor LNW EC, Cornwell PL, O'Connor SN, et al. Impact of nasogastric tubes on swallowing physiology in older, healthy subjects: a randomized controlled crossover trial. Clin Nutr 2015;34:572–8.

17. Huggins PS, Tuomi SK, Young C. Effects of nasogastric tubes on the young, normal swallowing mechanism. Dysphagia 1999;14(3):157–61.
18. Lord LM. Enteral access devices: types, function, care, and challenges. Nutr Clin Pract 2018;33(1):16–38.
19. Bloom L, Seckel MA. Placement of nasogastric feeding tube and postinsertion care review. AACN Adv Crit Care 2022;33(1):68–84.
20. Krenitsky J. Blind bedside placement of feeding tubes: treatment or threat? Practical Gastroenterol 2011;35(3):32–42.
21. Passier RHA, Davies AR, Ridley E, et al. Periprocedural cessation of nutrition in the intensive care unit: opportunities for improvement. Intensive Care Med 2013;39(7): 1221–6.
22. Uozumi M, Sanui M, Komuro T, et al. Interruption of enteral nutrition in the intensive care unit: a single-center survey. J Intens Care 2017;5(1).
23. Carey SK, Conchin S, Bloomfield-Stone S. A qualitative study into the impact of fasting within a large tertiary hospital in Australia–the patients' perspective. J Clin Nurs 2015;24(13–14):1946–54.
24. Segaran E. Returning to normal: the role of eating in recovery from a critical illness. Br J Neurosci Nurs 2006;2(3):141–8.
25. Chapple LS, Ridley EJ, Ainscough K, et al. Nutrition delivery across hospitalisation in critically ill patients with COVID-19: an observational study of the Australian experience. Aust Crit Care 2024;37(3):422–8.
26. Nematy M, O'Flynn JE, Wandrag L, et al. Changes in appetite related gut hormones in intensive care unit patients: a pilot cohort study. Crit Care 2006; 10(1):R10.
27. Ramsay P, Huby G, Merriweather J, et al. Patient and carer experience of hospital-based rehabilitation from intensive care to hospital discharge: mixed methods process evaluation of the RECOVER randomised clinical trial. BMJ Open 2016;6(8):e012041.
28. Field K, Prinjha S, Rowan K. 'One patient amongst many': a qualitative analysis of intensive care unit patients' experiences of transferring to the general ward. Crit Care 2008;12(1):R21.
29. Marshall AP, Takefala T, Williams LT, et al. Health practitioner practices and their influence on nutritional intake of hospitalised patients. Int J Nurs Sci 2019;6(2): 162–8.
30. Howson FFA, Robinson SM, Lin SX, et al. Can trained volunteers improve the mealtime care of older hospital patients? An implementation study in one English hospital. BMJ Open 2018;8(8):e022285.
31. Fazzini B, Markl T, Costas C, et al. The rate and assessment of muscle wasting during critical illness: a systematic review and meta-analysis. Crit Care 2023; 27(1):2.
32. Alvarez-Hernandez J, Matia-Martin P, Cancer-Minchot E, et al. Long-term outcomes in critically ill patients who survived COVID-19: the NUTRICOVID observational cohort study. Clin Nutr 2023;42(10):2029–35.
33. Johansson L, Fjellman-Wiklund A. Ventilated patients' experiences of body awareness at an intensive care unit. Adv Physiother 2009;7(4):154–61.
34. Merriweather JL, Griffith DM, Walsh TS. Appetite during the recovery phase of critical illness: a cohort study. Eur J Clin Nutr 2018;72(7):986–92.
35. Chapple LS, Weinel LM, Abdelhamid YA, et al. Observed appetite and nutrient intake three months after ICU discharge. Clin Nutr 2019;38(3):1215–20.
36. Hardy G, Camporota L, Bear DE. Nutrition support practices across the care continuum in a single centre critical care unit during the first surge of the COVID-19

pandemic - a comparison of VV-ECMO and non-ECMO patients. Clin Nutr 2022; 41(12):2887–94.

37. Thackeray M, Kotowicz MA, Pasco JA, et al. Changes in body composition in the year following critical illness: a case-control study. J Crit Care 2022;71:154043.
38. Larsen KL, Schjøtler B, Melgaard D. Patients' experiences eating in a hospital – a qualitative study. Clinical Nutrition ESPEN 2021;45:469–75.
39. McCray S, Maunder K, Krikowa R, et al. Room service improves nutritional intake and increases patient satisfaction while decreasing food waste and cost. J Acad Nutr Diet 2018;118(2):284–93.
40. Neaves B, Bell JJ, McCray S. Impact of room service on nutritional intake, plate and production waste, meal quality and patient satisfaction and meal costs: a single site pre-post evaluation. Nutr Diet 2022;79(2):187–96.
41. Duncan DG, Beck SJ, Hood K, et al. Using dietetic assistants to improve the outcome of hip fracture: a randomised controlled trial of nutritional support in an acute trauma ward. Age Ageing 2006;35(2):148–53.
42. Crowley J, Ball L, Hiddink GJ. Nutrition in medical education: a systematic review. Lancet Planet Health 2019;3(9):e379–89.
43. Chapple LA, Chapman M, Shalit N, et al. Barriers to nutrition intervention for patients with a traumatic brain injury: views and attitudes of medical and nursing practitioners in the acute care setting. JPEN - J Parenter Enter Nutr 2018;42(2):318–26.
44. Huang J, Yang L, Zhuang Y, et al. Current status and influencing factors of barriers to enteral feeding of critically ill patients: a multicenter study. J Clin Nurs 2019;28(3–4):677–85.
45. Heyland DK, Patel J, Compher C, et al. The effect of higher protein dosing in critically ill patients with high nutritional risk (EFFORT Protein): an international, multi-centre, pragmatic, registry-based randomised trial. Lancet 2023;401(10376): 568–76.
46. Chapman M, Peake SL, Bellomo R, et al. Energy-dense versus routine enteral nutrition in the critically ill. N Engl J Med 2018;379(19):1823–34.
47. Arabi YM, Aldawood AS, Haddad SH, et al. Permissive underfeeding or standard enteral feeding in critically ill adults. N Engl J Med 2015;372(25):2398–408.
48. Bear DE, Wandrag L, Merriweather JL, et al. The role of nutritional support in the physical and functional recovery of critically ill patients: a narrative review. Crit Care 2017;21(1):226.
49. Saurabh K, Sureshkumar S, Mohsina S, et al. Adapted ERAS pathway versus standard care in patients undergoing emergency small bowel surgery: a randomized controlled trial. J Gastrointest Surg 2020;24(9):2077–87.
50. Mohsina S, Shanmugam D, Sureshkumar S, et al. Adapted ERAS pathway vs. standard care in patients with perforated duodenal ulcer-a randomized controlled trial. J Gastrointest Surg 2018;22(1):107–16.
51. Rowles A, Langan A, Bear DE. SUN-P019: oral intake and appetite in the intensive care unit. Clin Nutr 2016;35:S51.

Navigating Nutrition Complexity in Critical Care

A Focus on Swallowing Function and Rehabilitation

Amy Freeman-Sanderson, BAppSc (Speech Pathology), PhD[a,b,c,d,*],
Nicola A. Clayton, BAppSc (Speech Pathology), MScMed, PhD[e,f,g],
Charissa J. Zaga, BSpPath, MPH, PhD[h,i,j,k],
Anna-Liisa Sutt, BA, MA, PhD[l,m,n], Martin B. Brodsky, PhD, ScM[o,p,q]

KEYWORDS

- Dysphagia • Deglutition disorders • Critical care • Critical illness • Nutrition
- Post-extubation dysphagia • Assessment • Rehabilitation

Continued

[a] Graduate School of Health, University of Technology Sydney, 100 Broadway, Chippendale, New South Wales 2008, Australia; [b] Royal Prince Alfred Hospital, Sydney, New South Wales, Australia; [c] Critical Care Division, The George Institute for Global Health, Faculty of Medicine, UNSW Sydney, Sydney, Australia; [d] Australian and New Zealand Intensive Care Research Centre (ANZIC-RC), School of Public Health and Preventive Medicine, Monash University, Melbourne, Australia; [e] Department of Speech Pathology, Concord Repatriation General Hospital, Hospital Road, Concord, Sydney, New South Wales 2139, Australia; [f] Faculty of Medicine and Health, University of Sydney, Sydney, New South Wales, Australia; [g] School of Health and Rehabilitation Sciences, University of Queensland, Brisbane, Queensland, Australia; [h] Department of Speech Pathology, Austin Health, Level 3, Lance Townsend Building, 145 Studley Road, Heidelberg, Victoria 3084, Australia; [i] Implementation Science Unit, Institute for Breathing and Sleep, Austin Health, Victoria, Australia; [j] Department of Critical Care, University of Melbourne, Victoria, Australia; [k] Department of Audiology and Speech Pathology, University of Melbourne, Victoria, Australia; [l] Critical Care Research Group, The Prince Charles Hospital, Brisbane, Australia; [m] Institute of Molecular Bioscience, University of Queensland, Brisbane, Australia; [n] Department of Speech and Language Therapy, The Royal London Hospital, Whitechapel Road, London E1 1FR, United Kingdom; [o] Department of Otolaryngology-Head and Neck Surgery, Cleveland Clinic, 9500 Euclid Avenue, Cleveland, OH 44195, USA; [p] Physical Medicine and Rehabilitation, John Hopkins University, Baltimore, MD, USA; [q] Pulmonary and Critical Care, Johns Hopkins University, Baltimore, MD, USA
* Corresponding author. Graduate School of Health, University of Technology Sydney, 100 Broadway, Chippendale, New South Wales 2008, Australia.
E-mail address: Amy.freeman-sanderson@uts.edu.au
Twitter: @DrAmyFS (A.F.-S.); @DrNicolaC_SP (N.A.C.); @CharissaZaga (C.J.Z.); @MsAnnaLiisaSutt (A.-L.S.); @MBBrodskyPhD (M.B.B.)

Crit Care Clin 41 (2025) 327–344
https://doi.org/10.1016/j.ccc.2024.11.001   **criticalcare.theclinics.com**
0749-0704/25/Crown Copyright © 2024 Published by Elsevier Inc. All rights reserved, including those for text and data mining, AI training, and similar technologies.

Continued

KEY POINTS

- Dysphagia is multifactorial and can impact the safety and efficiency of oral intake.
- Newly acquired dysphagia is common yet underdiagnosed and reported in critically ill patients.
- Accurate diagnosis is paramount to informing optimal management. Instrumental assessment should be considered beyond swallow screening.
- Interventions optimizing body structure, function, and activities with a person-centered focus are essential.
- Future research should focus on dysphagia phenotypes and causation to enable the design of effective and feasible treatments.

INTRODUCTION

Swallowing is the key antecedent to enable oral intake, the primary mode of nutrition for critically ill patients during their recovery process.[1,2] An effective swallow mechanism is vital to supporting oral nutrition and nutritional adequacy. Swallowing is a complex neurophysiologic and dynamic process, relying on the coordination of more than 30 muscles and 6 cranial nerves.[3,4] Swallow dysfunction (ie, dysphagia) occurs with critical illness due to several factors and is commonly underreported.[5] Critical illness dysphagia is an independent risk factor for increased morbidity and mortality.[6] Related sequelae can include short-term and long-term health, personal activity, and economic impacts.[7–11] Variability across study designs, assessment methods, and patient populations, make it challenging to analyze dysphagia risk factors.

We review recent literature describing the pathophysiology of dysphagia in adults with critical illness and synthesize the evidence across the continuum of assessment and management. Our focus emphasizes the importance of patient-centered outcomes and management using the International Classification of Functioning, Disability and Health Framework (ICF).[12]

Defining Swallowing and Dysphagia

Swallowing is comprised of 4 phases: (1) pre-oral, (2) oral, (3) pharyngeal, and (4) esophageal (**Fig. 1**). Whereas the oral preparatory and oral phases of swallowing are volitional, the pharyngeal and esophageal phases are reflexive; however, some

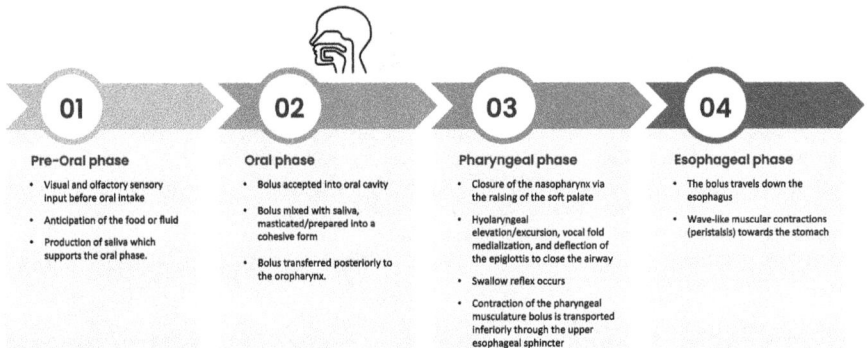

01 Pre-Oral phase
- Visual and olfactory sensory input before oral intake
- Anticipation of the food or fluid
- Production of saliva which supports the oral phase.

02 Oral phase
- Bolus accepted into oral cavity
- Bolus mixed with saliva, masticated/prepared into a cohesive form
- Bolus transferred posteriorly to the oropharynx.

03 Pharyngeal phase
- Closure of the nasopharynx via the raising of the soft palate
- Hyolaryngeal elevation/excursion, vocal fold medialization, and deflection of the epiglottis to close the airway
- Swallow reflex occurs
- Contraction of the pharyngeal musculature bolus is transported inferiorly through the upper esophageal sphincter

04 Esophageal phase
- The bolus travels down the esophagus
- Wave-like muscular contractions (peristalsis) towards the stomach

Fig. 1. Stages of swallowing. (Image from flaticon.com.)

endogenous and exogenous sensory inputs can influence the pharyngeal phase of swallowing (eg, a therapeutic swallowing maneuver or bolus volume).[13]

Swallowing is generally initiated in the post-inspiratory/expiratory phase, followed by a brief pause in breathing as the bolus passes through the oropharynx and pharynx followed by expiration.[14] Due to the shared passageway of the larynx and pharynx, intact swallowing function requires the passage of a saliva or food/fluid bolus with precision and coordination with airway protection. Dysphagia may impact both the safety and efficiency of the swallowing mechanism across swallow phases. Impact on safety includes airway compromise as laryngeal penetration and/or aspiration. The individual's response to laryngeal penetration or aspiration relies on intact sensory function and efficiency of the cough response in expelling the bolus from the airway. The adduction of the vocal folds, hyolaryngeal excursion and precise coordination of swallows with breathing, minimizes the risk of aspiration. Aspiration can be audible or silent, the latter defined as no clinical response (eg, gurgly voice, throat clearing, and cough) initiated in response to aspiration. Impact on swallow efficiency includes the ability to complete coordinated actions including chewing and bolus movement, with impairments often resulting in oral and/or pharyngeal residue post swallow. Dysphagia and resultant recommendation of nil oral intake, texture-modified diet and/or fluids, or reduced quantity of oral intake to account for swallow fatigue, or therapeutic swallowing strategies may result in nutritional inadequacy.

Swallowing and eating are inherently linked but different, with eating extending to a broader context often encapsulating social activities (eg, eating a meal with family and friends).[15] Both are important concepts in navigating the concepts of nutrition complexity during recovery from critical illness.

Dysphagia Prevalence and Pathophysiology in the Critically Ill

The prevalence of dysphagia during admission to the intensive care unit (ICU) ranges from 3% to 68% across multiple systematic reviews (**Table 1**).[16–19] Variability of dysphagia prevalence can be attributed to population studied (eg, neurologic, surgical) and method of assessment.[20–22]

Dysphagia pathophysiology is multifactorial and involves components related to both swallow safety and efficiency. The term ICU-acquired swallow disorder,[23] reflects the multi-component combination of body systems, environmental factors, concomitant medical diagnoses, and iatrogenic factors across the continuum of critical illness (**Fig. 2**). Six key mechanisms primarily contribute to the pathophysiology of dysphagia with critical illness.[24] These include (1) oropharyngeal and laryngeal trauma associated with the use of artificial airways (discussed in detail in the proceeding section), (2) neuromyopathy, (3) impaired laryngeal sensory function, (4) impaired sensory function across other areas of the neurologic system, (5) gastroesophageal reflux, and (6) impaired coordination of the breathing-swallow pattern. Additionally, reduced pre-ICU admission physical status,[25] a diagnosis of sepsis,[26] and increased size of the endotracheal tube[27] are associated with increased prevalence and protraction dysphagia.[5,18] Critical illness is recognized to profoundly impact the human body physiologically and systemically. Hypermetabolism or catabolism is evidenced in conditions including severe burn injury and other massive tissue loss conditions (eg, necrotizing fasciitis).[28] Hypermetabolism results in increased pressure to ensure that the patient receives adequate nutrition, whether it is via an oral or non-oral route. When dysphagia due to critical illness ensues, this can further complicate the management of the potentially already nutritionally compromised patient and is a factor to consider in optimizing rehabilitation.

Table 1
Prevalence of dysphagia and aspiration in patients post-extubation reported by systematic reviews

Reference	Population	Mean/Median Duration of Intubation	Dysphagia Prevalence	Aspiration Prevalence, Type	Number of Patients (Studies) Reported
Brodsky et al,[16] 2018 (SR)	Mixed ICU	Mean = 8.2 d	49%, range = 9%-67%		319 (4 studies)
Brodsky et al,[17] 2021 (SRMA)	Post-extubation from surgery	Mean = 410 min	43% (95% CI: 21%-68%)		94 (3 studies)
McIntyre et al,[18] 2021 (SRMA)	Mixed ICU	Overall ≤48 h >48 h	41% (95% CI: 33%-50%) 37% (95% CI: 8%-65%) 37% (95% CI: 27%-46%)	36% (95% CI: 22%-50%) silent	5798 (38 studies)
Skoretz et al,[19] 2010 (SR)	Mixed ICU	Mean = 167 h	12%, range = 3%-56%		2158 (8 studies)

Abbreviations: CI, confidence interval; ICU, intensive care unit; SR, systematic review; SRMA, systematic review with meta-analysis.

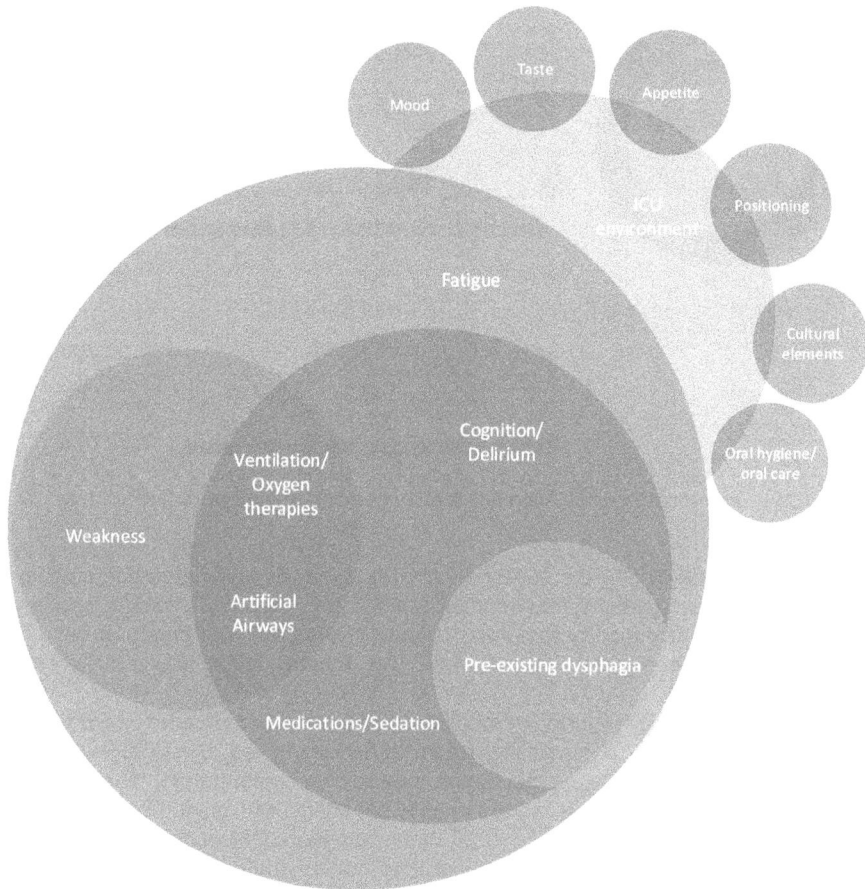

Fig. 2. Pathophysiological and environmental influences on swallowing.

Neurologic dysfunction is one of highest occurring diagnoses for patients diagnosed with ICU-acquired dysphagia.[23,29] One of the most prevalent reported sensory dysfunctions is silent aspiration.[5] Increased rates of silent aspiration occur with artificial airways,[18] with increased risk associated with an increased size of artificial airway.[27] Disruption to efferent neurologic pathways can also occur, resulting in reduced range of motion and strength of musculature contraction across all swallow phases. Beyond the head and neck musculature, trunk and upper limb weakness can impact upright seated postures, upper limb strength for self-feeding,[30] and strength of respiratory muscles required for effective cough strength.[31]

For effective oral intake, patients require an adequate level of alertness, attention, and awareness particularly for the oral stage of swallow. Delirium, altered mental status,[32] and polypharmacy[33] are associated with worse swallowing outcomes for adults with dysphagia, but causation has not been established.

Dysphagia Outcomes

An acquired critical care dysphagia is an independent predictor of all-cause mortality at 28 and 90-days postextubation.[20] With advancements in clinical care leading to higher ICU survival rates, mortality as a sole outcome is insufficient. Patients and

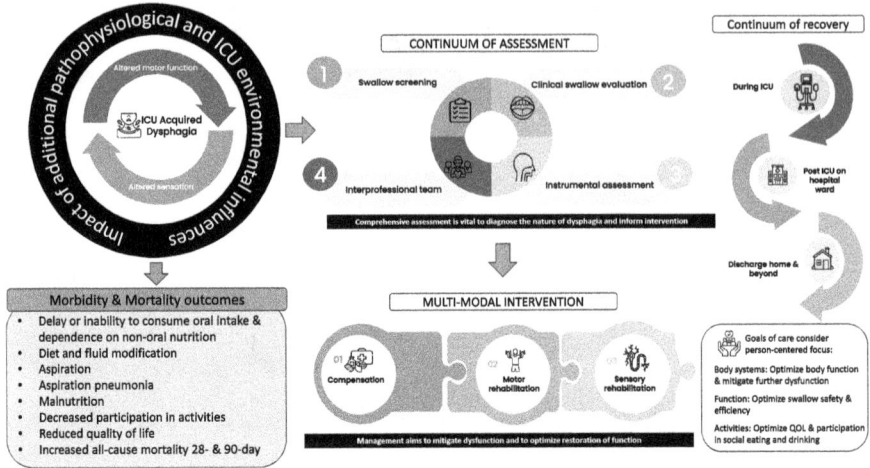

Fig. 3. ICU acquired dysphagia: Outcomes & management. (Image from flaticon.com.)

families consistently report the quality of survival, and their associated outcomes are the key. As informed by the ICF, outcomes can be conceptualized into body systems, activities, and participation across the continuum of care.[12] The timing of outcome measures varies across studies; however, 6 months after ICU admission is recommended.[34]

Outcomes commonly reported in studies include resolution of safety swallow outcomes (eg, penetration or aspiration), return to oral intake (eg, diet/fluid levels), and associated sequelae such as aspiration pneumonia, malnutrition, and mortality (**Fig. 3**).[6,35,36] Aspiration occurs in 29% to 56% of patients who are intubated with mechanical ventilation (**Table 2**).[21,25,27,37–39] With more than 30% of critically ill patients presenting with dysphagia at hospital discharge[31] and symptoms lasting as long as 5 years,[40] it is perhaps unsurprising that dysphagia is statistically associated with other body system disability including reduced mobility, dyspnea, and pain.[41] Patients with persistent dysphagia following critical illness are also less likely to be discharged home, highlighting the need for ongoing focused health support.[42]

Activities and participation refer to the related functions beyond swallowing, including independent feeding, eating, and drinking to enable dining out with family and friends. Return to eating and drinking is ranked as one of the highest functional goals for critical cares survivors,[43] reinforcing the ability to swallow and eat as core to quality of life. Beyond the individual patient outcomes, system outcomes such as hospitalization, use of resources, and cost are among the priority outcomes.[10,44]

Swallowing Across Ventilation Status

Endotracheal intubation

Dysphagia is common after endotracheal intubation with mechanical ventilation. If it is not caused by the underlying disease, critical care treatments such as endotracheal intubation with mechanical ventilation impact swallowing anatomy and physiology. Patients are usually orally intubated when mechanical ventilation commences. An endotracheal tube (ETT) traverses the oral cavity, larynx, and lower trachea. No airflow occurs above the ETT's cuff, disrupting taste and smell. Patients are often sedated and sometimes paralyzed, leading to infrequent (if any) swallow activity. In addition to reduced muscle mass, medications can cause dysphagia. One study found

Table 2
Prevalence of dysphagia and aspiration in patients post-extubation reported by studies with consecutive, nonreferral-based subject enrollment and instrumental evaluation confirmation

Reference	Population	Mean/Median Duration of Intubation	Aspiration Prevalence, Type	Number of Patients (Sites) Reported
Ajemian et al,[37] 2001	Medical, surgical ICU	*Overall duration not reported* • Nonaspirators mean = 7.7 d • Aspirators mean = 8 d	56% (n = 27) overall • 25% (n = 12) silent	48 (1 site)
El Solh, et al,[25] 2003	Medical ICU	*Aspiration* • <65 y median = 9.3 d • ≥65 y median = 7.8 d *No aspiration* • <65 y median = 7.7 d • ≥65 y median = 6.2 d	36% (n = 15) • 20% (n = 3) silent 52% (n = 22) • 36% (n = 8) silent N/A N/A	84 (1 site)
Krisciunas et al,[27] 2020	Mixed ICU	Median = 133 h	32% (n = 68) • 13.8% (n = 29) silent • 23.8% (n = 50) overt	210 (4 sites)
Leder et al,[38] 1998	Trauma	Median = 11 d	45% (n = 9)	20 (1 site)
Langmore et al,[39] 2021	Mixed ICU	Median = 126 h	33% (n = 70)	213 (4 sites)
Plowman et al,[21] 2023	Cardiac surgery	Mean = 38.3 h	29% (n = 53) • 53% (n = 28) silent	182 (1 site)

Abbreviation: ICU, intensive care unit.

morphine and midazolam are associated with increased pharyngeal dysfunction and breathing-swallow coordination difficulties.[45] ETTs (oral or nasal) can cause anatomic and functional impairments (eg, broken teeth, abrasions/lacerations, and laryngeal injury) during insertion and while *in situ* across the oral (or nasal), pharyngeal and laryngeal areas, with a systematic review reporting prevalence of laryngeal injuries at 83%.[16] Lack of airflow and damage from the ETT can lead to upper airway sensory deficits. Laryngeal adductor reflex was missing in 50% of patients post-ETT, which was associated with the presence of secretions and aspiration.[46] Whilst no routine tools are used to identify postextubation upper airway symptoms in clinical practice, the newly adapted Laryngeal Hypersensitivity Questionnaire-Acute appears to be promising.[47] Structural issues, sensory deficits, and muscle disuse atrophy all contribute to patients presenting with dysphagia after oral intubation.[16,48] The greater period the patient has been intubated, the more likely they will have difficulties, and the more severe the nature of these difficulties.[16]

Tracheostomy

Some patients cannot be safely extubated and consequently are converted from an oral (or nasal) endotracheal tube to a tracheostomy. Although the upper airway is freed from the ETT, ongoing mechanical ventilation requires insertion of a tracheostomy tube in the patient's neck with cuff inflation, continuing absent airflow in the upper airway. In addition to limited sensory information, no airflow via the glottis also means no subglottic pressures can develop during swallowing.[49,50] This results in the absence of a typical airway protective mechanisms during and after swallowing (eg, cough).

The frequency of dysphagia in patients with a tracheostomy is high, but causality has not been confirmed.[29] One also needs to consider the potential injuries from ETT that precede most tracheostomies. If oral intake with the tracheostomy cuff inflated is suggested, an instrumental swallowing assessment should be conducted to ensure safety and efficiency given the risk for silent aspiration.[51] While the tracheostomy cuff is inflated, the mode of mechanical ventilation via the tracheostomy has little impact on the swallow as the usual shared pathways for breathing and swallowing are separated. As soon as cuff deflation can be achieved safely, airflow may occur via the upper airway (absent stenosis), but challenges to laryngeal closure will persist with an open system.[52] To facilitate more coordinated and natural airflow movement and swallowing, a one-way valve should be placed on the tracheostomy following cuff deflation,[49,53] once upper airway patency has been established.[54] Although the mode of mechanical ventilation may change, the dynamics of the swallow, it is likely that the underlying disease process has a bigger impact on the swallow than the tracheostomy tube or the mode of ventilation being delivered.[55,56]

Non-invasive ventilation

Many ICU patients receive noninvasive ventilation (NIV), either as a step-down from being mechanically ventilated or as a step-up from inability to manage with spontaneous breathing. NIV can be delivered via nasal cannula, masks, or hood. The oxygen delivery route impacts the patient's ability to consume oral intake. Anything that covers the patient's mouth reduces their ability to eat and drink regardless of the presence or severity of dysphagia. The pressures and flows delivered differ depending on the method of NIV (eg, high-flow nasal cannula, Bi-Level positive air pressure); however, these are generally lower than pressures and flows from modes of invasive mechanical ventilation. Data show that NIV can affect the swallow.[57–59] Advantages of NIV have been demonstrated, including the positive impact of the humidity of high-flow on secretions[60] and increases in laryngeal vestibular closure duration without impact on airway invasion with increasing airflow. However, the impact of high-flow nasal oxygen delivery on swallowing remains unclear, with contrasting findings in studies mostly conducted on healthy volunteers, and requires further investigation, especially in patient populations.[61]

Assessment of Swallowing

Accurate assessment of swallowing is key to establishing dysphagia pathophysiology and intervention pathways. Assessment approaches span across screening, noninstrumental (eg, clinical swallow evaluation [CSE]) and instrumental modalities (see **Fig. 3**), each varying in their discriminative ability, validity, and reliability. Models of care for swallowing assessment vary across ICUs,[62] generally with speech-language pathologists leading overall management; however there is agreed consensus that various interprofessional team members should be trained in swallow screening.[63] Central to the assessment process is the patient. Critical care communication disability can impact patients' ability to comprehensively report symptoms and participate in care decisions. Restoring effective patient–provider communication is pivotal to optimizing assessment and outcomes.[64]

Internationally, most clinicians agree that assessment of swallowing post-extubation should be the standard practice; however, a gap remains between ideal agreed practice and reality.[65,66] This gap is driven by a variety of factors including lack of consensus on a singular assessment tool, lack of protocols, the need for both noninstrumental and instrumental assessment across critically ill populations and resource limitations.[22,65,67]

Swallow screening

The primary goal of swallow screening is to determine patient risk. Risk is categorized across (1) commencement of oral intake, and (2) need for further detailed assessment. Swallow screening is quick and can be conducted by different health professionals.[68] Since 2018, there has been an increase in establishing valid and reliable screening tools and algorithms specific to critical care.

Four tools have been validated for the ICU population: (1) Post-extubation Dysphagia Screening tool,[69] (2) Yale Swallow Protocol,[70] (3) GUSS-ICU,[71] (4) and the Modified Volume-Viscosity Test (mV-VST).[72] Dysphagia algorithms including the Bernese ICU dysphagia[67] and Moss algorithm[73] also offer structured systems for swallow screening.

Whilst screening tools offer an initial evaluation of dysphagia risk, use of screening tools in isolation are inadequate for accurate diagnostic assessment of swallowing physiology.[63]

Clinical swallow evaluation and adjunct assessment

CSE commonly comprises of medical history, current medical status, oromotor exam, and trial of fluids and food.[74] Beyond screening, CSEs are conducted by SLPs as the initial mode of swallowing assessment, informing management decisions including need for instrumental assessment. Variability exists in the sensitivity and specificity of CSEs to detect aspiration across bolus consistencies; with CSE yielding a higher sensitivity and lower specificity when compared to swallow screening.[75] Additional adjunct assessments such as cervical auscultation can be used by trained healthcare professionals.[76]

Instrumental swallowing assessment

Instrumental assessments are considered reference standards for swallow assessment and include videofluorosocopy, endoscopy, scintigraphy, and manometry. Each offers complementary diagnostic information on swallowing anatomy and physiology. Flexible Endoscopic Evaluation of Swallowing (FEES) is commonly used for critically ill patients due to its portability, repeatability, and applicability across dysphagia assessment and evaluation of intervention[62,67,77] but may not be easily accessible.[78] Briefly, FEES involves passing a small flexible scope transnasally to the pharynx. Anatomic and physiologic assessment of the nasopharynx, oropharynx and laryngopharynx are conducted, followed by oral trials. Accuracy in the detection of safety (eg, aspiration) and efficiency (eg, residue) of the swallow and the subsequent efficacy of intervention for a patient is higher when compared to both CSE and swallow screening, and fluoroscopy.[79] Use of FEES can lead to improved safety outcomes for patients following endotracheal extubation and tracheostomy insertion.[80]

Dysphagia Management

Recovery of dysphagia in patients with critical illness can be lengthy and expensive. Following mechanical ventilation, patients diagnosed with dysphagia compared to those without had a 93% increased median cost.[10] It is advantageous to establish the presence of dysphagia in a timely manner postextubation. Costs are associated with increased ICU length of stay,[10] higher rates of reintubation, pneumonia, and feeding tube placement.[11,81]

Current dysphagia treatment practices are largely compensatory or behavioral,[24,82] with little evidence to guide interventions that include active dysphagia rehabilitation[35] and equally consider sensory dysfunction.[83] Systematic reviews of swallowing interventions in ICU report nil significant impact on time to return to oral intake, aspiration following treatment, or swallowing related quality of life; however, they do cite reduced rates of pneumonia.[36,84]

Minimising atrophy and improving strength in ICU is the core focus of many physical allied health treatments (see **Fig. 3**). This is achieved through early active and passive range of movement, early mobilization, and other techniques such as neuromuscular electrical stimulation.[85,86] Such strategies may be applied generally in many contexts for patients intubated with mechanical ventilation; however, most are unsuitable for swallowing because of the presence of an ETT within the oropharynx and larynx. Doing so may further injure swallowing structures. Consequently, the patient needs to be extubated or tracheotomised to enable active swallowing rehabilitation. The exception is pharyngeal electrical stimulation (PES), which provides sensory stimulation to the oropharynx, targeting sensory nerves and exciting the motor cortex toward reorganization of damaged pathways using principles of neuroplasticity. Emerging data suggest that the use of PES results in the reduction of extubation failure and dysphagia severity for acute stroke patients at high dysphagia risk.[87] Other dysphagia treatments proposed but not specifically tested in the critically ill population are repetitive transcranial magnetic stimulation (rTMS), transcranial direct current stimulation (tDCS) and neuromuscular electrical stimulation (NMES). Whilst these techniques may be beneficial, the underlying mechanism for each of these treatments on how they improve swallowing ability is not well understood; they are not widely available for use nor are they proven to be of benefit in critical illness.[88]

Many critically ill patients may experience ICU-acquired weakness (ICUAW), a severe complication caused by neuromuscular disorders, namely critical illness, myopathy, and critical illness polyneuropathy. The predominant feature is profound neuromuscular weakness and may involve either or both the proximal or distal musculature. The application of a multimodal rehabilitation program can facilitate expeditious weaning from the ventilator and improved functional status.[89] Thus, rehabilitation programs should be multimodal, with the primary focus to improve muscular strength and cardiopulmonary endurance, as key principles for success.

It is reasonable to suggest with oropharyngeal weakness that a multimodal strength-based rehabilitation training program may be beneficial to facilitate faster transition to oral intake and resolution of dysphagia. Although some swallowing and nonswallowing techniques are potentially beneficial,[24,36,90] the evidence specifically in the ICU or with ICUAW is limited. Active swallowing exercises proposed specifically for this clinical population have included volitional swallowing, effortful swallow, tongue hold maneuver,[90] and Mendelsohn maneuver.[24] These studies indicate that swallowing does improve with treatment; however, each exercise has not been specifically tested in isolation or as part of a program for the patient with ICUAW. To date, active swallowing exercises in the patient with ICUAW have been purely suggested as potentially beneficial[24] and/or have been recommended in concordance with results on FEES.[90]

Given sensory dysfunction is also common with dysphagia[83]; interventions that aim to restore sensation have shown positive effects on swallow function. Specific to patients with tracheostomy, return of laryngeal airflow and/or restoration of laryngopharyngeal pressures can mitigate aspiration.[91,92] Optimizing sensation is hypothesised to result in improving the motor response; however, future research is needed to determine exact associations.

A strong evidence base exists for the application of inspiratory muscle strength training in the critical care environment, with emerging evidence for expiratory muscle strength training (EMST).[93] EMST uses a device designed to strengthen expiratory musculature against a physiologic load. Its proposed mechanism of action in swallowing rehabilitation is that forceful expiration engages the supralaryngeal musculature (muscles necessary for enabling hyolaryngeal excursion), facilitating epiglottic deflection to allow airway closure, which is a key component to successful swallowing. Further to this, EMST has also been described as having a positive impact on expiratory force-generating capacity; this translates to improved voice and cough strength, the latter critical to airway protection and airway clearance in the critically ill or dysphagic individual.[93] A published case series with 2 critically ill patients showed positive results with improved swallowing and respiratory function with no reported adverse events.[94] Results from a recent pilot study conducted in Australia (n = 13), support the safety and feasibility of EMST after prolonged invasive ventilation and demonstrate positive respiratory and swallowing outcomes, although nutritional requirements increase as indicated by indirect calorimetry data.[95]

Future Directions for Research/Clinical Implementation

The detrimental impact of ICU-acquired dysphagia is apparent. Focused research efforts using rigorous systematic methods need to investigate the nature of dysphagia across the critical care continuum, enabling further insights into the neural, anatomic, and physiologic swallowing mechanisms. This is essential to inform effective person-centered interventions.

Other future directions include identifying the optimal timing, intensity, dosage, and frequency of swallowing rehabilitation programs. This should be considered with active engagement with patients and families in codesigned research. Most literature to date has focused on dysphagia post-extubation but needs to extend to all critically ill populations. A focused lens on the prevalence, targeted rehabilitation and/or maintenance needs of patients requiring noninvasive ventilation and high-flow oxygen therapy is also needed. Importantly, the translation of existing knowledge and best available evidence on swallow screening and use of instrumental swallowing evaluations should be implemented in routine clinical practice. Emerging assessment and therapeutic interventions such as the use of ultrasound[96] and PES[97] should advance with research methodology and translation into critical care practice.

SUMMARY

Dysphagia can occur as a consequence of critical illness and critical care treatments. The etiology is multifactorial and requires early identification and treatment to ameliorate significant impacts on patient morbidity and mortality. Accurate diagnoses spanning the stages of the swallowing mechanism that include both sensory and motor function are key to establishing evidence-based multimodal management plans to optimize function and nutritional outcomes.

CLINICS CARE POINTS

- Dysphagia can involve impairments in sensory and/or motor function across one or multiple phases of the swallow (including the oral, pharyngeal, or esophageal phases). This can impact the safety and/or efficiency of the swallowing process, with consequences to nutrition, quality of life, morbidity, and mortality.
- The etiology of dysphagia for adults with critical illness is multifactorial. Use and duration of artificial airways and other ventilation therapies has been linked to an increased prevalence of dysphagia.
- A proactive approach to identifying dysphagia is recommended. This framework may involve at a minimum, swallowing screening and further referral for instrumental assessment of swallow function and nutritional intake.
- Access to early multifaceted rehabilitation of swallow function should be enabled for critically ill adults to mitigate further nutrition deficits and morbidity, to optimize swallow recovery, and to enhance health-related quality of life.

DISCLOSURES

Nicola Clayton is a consultant and speaker for Main Medical, Sydney Australia. The other authors have no disclosures to report.

REFERENCES

1. Ridley EJ, Chapple LS, Ainscough K, et al. Nutrition care processes across hospitalisation in critically ill patients with COVID-19 in Australia: a multicentre prospective observational study. Aust Crit Care 2023;36(6):955–60.
2. Ridley EJ, Parke RL, Davies AR, et al. What happens to nutrition intake in the post-intensive care unit hospitalization period? An observational cohort study in critically ill adults. JPEN - J Parenter Enter Nutr 2019;43(1):88–95.
3. Humbert IA, German RZ. New directions for understanding neural control in swallowing: the potential and promise of motor learning. Dysphagia 2013;28(1):1–10.
4. Matsuo K, Palmer JB. Anatomy and physiology of feeding and swallowing: normal and abnormal. Phys Med Rehabil Clin 2008;19(4):691–707.
5. Brodsky MB, Nollet JL, Spronk PE, et al. Prevalence, pathophysiology, diagnostic modalities, and treatment options for dysphagia in critically ill patients. Am J Phys Med Rehabil 2020;99(12):1164–70.
6. Zuercher P, Moser M, Waskowski J, et al. Dysphagia post-extubation affects long-term mortality in mixed adult ICU patients-data from a large prospective

observational study with systematic dysphagia screening. Crit Care Explor 2022; 4(6):e0714.

7. Barker J, Martino R, Reichardt B, et al. Incidence and impact of dysphagia in patients receiving prolonged endotracheal intubation after cardiac surgery. Research Support, Non-U.S. Gov't. Can J Surg 2009;52(2):119–24.

8. Mirzakhani H, Williams J-N, Mello J, et al. Muscle weakness predicts pharyngeal dysfunction and symptomatic aspiration in long-term ventilated patients. Anesthesiology 2013;119(2):389–97.

9. Daly E, Miles A, Scott S, et al. Finding the red flags: swallowing difficulties after cardiac surgery in patients with prolonged intubation. J Crit Care 2016;31(1): 119–24.

10. McIntyre ML, Chimunda T, Murray J, et al. The prevalence of post-extubation dysphagia in critically ill adults: an Australian data linkage study. Crit Care Resusc 2022;24(4):352–9.

11. Macht M, Wimbish T, Clark BJ, et al. Postextubation dysphagia is persistent and associated with poor outcomes in survivors of critical illness. Crit Care 2011; 15(5):R231.

12. World Health Organization. ICF: international classification of functioning, disability and health. 2001.

13. Mulheren RW, Humbert IA. The effect of swallowing cues in healthy individuals: an exploratory study. Dysphagia 2023;38(1):260–7.

14. Hopkins-Rossabi T, Curtis P, Temenak M, et al. Respiratory phase and lung volume patterns during swallowing in healthy adults: a systematic review and meta-analysis. J Speech Lang Hear Res 2019;62(4):868–82.

15. Ekberg O, Hamdy S, Woisard V, et al. Social and psychological burden of dysphagia: its impact on diagnosis and treatment. Dysphagia. Spring 2002; 17(2):139–46.

16. Brodsky MB, Levy MJ, Erin J, et al. Laryngeal injury and upper airway symptoms after oral endotracheal intubation with mechanical ventilation during critical care: a systematic review. Crit Care Med 2018;46(12):2010–7.

17. Brodsky MB, Akst LM, Jedlanek E, et al. Laryngeal injury and upper airway symptoms after endotracheal intubation during surgery: a systematic review and meta-analysis. Anesth Analg 2021;132(4):1023–32.

18. McIntyre M, Doeltgen S, Dalton N, et al. Post-extubation dysphagia incidence in critically ill patients: a systematic review and meta-analysis. Aust Crit Care 2021; 34(1):67–75.

19. Skoretz SA, Flowers HL, Martino R. The incidence of dysphagia following endotracheal intubation: a systematic review. Chest 2010;137(3):665–73.

20. Schefold JC, Berger D, Zurcher P, et al. Dysphagia in mechanically ventilated ICU patients (DYnAMICS): a prospective observational trial. Crit Care Med 2017;45(12):2061–9.

21. Plowman EK, Anderson A, York JD, et al. Dysphagia after cardiac surgery: prevalence, risk factors, and associated outcomes. J Thorac Cardiovasc Surg 2023; 165(2):737–746 e3.

22. Freeman-Sanderson A, Hemsley B, Thompson K, et al. Dysphagia in adult intensive care patients: results of a prospective, multicentre binational point prevalence study. Aust Crit Care 2023;36(6):961–6.

23. Macht M, Wimbish T, Bodine C, et al. ICU-acquired swallowing disorders. Crit Care Med 2013;41(10):2396–405.

24. Zuercher P, Moret CS, Dziewas R, et al. Dysphagia in the intensive care unit: epidemiology, mechanisms, and clinical management. Crit Care 2019;23(1):103.

25. El Solh A, Okada M, Bhat A, et al. Swallowing disorders post orotracheal intubation in the elderly. Intensive Care Med 2003;29(9):1451–5.
26. Zielske J, Bohne S, Brunkhorst FM, et al. Acute and long-term dysphagia in critically ill patients with severe sepsis: results of a prospective controlled observational study. Eur Arch Oto-Rhino-Laryngol 2014;271(11):3085–93.
27. Krisciunas GP, Langmore SE, Gomez-Taborda S, et al. The association between endotracheal tube size and aspiration (during flexible endoscopic evaluation of swallowing) in acute respiratory failure survivors. Crit Care Med 2020;48(11):1604–11.
28. Singer P, Blaser AR, Berger MM, et al. ESPEN guideline on clinical nutrition in the intensive care unit. Clinical nutrition (Edinburgh, Scotland) 2019;38(1):48–79.
29. Skoretz SA, Riopelle SJ, Wellman L, et al. Investigating swallowing and tracheostomy following critical illness: a scoping review. Crit Care Med 2020;48(2):e141–51.
30. Naithani S, Whelan K, Thomas JE, et al. Multiple morbidity is associated with increased problems of food access in hospital: a cross-sectional survey utilising the Cumulative Illness Rating Scale. J Hum Nutr Diet 2010;23(6):575–82.
31. Schefold JC, Wollersheim T, Grunow JJ, et al. Muscular weakness and muscle wasting in the critically ill. J Cachexia Sarcopenia Muscle 2020;11(6):1399–412.
32. Cheng H, Song S, Tang Y, et al. Does ICU admission dysphagia independently contribute to delirium risk in ischemic stroke patients? Results from a cohort study. BMC Psychiatr 2024;24(1):65.
33. Matsumoto A, Yoshimura Y, Nagano F, et al. Polypharmacy and its association with dysphagia and malnutrition among stroke patients with sarcopenia. Nutrients 2022;14(20). https://doi.org/10.3390/nu14204251.
34. Angus DC, Carlet J, Brussels Roundtable P. Surviving intensive care: a report from the 2002 Brussels Roundtable. Intensive Care Med 2003;29(3):368–77.
35. Chen L, Liu C, Yuan M, et al. Interventions for postextubation dysphagia in critically ill patients: a systematic review and meta-analysis. Dysphagia 2024. https://doi.org/10.1007/s00455-024-10695-1.
36. Duncan S, McAuley DF, Walshe M, et al. Interventions for oropharyngeal dysphagia in acute and critical care: a systematic review and meta-analysis. Intensive Care Med 2020;46(7):1326–38.
37. Ajemian MS, Nirmul GB, Anderson MT, et al. Routine fiberoptic endoscopic evaluation of swallowing following prolonged intubation - implications for management. Arch Surg 2001;136(4):434–7.
38. Leder SB, Cohn SM, Moller BA. Fiberoptic endoscopic documentation of the high incidence of aspiration following extubation in critically ill trauma patients. Dysphagia. Fall 1998;13(4):208–12.
39. Langmore SE, Krisciunas GP, Warner H, et al. Correction to: abnormalities of aspiration and swallowing function in survivors of acute respiratory failure. Dysphagia 2021;36(5):842–53.
40. Brodsky MB, Huang M, Shanholtz C, et al. Recovery from dysphagia symptoms after oral endotracheal intubation in acute respiratory distress syndrome survivors. A 5-year longitudinal study. Ann Am Thorac Soc 2017;14(3):376–83.
41. Dawson C, Clunie G, Evison F, et al. Prevalence of swallow, communication, voice and cognitive compromise following hospitalisation for COVID-19: the PHOSP-COVID analysis. BMJ Open Respir Res 2023;10(1):e001647.
42. Macht M, King CJ, Wimbish T, et al. Post-extubation dysphagia is associated with longer hospitalization in survivors of critical illness with neurologic impairment. Crit Care 2013;17(3):R119.

43. Dubin R, Veith JM, Grippi MA, et al. Functional outcomes, goals, and goal attainment amongst chronically critically ill long-term acute care hospital patients. Ann Am Thorac Soc 2021. https://doi.org/10.1513/AnnalsATS.202011-1412OC.

44. Pagnamenta E, Longhurst L, Breaks A, et al. Research priorities to improve the health of children and adults with dysphagia: a National Institute of Health Research and Royal College of Speech and Language Therapists research priority setting partnership. BMJ Open 2022;12(1):e049459.

45. Hardemark Cedborg AI, Sundman E, Boden K, et al. Effects of morphine and midazolam on pharyngeal function, airway protection, and coordination of breathing and swallowing in healthy adults. Anesthesiology 2015;122(6):1253–67.

46. Borders JC, Fink D, Levitt JE, et al. Relationship between laryngeal sensation, length of intubation, and aspiration in patients with acute respiratory failure. Dysphagia 2019;34(4):521–8.

47. Brodsky MB, Friedman LA, Colantuoni E, et al. Instrument adaptation and preliminary validation study of the Laryngeal Hypersensitivity Questionnaire used for assessment of laryngeal symptoms in patients with artificial airways. Aust Crit Care 2023. https://doi.org/10.1016/j.aucc.2023.09.005.

48. Brodsky M, De I, Chilukuri K, et al. Coordination of pharyngeal and laryngeal swallowing events during single liquid swallows after oral endotracheal intubation for patients with acute respiratory distress syndrome. Dysphagia 2018;33(6):768–77.

49. Eibling DE, Gross RD. Subglottic air pressure: a key component of swallowing efficiency. Review. Ann Otol Rhinol Laryngol 1996;105(4):253–8.

50. Gross RD, Mahlmann J, Grayhack JP. Physiologic effects of open and closed tracheostomy tubes on the pharyngeal swallow. Ann Otol Rhinol Laryngol 2003;112(2):143–52.

51. Goff D, Patterson J. Eating and drinking with an inflated tracheostomy cuff: a systematic review of the aspiration risk. Int J Lang Commun Disord 2019;54(1):30–40.

52. Shaker R, Milbrath M, Ren J, et al. Deglutitive aspiration in patients with tracheostomy: effect of tracheostomy on the duration of vocal cord closure. Research Support, U.S. Gov't, Non-P.H.S.Research Support, U.S. Gov't, P.H.S. Gastroenterology 1995;108(5):1357–60.

53. Wallace S, McGowan S, Sutt AL. Benefits and options for voice restoration in mechanically ventilated intensive care unit patients with a tracheostomy. J Intensive Care Soc 2023;24(1):104–11.

54. Sutt A-L, Wallace S, Egbers P. Upper airway assessment for one-way valve use in a patient with a tracheostomy. Am J Speech Lang Pathol 2021;30(6):2716–7.

55. Kang J, Choi K, Yun G, et al. Does removal of tracheostomy affect dysphagia? A kinematic analysis. Dysphagia 2012;27(4):498–503.

56. Galli J, Marchese MR, Di Cesare T, et al. Impact of tracheal tube on swallowing in post-operative head and neck cancer patients: scintigraphic analysis. Dysphagia 2021;36(6):953–8.

57. Vergara J, Brenner MJ, Skoretz SA, et al. Swallowing during provision of helmet ventilation: review and provisional multidisciplinary guidance. J Intensive Care Soc 2024. 17511437241231704.

58. Rattanajiajaroen P, Kongpolprom N. Effects of high flow nasal cannula on the coordination between swallowing and breathing in postextubation patients, a randomized crossover study. Crit Care 2021;25(1):365.

59. Graf AE, Mehl A, De Costa A, et al. Assessment of swallowing function in healthy adults while using high-flow nasal cannula. Otolaryngol Head Neck Surg 2024; 170(5):1372–9.

60. Coghlan K, Skoretz SA. Breathing and swallowing with high flow oxygen therapy. Perspect ASHA Spec Interest Groups 2017;2(13):74–81.

61. Gutierrez-Arias R, Salgado-Maldonado G, Valdivia PL, et al. Assessing swallowing disorders in adults on high-flow nasal cannula in critical and non-critical care settings. A scoping review protocol. PLoS One 2023;18(10):e0291803.

62. Spronk PE, Spronk LEJ, Egerod I, et al. Dysphagia in intensive care evaluation (DICE): an international cross-sectional survey. Dysphagia 2022;37(6):1451–60.

63. Likar R, Aroyo I, Bangert K, et al. Management of swallowing disorders in ICU patients - a multinational expert opinion. J Crit Care 2024;79:154447.

64. Freeman-Sanderson AL, Togher L, Elkins M, et al. Quality of life improves for tracheostomy patients with return of voice: a mixed methods evaluation of the patient experience across the care continuum. Intensive Crit Care Nurs 2018; 46:10–6.

65. Nielsen AH, Kaldan G, Gade LM, et al. Postextubation dysphagia management in Danish intensive care units: a national survey. Acta Anaesthesiol Scand 2024. https://doi.org/10.1111/aas.14438.

66. Spronk PE, Spronk LEJ, Egerod I, et al. Dysphagia in intensive care evaluation (DICE): an international cross-sectional survey. Dysphagia 2022. https://doi.org/10.1007/s00455-021-10389-y.

67. Zuercher P, Dziewas R, Schefold JC. Dysphagia in the intensive care unit: a (multidisciplinary) call to action. Intensive Care Med 2020;46(3):554–6.

68. Perren A, Zurcher P, Schefold JC. Clinical approaches to assess post-extubation dysphagia (PED) in the critically ill. Dysphagia 2019;34(4):475–86.

69. Johnson KL, Speirs L, Mitchell A, et al. Validation of a postextubation dysphagia screening tool for patients after prolonged endotracheal intubation. Am J Crit Care 2018;27(2):89–96.

70. Leder SB, Warner HL, Suiter DM, et al. Evaluation of swallow function post-extubation: is it necessary to wait 24 hours? Ann Otol Rhinol Laryngol 2019; 128(7):619–24.

71. Troll C, Trapl-Grundschober M, Teuschl Y, et al. A bedside swallowing screen for the identification of post-extubation dysphagia on the intensive care unit - validation of the Gugging Swallowing Screen (GUSS)-ICU. BMC Anesthesiol 2023; 23(1):122.

72. Martinez de Lagran Zurbano I, Laguna LB, Soria CV, et al. Utility of the modified Volume-Viscosity Swallow Test for bedside screening of dysphagia in critically ill patients. Clin Nutr ESPEN 2023;53:214–23.

73. Moss M, White SD, Warner H, et al. Development of an accurate bedside swallowing evaluation decision tree algorithm for detecting aspiration in acute respiratory failure survivors. Chest 2020;158(5):1923–33.

74. Brodsky MB, Mayfield EB, Gross RD. Clinical decision making in the ICU: dysphagia screening, assessment, and treatment. Semin Speech Lang 2019; 40(3):170–87.

75. Lynch YT, Clark BJ, Macht M, et al. The accuracy of the bedside swallowing evaluation for detecting aspiration in survivors of acute respiratory failure. J Crit Care 2017;39:143–8.

76. Jaghbeer M, Sutt AL, Bergstrom L. Dysphagia management and cervical auscultation: reliability and validity against FEES. Dysphagia 2023;38(1):305–14.

77. Dziewas R, Warnecke T, Labeit B, et al. Systematic approach to contextualize findings of flexible endoscopic evaluation of swallowing in neurogenic dysphagia– towards an integrated FEES report. Neurol Res Pract 2024;6(1):26.

78. Macht M, Wimbish T, Clark BJ, et al. Diagnosis and treatment of post-extubation dysphagia: results from a national survey. J Crit Care 2012;27(6):578–86.

79. Giraldo-Cadavid LF, Leal-Leano LR, Leon-Basantes GA, et al. Accuracy of endoscopic and videofluoroscopic evaluations of swallowing for oropharyngeal dysphagia. Laryngoscope 2017;127(9):2002–10.

80. Morris K, Taylor NF, Freeman-Sanderson A. Safety-related outcomes for patients with a tracheostomy and the use of flexible endoscopic evaluation of swallowing (FEES) for assessment and management of swallowing: a systematic review. Int J Speech Lang Pathol 2024;1–11. https://doi.org/10.1080/17549507.2023.2293633.

81. Omura K, Komine A, Yanagigawa M, et al. Frequency and outcome of post-extubation dysphagia using nurse-performed swallowing screening protocol. Nurs Crit Care 2019;24(2):70–5.

82. Speyer R, Cordier R, Sutt AL, et al. Behavioural interventions in people with oropharyngeal dysphagia: a systematic review and meta-analysis of randomised clinical trials. J Clin Med 2022;11(3). https://doi.org/10.3390/jcm11030685.

83. Steele CM, Miller AJ. Sensory input pathways and mechanisms in swallowing: a review. Dysphagia 2010;25(4):323–33.

84. Kuriyama A, Watanabe S, Katayama Y, et al. Dysphagia rehabilitation in dysphagic patients with acute or critical illness: a systematic review and meta-analysis. Dysphagia 2024. https://doi.org/10.1007/s00455-024-10700-7.

85. Kress JP, Hall JB. ICU-acquired weakness and recovery from critical illness. N Engl J Med 2014;370(17):1626–35.

86. Maffiuletti NA, Roig M, Karatzanos E, et al. Neuromuscular electrical stimulation for preventing skeletal-muscle weakness and wasting in critically ill patients: a systematic review. BMC Med 2013;11(1):137.

87. Muhle P, Claus I, Labeit B, et al. Pharyngeal Electrical Stimulation prior to extubation - reduction of extubation failure rate in acute stroke patients? J Crit Care 2024;82:154808.

88. Cheng I, Hamad A, Sasegbon A, et al. Advances in the treatment of dysphagia in neurological disorders: a review of current evidence and future considerations. Neuropsychiatr Dis Treat 2022;18:2251–63.

89. Verceles AC, Wells CL, Sorkin JD, et al. A multimodal rehabilitation program for patients with ICU acquired weakness improves ventilator weaning and discharge home. J Crit Care 2018;47:204–10.

90. Ponfick M, Linden R, Nowak DA. Dysphagia–a common, transient symptom in critical illness polyneuropathy: a fiberoptic endoscopic evaluation of swallowing study. Crit Care Med 2015;43(2):365–72.

91. Marvin S, Thibeault SL. Predictors of aspiration and silent aspiration in patients with new tracheostomy. Am J Speech Lang Pathol 2021;30(6):2554–60.

92. Mills CS, Cuthbertson BH, Michou E. What's new in reducing the impact of tracheostomy on communication and swallowing in the ICU. Intensive Care Med 2023. https://doi.org/10.1007/s00134-023-07064-1.

93. Brooks M, McLaughlin E, Shields N. Expiratory muscle strength training improves swallowing and respiratory outcomes in people with dysphagia: a systematic review. Int J Speech Lang Pathol 2019;21(1):89–100.

94. Clayton NA, Ward EC, Nicholls C, et al. The addition of respiratory muscle strength training to facilitate swallow and pulmonary rehabilitation following

massive tissue loss and severe deconditioning: a case series. Aust Crit Care 2022;35(2):210–6.

95. Clayton N, Ward E, Place C, et al. Early dysphagia rehabilitation in critical care: a pilot study of feasibility, safety and effectiveness of a strength-based dysphagia treatment protocol for patients with ICU acquired weakness. Aust Crit Care 2024; 37:S20.

96. Allen JE, Clunie GM, Slinger C, et al. Utility of ultrasound in the assessment of swallowing and laryngeal function: a rapid review and critical appraisal of the literature. Int J Lang Commun Disord 2020;56(1):174–204.

97. Dziewas R, Stellato R, van der Tweel I, et al. Pharyngeal electrical stimulation for early decannulation in tracheotomised patients with neurogenic dysphagia after stroke (PHAST-TRAC): a prospective, single-blinded, randomised trial. Lancet Neurol 2018;17(10):849–59.

Critical Care Nutrition for Children – Where are we now?

Jacinta Winderlich, BNutDietet, MClinRes[a,b,c,]*,
Georgia Brown, MBBS, MD[d,e,f], Andrew A. Udy, FCICM, PhD[a,g],
Emma J. Ridley, BNutriDietet, PhD[a,h]

KEYWORDS

- Pediatric • Critical care • Nutrition • Dietitians • Nutritional support
- Enteral nutrition

KEY POINTS

- Nutrition has emerged as a key consideration in pediatric critical care management; this is reflected via increased research activity, with more recent studies focusing on early enteral nutrition, protein intake, and short- and long-term outcomes.
- There is limited high-level evidence; however, published practice guidelines provide a framework for nutrition management, incorporating expert consensus where evidence gaps remain.
- Emerging areas of research which may inform future standard practice include skeletal muscle ultrasound, bioelectrical impedance analysis, and the role of the microbiome (including pre- and pro-biotics).

INTRODUCTION

Since the establishment of the first pediatric intensive care unit (PICU) in Sweden in 1955[1] and advances in nutrition therapies including parenteral nutrition in the 1960s and 1970s,[2] the nutritional management of the critically-ill child has emerged as a key focus. As reflected by the increasing number of publications and dedicated

[a] Australian and New Zealand Intensive Care Research Centre, School of Public Health and Preventive Medicine, Monash University, Melbourne, VIC, Australia; [b] Department of Nutrition and Dietetics, Monash Children's Hospital, Melbourne, VIC, Australia; [c] Paediatric Intensive Care Unit, Monash Children's Hospital, Melbourne, VIC, Australia; [d] Paediatric Intensive Care Unit, The Royal Children's Hospital, Melbourne, VIC, Australia; [e] Murdoch Children's Research Institute, Melbourne, VIC, Australia; [f] Department of Critical Care, The University of Melbourne, Melbourne, VIC, Australia; [g] Department of Intensive Care and Hyperbaric Medicine, The Alfred, Melbourne, VIC, Australia; [h] Department of Dietetics and Nutrition, Alfred Health, Melbourne, VIC, Australia
* Corresponding author. Monash Children's Hospital, 246 Clayton Road, Clayton, VIC 3168, Australia.
E-mail address: jacinta.winderlich@monash.edu

Crit Care Clin 41 (2025) 345–361
https://doi.org/10.1016/j.ccc.2024.11.003
0749-0704/25/© 2024 Elsevier Inc. All rights reserved, including those for text and data mining, AI training, and similar technologies.
criticalcare.theclinics.com

research groups, nutrition has experienced an increased profile in pediatric critical care in recent decades.[3] Most recently, research activity has focused on early enteral nutrition (EN), protein intake, and short and long-term outcomes.

Despite this, many practice guidelines remain based on low-level evidence and expert consensus, and investigation has largely been confined to specific groups including major burns, congenital heart disease (CHD), head trauma, and bronchiolitis.[4] The relatively limited number of randomized controlled trials (RCTs) to date is potentially partially explained by the additional challenges inherent to trials of nutrition interventions when compared to, for example, drug trials.[5] Additional considerations in nutrition intervention trials include: (a) What is an ethical and meaningful control? (b) Will other aspects of the diet or nutrition provision be displaced by the intervention, and will this confound the findings? and (c) Will the baseline nutritional status of the participants affect the effectiveness of the intervention? Moreover, in the intensive care setting, nutrition research must also consider the implications of the 3 phases of critical illness, namely the acute, stable, and recovery periods.[6,7] In each phase, it is highly plausible that patient nutritional needs are very different, and the potential impact of nutrition may also vary. Pediatric studies must also take into account growth and development, including their effect on nutritional requirements and as an area potentially impacted following critical illness.

In this review, we outline key practical components of the nutritional management of critically-ill children (refer **Box 1** and **Fig. 1**) in the context of the current peer reviewed literature and identify vital knowledge gaps for further investigation.

KEY PRACTICE RESOURCES

Fundamental resources to support nutrition management in the PICU include the 2017 Society of Critical Care Medicine (SCCM)/American Society for Parenteral and Enteral Nutrition (ASPEN) guidelines and the European Society for Pediatric and Neonatal Intensive Care (ESPNIC) 2020 clinical recommendations.[8,9] The 2021 European Society for Paediatric Gastroenterology, Hepatology and Nutrition (ESPGHAN) position paper provides an overview specifically on the critically ill neonate.[10] These publications reinforce the importance of nutrition as a key element in a critically-ill child's overall care. As a reflection of the limited evidence available, a substantial proportion

---

Box 1
Recommended practical considerations for nutrition management in the pediatric intensive care unit

Strategy
- Refer to key published guidelines.[8,9]
- Establish a collaborative multidisciplinary approach to nutrition care, including the implementation of local guidelines and algorithms.
- Consider the phases of critical illness to guide appropriate nutrition prescription.[6,7]
- Commence enteral nutrition within 24 hours unless contraindicated.
- Aim for nutrition provision to initially meet resting energy expenditure (determined via indirect calorimetry or estimation via Schofield equation) and 1.5 g/kg protein.
- Gradually increase nutrition provision as tolerated and as appropriate for the phase of critical illness.
- Consider the energy to protein ratio of prescribed nutrition to ensure appropriate provision of both components.
- Avoid unnecessary gastric residual volume monitoring unless deemed at high risk of vomiting or aspiration.
- Avoid supplemental parenteral nutrition in the first week of critical illness.

Optimal Nutrition Facilitators:

Multi-disciplinary roles in nutrition care

Automatic referral to nutrition specialists

Local nutrition guidelines

Enteral feeding algorithms

Nutrition champions

Nutrition quality initiatives

Barriers to Optimal Nutrition:

Lack of local guidelines and protocols

Culture where nutrition is not a priority

Team lacking nutrition knowledge

Limited nutrition specialist resources

Prolonged unnecessary fasting

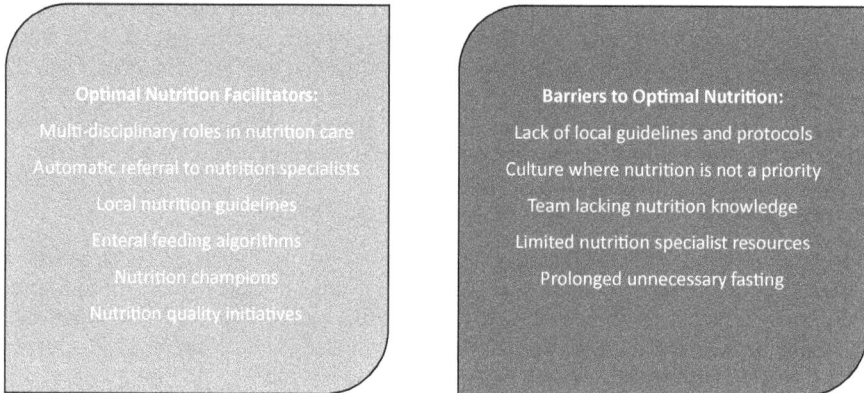

Fig. 1. Enablers and barriers to optimal nutrition provision in the pediatric intensive care unit (PICU).

of these documents are based upon observational data and expert consensus. Nonetheless, when combined with clinical judgment, reference to these guides ensures that an individualized nutrition assessment and intervention plan has considered the available evidence and expert consensus. Checklists outlining practical strategies for PICU medical, nursing, and dietetics staff have been published to facilitate implementation of these guidelines.[11] The evolution of the ASPEN guidelines since their initial edition in 2009 signals the increase in pediatric critical care nutrition research and body of evidence. Ongoing expansion of the evidence base is anticipated to be reflected in the updated version of the SCCM/ASPEN guidelines, currently under review.[12]

ROLE OF THE MULTIDISCIPLINARY TEAM IN NUTRITION CARE

All members of the PICU multidisciplinary team can influence a child's nutrition by optimizing opportunities for adequate provision and minimizing instances where delivery is reduced or delayed. The medical team advise on early EN and minimize fasting; nursing staff identify opportunities to fine tune an EN regimen and facilitate oral intake; dietitians undertake a comprehensive nutrition assessment and devise a tailored nutrition prescription; pharmacists optimize oral and enteral medication delivery and contribute to parenteral nutrition prescription; speech pathologists undertake a swallow assessment and advise on modified oral diet and fluids; and the occupational therapist ensures optimal positioning for safe and comfortable oral intake. Additional services including child life, art, and music therapy may also indirectly inform nutrition care for those alert and capable of some oral intake via their overall supportive interventions.

Research is increasingly demonstrating the benefits of such collaborative nutrition care in the critical care setting. Multidisciplinary nutrition management models have been shown to improve nutritional indices and reduce intensive care unit (ICU) length-of-stay when compared to a traditional management model, and improve nutrition provision in a trauma ICU.[13,14] In a low resource PICU, an EN protocol developed and implemented by a multidisciplinary nutrition support team has been demonstrated to lead to improved energy and protein delivery, and less time to commencement and interruptions.[15]

Although the role can vary between locations, dietitians are well-equipped to provide specialized nutrition expertise and lead nutrition service development. Data are lacking though to define current dietetics resources and guide ideal staffing. A study conducted by our group across Australia and New Zealand found a median 0.03 (inter-quartile range [IQR] 0.02, 0.04) dietetics full time equivalent (FTE) per funded bed.[16] A recent survey in the United Kingdom (UK) and Ireland identified that children in PICUs well-resourced with dietetics FTE were more likely to be reviewed by a dietitian without a referral, which may translate into improved nutrition outcomes.[17]

NUTRITION SCREENING AND DIAGNOSIS OF MALNUTRITION

Nutrition screening tools (NSTs) identify malnourished individuals or those at risk of malnutrition. Identification allows for early nutrition intervention and prioritization where resources are limited in order to direct further assessment to those most likely to benefit. To date there are no validated NSTs established in the pediatric critical care setting. A 2022 systematic review assessed inpatient pediatric NSTs against criteria deemed to be essential for critically-ill children; these included clinical, nutritional status, laboratory, and dietary intake variables.[18] The authors concluded that none of the 19 included studies were suitable for the pediatric critical care setting, and that a new NST should be developed for this population, which was predictive of meaningful outcomes including nutritional status deterioration and PICU length-of-stay.

Nutrition assessment is recommended on admission to the PICU to diagnose malnutrition and other nutrition-related issues, and allow for the implementation of an individualized nutrition intervention plan.[8,9] As in all clinical areas, nutrition assessment in critically-ill children must encompass current nutritional status, dietary intake, clinical factors, and a nutrition-focused physical examination. In the absence of a biomarker or validated 'nutrition score', nutritional status in the PICU is generally defined by anthropometric z-scores. Weight, height or length, and body mass index z-scores for age can be categorized and also allow for determining change over time. Anthropometric measures must, however, be interpreted with caution given potential issues associated with measurement error and fluid status, both of which are arguably more likely in the critical care setting.

ENERGY AND PROTEIN

Energy and protein provision during critical illness is intended to meet basal metabolic requirements and support recovery whilst avoiding the complications associated with excess delivery. 'Adequate' energy and protein intake have been associated with decreased mortality and morbidity. However, measurement of energy and protein balance is challenging, and the evidence to support current definitions of 'adequate' energy and protein provision is limited. This is in the context of the heterogeneous PICU population and factors impacting upon requirements including age, pre-existing nutritional status, clinical condition, management and interventions, and phase of illness. The 3 phases of the acute stress response provide an important framework to guide appropriate nutrition support; acute, stable, and recovery.[6,7] Care must be taken during the acute phase where the risk of overfeeding is highest.

Energy Requirements

Energy requirements may vary significantly over the course of critical illness. Indirect calorimetry (IC) is therefore recommended to measure resting energy expenditure. However, this is not possible if a unit does not possess the equipment and technical expertise. Guidelines have been published to aid clinicians in the acquisition and implementation of IC.[19] Additionally, some children may not be eligible for IC due to a range of factors including chest drain tube leaks or requirement for extracorporeal membrane oxygenation (ECMO).[20] In the absence of IC, the Schofield equation is recommended to estimate resting energy expenditure.[21] Expert consensus states that this should not be exceeded in the acute phase, to avoid the risk of overfeeding and resulting hyperglycaemia and difficulties weaning respiratory support.[22]

In practice, as clearly outlined by Joosten and colleagues, nutrition provision should aim to meet resting energy expenditure (as determined by IC or estimated via the Schofield equation) and then be gradually increased as tolerated.[6] During the recovery phase, at least twice the resting energy expenditure is generally required to support rehabilitation and achieve catch-up weight gain.[7] The nutrition prescription should be adjusted according to ongoing reviews of tolerance and anthropometric measurement trends.

Protein Requirements

Two systematic reviews have investigated protein intake in critically-ill children and found that a minimum intake of 1.5 g/kg/day was associated with a positive protein balance and lower mortality.[23,24] It should be noted that ASPEN 2017 guidelines advise that the optimal dose may be higher in critically ill infants and young children, whilst the ESPNIC 2020 guideline acknowledges that there is currently insufficient evidence to support the provision of additional protein during the acute phase of illness.[8,9] Studies exploring protein adequacy using longitudinal measurements of total urinary nitrogen are lacking. A systematic review by a European and UK author group plans to explore the effectiveness of high versus low enteral protein intake on clinical outcomes in critically ill children, whilst importantly considering energy intake.[25]

Once again, as per the published international recommendations[8,9] and well-defined guidance of Joosten and colleagues,[6,7] in practice nutrition prescriptions should aim to provide a minimum of 1.5 g/kg in the acute phase. This should then be gradually increased as tolerated up toward 3 g/kg by the stage of recovery. Attention should be paid to the energy to protein ratio of prescribed nutrition to ensure appropriate provision of both components.

ORAL NUTRITION

There is logically a focus of PICU nutrition practice guidelines and research on enteral and parenteral nutrition provision given the requirement of many critically-ill children to receive artificial nutrition provision; however, a proportion remain capable of managing oral intake. This group requires practical consideration in PICU food service operations and daily routines in the unit to support and facilitate eating and drinking, in addition to the clinical and academic considerations of nutrition provision from oral consumption. Facilitation of oral intake can reduce reliance on artificial nutrition interventions, which are associated with increased risk of complications and costs. Perhaps most important overall, is acknowledging that eating and drinking can provide children in the PICU a sense of comfort, normality, and enjoyment.

Breastfeeding and Expressing

Human milk should be provided where available given the multitude of benefits, with support of immune function particularly important for critically-ill infants.[26] Human milk has also been established as beneficial for infants at increased risk of necrotising enterocolitis, meaning that donor milk should also be considered where the option is available.

In a 2023 UK qualitative study of sick breastfed children in hospital, mothers described breastfeeding as emotionally and immunologically meaningful; however, challenges to doing so included gaps in staff knowledge and clinical environments not conducive to breastfeeding or expressing.[27] A systematic review by the same group exploring challenges of medically complex breastfed children identified key themes including practical and psychological challenges in the hospital setting, lack of specialist breastfeeding support and equipment, and complications of the child's condition making breastfeeding difficult.[28] In order to support breastfeeding and expressing mothers, units should review their processes and resources in order to identify areas for improvement.

ENTERAL NUTRITION
When to Provide Enteral Nutrition?

EN is the preferred mode of artificial nutrition support for children unable to manage oral intake due to both the effects of their critical illness and its management. Practice guidelines recommend commencement of early EN where there are nil contraindications.[8,9] Definitions vary though this generally refers to EN commenced within 24 to 48 h of PICU admission. These same guidelines advise caution in feeding those with severe burns, CHD and shock, and recommend a cautious approach and close monitoring due to the risk of necrotising enterocolitis (NEC). A recent review identified benefits associated with early EN to include attainment of energy and protein targets, increased ventilator free days, decreased length-of-stay, reduced cost, and reduced mortality.[29] However, it was highlighted that due to the data being mainly derived from observational studies with heterogenous populations, the suggestion of improved outcomes may reflect greater feasibility of providing EN to those with lower severity critical illness. When considering the timing of progression toward targets, large observational studies have demonstrated a cumulative mean energy intake of 60% to 70% up to the first 10 d in PICU to be associated with reduced mortality.[30] An improved protein intake has also been found to be associated with reduced mortality.[31]

How to Provide Enteral Nutrition?

Route
EN via the gastric route is physiologic and generally the preferred route. However, delayed gastric emptying associated with critical illness may increase the risk of feeding intolerance and aspiration, leading to a requirement for post-pyloric administration of EN. A nursing competency package for bedside post-pyloric feeding tube placement has found the practice to be safe and feasible.[32]

Method
A range of options exist for administration of EN: continuous (via pump over 24 h), cyclic (via pump over <24 h), intermittent (via pump multiple times per day over approximately 20–60 min, and bolus (via syringe or gravity drip).[33] Unless a child is reliant on post-pyloric feed delivery, which requires continuous or cyclic administration, clinicians must determine if intermittent or bolus may be preferable over continuous or cyclic for children receiving gastric feeding. The method ultimately used generally depends upon individual patient factors and local resources (including staffing ratios and equipment);[34] however, there are some limited evidence to suggest that bolus feeding improves attainment of nutrition targets. A randomized trial of 25 mechanically ventilated children comparing bolus versus continuous nasogastric feeding found that bolus feeding resulted in improved EN delivery with a comparable safety profile.[35] An RCT has also explored 24 h continuous versus intermittent feeding with an overnight fast ('ContInNuPIC'); however, further research is required to determine if there are clinically relevant benefits related to an overnight fast and to establish non-inferiority in regards to achieving calorie targets.[36]

Gastric residual volumes monitoring

A practice associated with enteral feeding that is relatively common is the monitoring of gastric residual volumes (GRVs) as a measure of feed tolerance. A comparison study has demonstrated that not undertaking routine monitoring is not associated with increased vomits, aspiration pneumonia events or necrotising enterocolitis.[37] This practice is being explored via the GASTRIC-PICU trial, which is seeking to determine non-inferiority of no routine GRV monitoring compared to at least 6 hourly GRV monitoring in terms of health and economic outcomes.[38] In the meantime, units should define and review their current local practice to ensure consistency and identify potentially unnecessary GRV monitoring in children not deemed to be at high risk of vomiting and aspiration.

What to Administer as Enteral Nutrition?

Perhaps the area of EN that has been explored least is the 'what' to provide as EN. As previously discussed, human milk should be provided where available; however, standard EN options are otherwise generally accepted to be infant formula, or age-appropriate complete enteral formulas for older children and adolescents. A study completed by our group found that expressed breast milk is provided as EN in over 50% of children aged less than 2 y admitted to PICUs in our region, and when this was fortified this was achieved with the addition of standard infant formula powder.[39]

The use of increased energy and protein density options amongst infants and young children with CHD is the group with the most evidence to date. A systematic review and meta-analysis found that 'enriched' post-operative EN improved attainment of energy and protein targets, and was associated with reduced duration of ventilation, maintenance of weight, and reduced PICU and hospital length-of-stay.[40] Our group is exploring the use of feed modification to optimize energy and protein provision via feed modification in a scoping review, which will determine the extent of evidence beyond this patient group.[41] A peptide-based energy-dense formula has been explored in a retrospective observational study[42]; it was found to be feasible, well-tolerated and suitable to meet nutrition targets; however, further trials are required to determine potential benefits and patient groups.

Enteral Nutrition Considerations for Infants with Congenital Heart Disease

Infants with CHD and duct-dependant circulations are at risk of systemic, and therefore, mesenteric hypoperfusion. Necrotising enterocolitis is much more prevalent in neonates with CHD and as a consequence, many institutions withhold enteral nutrition in the pre-operative period.[43,44] However, a recent meta-analysis determined no association between NEC and pre-operative feeding status in neonates awaiting cardiac surgery.[45] Additionally, some retrospective studies show an exclusive unfortified human milk diet was associated with a significantly lower risk of preoperative NEC, but that feed volumes greater than 100 mL/kg/day may significantly increase the risk.[46] Cautious initiation of enteral breast milk, where available, in this population may confer some immunologic and antimicrobial benefit, in addition to reducing the risk of NEC.

PARENTERAL NUTRITION

Parenteral nutrition is generally indicated when enteral nutrition is anticipated to not be possible or inadequate for an extended period of time. Following the PEPaNIC trial, guidelines now advise against the administration of supplemental parenteral nutrition (PN) in the first week of critical illness.

The PEPaNIC study explored early versus late parenteral nutrition in 1440 children.[47] PN commenced on Day 8 rather than within the first 24 h of admission was found to be associated with multiple superior outcomes including less new infections and a reduced PICU length-of-stay. It has been suggested that early administration of amino acids may provide an explanation for the potential harm.[48] Limitations have been discussed, including that PN was initiated based on a nutrition risk score potentially resulting in overuse and enteral nutrition was limited rather than advanced.[49] It appears to remain valid that PN should be commenced in those anticipated to be substantially reliant on parenteral nutrition support beyond a few days once stable, where EN will be inadequate for a prolonged period.[50]

In those that do appear suitable for PN provision, careful consideration must be given to the phase of critical illness the child is experiencing to avoid under or overfeeding. Guidelines are available to facilitate appropriate prescription of parenteral macronutrients, electrolytes and minerals, and micronutrients in the PICU setting.[51,52]

NUTRITION MANAGEMENT IN THE SETTING OF CRITICAL CARE INTERVENTIONS

The impact of clinical interventions on nutritional requirements and optimal nutrition delivery should always be considered. In the critical care setting, ECMO and renal replacement therapy (RRT) are the 2 major therapies to consider in nutrition care planning. Children requiring these advanced intensive care interventions are typically among the most unwell. This often means they experience prolonged stays in the PICU, higher rates of morbidity, and extended rehabilitation periods, all which emphasize the importance of careful nutrition management.

Extracorporeal membrane oxygenation

Metabolic changes from illness, barriers to starting nutrition therapy, and interruptions to feeding put those requiring ECMO at risk of receiving inadequate nutrition.[53] Current ECMO nutrition practice recommendations are predominantly based on observational data and expert consensus. A recent literature review identified that no RCTs have been conducted on enteral nutrition in ECMO.[54]

Determining nutritional requirements
Determining nutritional requirements during ECMO is challenging. ECMO involves the diversion of blood outside the body to a machine that oxygenates it and removes carbon dioxide before returning it to the patient. This process bypasses the patient's lungs, altering the gas exchange dynamics nutritional assessment methods rely upon. A modified IC method has been proposed, combining traditional IC via the ventilator plus calculations of oxygen consumption and carbon dioxide production derived from pre- and post-ECMO membrane blood gas analyses.[55–57] In a prospective pilot study of resting energy expenditure (REE) of children on ECMO, wide variability in metabolic demand was observed, with some patients, particularly those with septic shock, exhibiting REE levels substantially higher than aforementioned predicted values.[57] Using an alternative method, respiratory mass spectroscopy, the calculated REE of children on ECMO was similar to basal metabolic rate, contrary to traditional beliefs of hypermetabolism during critical illness with ECMO.[58] These studies show that modified assessment methods are possible but highlight the need for further validation and individualized assessment.

Nutrition delivery during extracorporeal membrane oxygenation
Despite potential concern for children receiving ECMO to develop enterocolitis and gut ischemia due to vasoactive medication and hemodynamic instability, guidelines

recommend early commencement of nutrition therapy.[9] Early enteral nutrition, defined as within 24 h, is recommended for children once stable on ECMO. A recent systematic review and meta-analysis on ECMO-treated children and adolescents receiving EN revealed heterogeneity in population and nutrition management. Despite variations, most studies suggest EN decreases mortality compared to PN. A large observational study found early EN was not associated with respiratory complications or bowel ischemia compared with delayed EN (>48 h after admission), dispelling some of the perceived barriers to initiation of feeding in this population.[59] Although patients may experience feed intolerance, it appears safe overall, emphasizing the importance of early initiation or transition to EN when clinically feasible.[60]

Targeted efforts to avoid prolonged nutritional deficits is paramount, for example, the use of nutrition protocols to target volumes, gradual increase of nutrient supply, use of concentrated formulas, avoidance of feeding interruptions, and consideration of post-pyloric feeding in patients with unavoidable interruptions, gastric feeding intolerance, or high-risk of aspiration.[61]

Acute Renal Replacement Therapy

A significant proportion of children with acute kidney injury (AKI) in the PICU are at risk of acute malnutrition, and the majority of those are likely already chronically malnourished.[62] The nutritional management of children requiring continuous RRT (CRRT) represents a complex scenario, intersecting critical illness and AKI diet therapy. In addition to the underlying pathology, nutrition prescriptions must consider medications, filter types, ultrafiltration and dialysate flow rates, effluent losses, and heat loss, all of which will vary depending on the CRRT modality. CRRT also poses challenges to IC by removing CO_2 as bicarbonate, underestimating energy needs. Additionally, citrate (used as an anticoagulant for RRT) has metabolic effects and may increase REE.[63]

Evidence is lacking in the nutrition management of children with AKI; however, clinical practice recommendations have recently been published by the Pediatric Renal Nutrition Taskforce.[64] These have been interpreted in the context of the PICU,[65] and sensibly highlight that when devising a nutrition prescription potassium is generally the primary determinant of the plan closely followed by fluid allowance. Whilst the optimal protein dose in the PICU remains unknown, further research is also required to confirm this in children with AKI. It is therefore suggested that a pragmatic starting point may be to aim for an additional 10% to 20% to account for effluent losses.

Additional important AKI nutrition management considerations flagged include a reminder of the relatively low renal solute load of human milk.[66] Increased concentration oral and enteral feeds in fluid restricted children with renal failure for improved nutrition delivery may be beneficial. However, this should be carefully balanced with the increased risk of gastrointestinal issues with these increased osmolality feeds, especially in children with short bowel syndrome or at high-risk of necrotising enterocolitis (both not uncommon in the critical care setting). In practice, a combination of feed types may provide the best composition to optimize nutritional intake without exacerbating issues related to the AKI. For example, a feeding plan comprising 50:50 expressed breast milk (EBM) or infant formula and a low potassium renal-specific formula may provide an appropriate balance of energy, protein, and electrolytes. Ultimately, the importance of multidisciplinary collaboration is emphasized in the care of a critically-ill child receiving CRRT, with the optimal management plan requiring input from the intensive care, nephrology, and nutrition support experts.

WHERE TO NEXT?

Overall, there is significant enthusiasm for PICU nutrition research, with increasing research activity, collaborations, and numerous avenues of enquiry. Collaborative studies focused on clinical interventions, treatments, and outcomes have been deemed priorities. A multidisciplinary consensus derived list of PICU nutrition research priorities was established in 2018 and includes protein intake, effects of mobilization, targeted-nutrition therapy, and development of a validated nutrition risk score.[67] Priorities of consumer stakeholders are yet to be determined. Key areas are outlined later and summarized in **Fig. 2**.

Point-of-care Ultrasonography for Skeletal Muscle Assessment

Multiple factors inherent to critical illness and its management can negatively impact upon muscle mass, and sub-optimal nutrition provision exacerbates wasting. Bedside ultrasonography has been used to assess skeletal muscle in adults and is being increasingly studied in critically-ill children due to its hypothesized association with functional outcomes.[68] A recent prospective study demonstrated that point-of-care ultrasonography of the quadriceps femoris can identify muscle atrophy in mechanically ventilated children. Increasing age, cumulative energy, and protein deficit, highest C-reactive protein value, exposure to neuromuscular blockers, and prolonged PICU admission were all predictive of greater decrease in thickness.[69] A further recent study in the UK also confirmed muscle wasting during pediatric critical illness, although nil significant associations were identified, the authors have acknowledged the limited sample size and highlighted the need for a systematic review and meta-analysis to guide future research.[70]

Potential Use of Bioelectrical Impedance for Fluid Management and Body Composition Monitoring

Bioelectrical impedance analysis (BIA) is another example of how technology may play a future role in nutrition-related management in the PICU. There is minimal evidence at present; however, a recent scoping review highlighted the emerging use of BIA in the NICU. BIA was identified to be used for fluid status evaluation and as a measure of

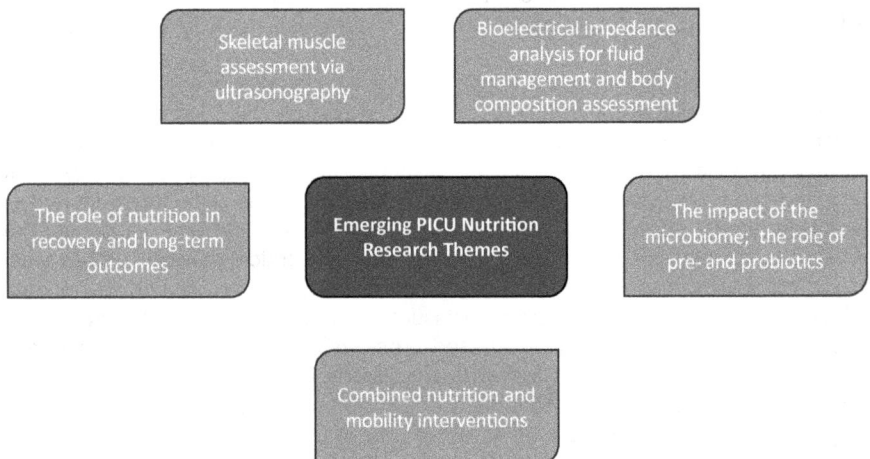

Fig. 2. Emerging areas of pediatric critical care nutrition research.

nutritional adequacy and growth in those with stable fluid balance.[71] Research is required though to establish BIA for these purposes in the pediatric critical care setting.

Combined Mobility and Nutrition Therapies

Given the bi-directional relationship of nutrition and physical function, it would be futile to optimize 1 aspect of care without the other. It is therefore only logical for nutrition and mobility to be researched collectively. A pilot feasibility RCT ('PROXIMUS') is currently underway in the United States (US), exploring high protein intake combined with individualized versus standard management during the acute phase in the PICU.[72] The investigators aim to determine preservation of muscle mass and functional status at 1- and 6-mo post-randomization. Following in the footsteps of adult colleagues, this is likely to be one of the first of many studies exploring the synergistic effect of these 2 areas of intervention.

The Microbiome and Use of Pre- and Probiotics

The gut microbiome is essential to the functioning of the gastrointestinal tract. Many aspects of pediatric critical care, including medications and fasting, interrupt the microbiome;[73,74] however, nutrition is a modifiable factor. It is anticipated that future research will identify associations between the gut microbiome and outcomes, and generate evidence to guide targeted-nutrition therapy.[75] Studies are required to determine potential benefits, safety, and cost-effectiveness.[76] An emerging area of research in the PICU includes exploring the effect of food-based fibre-containing enteral formula on antibiotic-related feed intolerance in critically-ill children with sepsis.[77] As this area of research expands, it is likely that practice guidelines will evolve to include recommendations on administration of pre- and pro-biotics, including fibre-containing enteral formulas.

Longer Term Outcomes—the Role of Nutrition in Rehab and Recovery?

Modifying patient-centred long-term outcomes through PICU interventions has been highlighted as the ultimate goal of PICU trials.[78] As pediatric critical care research increasingly focuses on long-term outcomes, questions arise regarding the role of nutrition interventions. Theoretically, it is expected that nutrition plays an important role in rehabilitation and recovery; however, this needs to be established. Unlike adults, physical and psychosocial development is at stake for children and nutrition is already accepted to play an important role in overall health and well-being. Minimization of deconditioning has been identified as a priority for clinical care and research in a study of the impact of pediatric critical illness on health-related quality-of-life.[79] Our group has recently described the modes of required nutrition support on the ward following discharge from the PICU, and identified that gaps remain between nutrition targets and actual provision as late as 28 days following PICU admission.[80] The PEPaNIC trial has demonstrated incorporating long-term follow-up of nutrition intervention on developmental outcomes.[81]

New Frameworks for Future Research

Future studies should consider the multi-stakeholder overall PICU core outcome set, which consists of 4 Global Domains (cognitive, emotional, physical, and overall health), and 4 Specific Outcomes (child health-related quality-of-life, pain, survival, and communication).[82] A set specific to nutrition is yet to be developed, which would ideally include outcome domains of nutrition efficiency, nutrition tolerance, and non-nutrition pediatric intensive care outcomes.[83] Additionally, the recently developed consensus definition for acute pediatric critical illness should be used to facilitate a consistent approach to global research across resource-variable settings[84]

SUMMARY

Pediatric critical care nutrition-focused clinicians and researchers eagerly await to see what directions current and future studies take and how PICU nutrition therapy may evolve over the next decade. Much is yet to be further understood regarding fundamentals including optimal energy and protein provision. Hypotheses related to nutrition in the PICU must be tested in well-designed trials. There are many exciting developments in areas including body composition monitoring via skeletal muscle ultrasound, tailoring nutrition provision to influence the microbiome, and combining nutrition and mobility interventions. Future studies must consider new frameworks, established consensus priorities and patient-reported outcomes with the shared ultimate goal of improving short- and long-term outcomes of critically ill children via nutrition interventions.

CLINICS CARE POINTS

- Nutrition prescriptions should take into account the phase of critical illness.
- Nutrition provision should aim to initially meet estimated resting energy expenditure and a minimum of 1.5 g/kg protein.
- Commence enteral nutrition early unless contraindicated.
- Avoid supplemental parenteral nutrition in the first week of PICU admission.
- Consider 'feed modification' to increase energy and protein provision via feed fortification (including fortified expressed breast milk), increased powdered formula concentration or use of increased nutrient density liquid formulas.

AUTHORS CONTRIBUTIONS (CREDIT STATEMENT)

J. Winderlich: Conceptualization, Writing – Original Draft, Writing – Editing and Reviewing, Project Administration. G. Brown: Writing – Original Draft, Writing – Editing and Reviewing. A.A Udy and E.J. Ridley: Conceptualization, Writing – Original Draft, Writing – Editing and Reviewing, Supervision.

FUNDING

This review did not receive any specific grant from funding agencies in the public, commercial, or not-for-profit sectors.

DISCLOSURE

The authors have no conflicts of interest to declare.

REFERENCES

1. Epstein D, Brill JE. A history of pediatric critical care medicine. Pediatr Res 2005; 58(5):987–96.
2. Kleinman RE, Barness LA, Finberg L. History of pediatric nutrition and fluid therapy. Pediatr Res 2003;54(5):762–72.
3. Iping R, Hulst JM, Joosten KFM. Research developments in pediatric intensive care nutrition: a research intelligence review. Clin Nutr ESPEN 2022;50:1–7. PubMed Central PMCID: 35871909.

4. Tume LN, Verbruggen SCAT, Valla F. The current state of knowledge and research required around nutrition in pediatric critical illness. Pediatric Medicine 2020;3.
5. Weaver CM, Miller JW. Challenges in conducting clinical nutrition research. Nutr Rev 2017;75(7):491–9.
6. Joosten KFM, Kerklaan D, Verbruggen SCAT. Nutritional support and the role of the stress response in critically ill children. Curr Opin Clin Nutr Metab Care 2016;19(3):226–33.
7. Joosten KFM, Eveleens RD, Verbruggen SCAT. Nutritional support in the recovery phase of critically ill children. Curr Opin Clin Nutr Metab Care 2019;22(2):152–8.
8. Mehta NM, Skillman HE, Irving SY, et al. Guidelines for the provision and assessment of nutrition support therapy in the pediatric critically ill patient: society of critical care medicine and American Society for Parenteral and Enteral Nutrition. J Parenter Enteral Nutr 2017;41(5):706–42. PubMed Central PMCID: 28686844.
9. Tume LN, Valla FV, Joosten K, et al. Nutritional support for children during critical illness: European Society of Pediatric and Neonatal Intensive Care (ESPNIC) metabolism, endocrine and nutrition section position statement and clinical recommendations. Intensive Care Med 2020;46(3):411–25. PubMed Central PMCID: 32077997.
10. Moltu SJ, Bronsky J, Embleton N, et al. Nutritional management of the critically ill neonate: a position paper of the ESPGHAN committee on nutrition. J Pediatr Gastroenterol Nutr 2021;73(2):274–89.
11. Tume LN, Ista E, Verbruggen S, et al. Practical strategies to implement the ESPNIC Nutrition Clinical recommendations into PICU practice. Clin Nutr ESPEN 2021;42:410–4.
12. (SCCM) ASoPaENAaSoCCM. ASPEN/SCCM pediatric critical care nutrition guideline: protocol. 2024. Available at: https://www.nutritioncare.org/uploadedFiles/Documents/Guidelines_and_Clinical_Resources/PediatricCriticalCareProtocol.pdf.
13. Shunxia S, Jin Y, Xiaoling T, et al. Effect of a multidisciplinary nutrition management model in patients with critical illness: a randomized trial. Nurs Crit Care 2024;29(2):417–26.
14. Oh E, Shim H, Yon HJ, et al. Effectiveness of a multidisciplinary team for nutrition support in a trauma intensive care unit. Acute Crit Care 2020;35(3):142–8.
15. Zeeshan A, Nairn QuA, Jawwad M, et al. Impact of nutrition support team in achieving target calories in children admitted in pediatric intensive care unit. J Pediatr Gastroenterol Nutr 2022;74(6):830–6.
16. Winderlich J, Little B, Oberender F, et al. Dietitian and nutrition-related practices and resources in Australian and New Zealand PICUs: a clinician survey. Aust Crit Care 2023. https://doi.org/10.1016/j.aucc.2023.03.003.
17. Meah S, Kidd C, Rothman B, et al. Exploring paediatric dietetic resources available for critically ill children in the UK and Ireland: a multicentre survey. J Hum Nutr Diet : the official journal of the British Dietetic Association 2024;37(2):459–63.
18. Ventura JC, Silveira TT, Bechard L, et al. Nutritional screening tool for critically ill children: a systematic review. Nutr Rev 2022;80(6):1392–418.
19. Ladd AK, Skillman HE, Haemer MA, et al. Preventing underfeeding and overfeeding: a clinician's guide to the acquisition and implementation of indirect calorimetry. Nutr Clin Pract 2018;33(2):198–205.
20. Beggs MR, Garcia Guerra G, Larsen BMK. Do PICU patients meet technical criteria for performing indirect calorimetry? Clin Nutr ESPEN 2016;15:80–4.
21. Schofield WN. Predicting basal metabolic rate, new standards and review of previous work. Hum Nutr Clin Nutr 1985;39(Suppl 1):5–41.

22. Veldscholte K, Joosten K, Jotterand Chaparro C. Energy expenditure in critically ill children. Pediatric Medicine 2020;3.

23. Bechard LJ, Parrott JS, Mehta NM. Systematic review of the influence of energy and protein intake on protein balance in critically ill children. J Pediatr 2012; 161(2):333–9.e1.

24. Hauschild DB, Ventura JC, Mehta NM, et al. Impact of the structure and dose of protein intake on clinical and metabolic outcomes in critically ill children: a systematic review. Nutrition 2017. https://doi.org/10.1016/j.nut.2017.04.013.

25. Jotterand Chaparro C, Bertoni Maluf V, Moullet C, et al. Effectiveness of high vs lower enteral protein intake, considering energy intake, on clinical outcomes in critically ill children: a systematic review protocol. JBI Evid Synth 2023;21(6): 1251–8.

26. Nagel EM, Elgersma KM, Gallagher TT, et al. Importance of human milk for infants in the clinical setting: updates and mechanistic links. Nutr Clin Pract 2023;38(S2): S39–55.

27. Hookway L, Brown A, Grant A. Breastfeeding sick children in hospital: exploring the experiences of mothers in UK paediatric wards. Matern Child Nutr 2023; 19(2):e13489.

28. Hookway L, Lewis J, Brown A. The challenges of medically complex breastfed children and their families: a systematic review. Matern Child Nutr 2021;17(4): e13182.

29. Fell DM, Bitetto EA, Skillman HE. Timing of enteral nutrition and parenteral nutrition in the PICU. Nutr Clin Pract 2023;38(S2):S174–212.

30. Mehta NM, Bechard LJ, Cahill N, et al. Nutritional practices and their relationship to clinical outcomes in critically ill children-An international multicenter cohort study. Crit Care Med 2012;40(7):2204–11.

31. Mehta NM, Bechard LJ, Zurakowski D, et al. Adequate enteral protein intake is inversely associated with 60-d mortality in critically ill children: a multicenter, prospective, cohort study. Am J Clin Nutr 2015;102(1):199–206.

32. Turner AD, Hamilton SM, Callif C, et al. Bedside postpyloric tube placement and enteral nutrition delivery in the pediatric intensive care unit. Nutr Clin Pract 2020; 35(2):299–305.

33. Ichimaru S. Methods of enteral nutrition administration in critically ill patients: continuous, cyclic, intermittent, and bolus feeding. Nutr Clin Pract 2018;33(6): 790–5.

34. Littler H, Tume LN. Is bolus or continuous enteral feeding better in critically ill children: an evidence-based review. Nurs Crit Care 2023;28(1):36–9.

35. Brown AM, Fisher E, Forbes ML. Bolus vs continuous nasogastric feeds in mechanically ventilated pediatric patients: a pilot study. JPEN J Parenter Enteral Nutr 2019;43(6):750–8.

36. Veldscholte K, Cramer ABG, de Jonge RCJ, et al. Intermittent feeding with an overnight fast versus 24-h feeding in critically ill neonates, infants, and children: an open-label, single-centre, randomised controlled trial. Clin Nutr 2023;42(9): 1569–80.

37. Tume LN, Bickerdike A, Latten L, et al. Routine gastric residual volume measurement and energy target achievement in the PICU: a comparison study. Eur J Pediatr 2017;176(12):1637–44.

38. Tume L. No routine measurement of gastric residual volume in paediatric critical care. 2024. Available at: https://www.isrctn.com/ISRCTN79668198. Accessed May 28, 2024.

39. Winderlich J, Little B, Oberender F, et al. Characteristics of enteral and oral nutrition support among infants and young children in the pediatric intensive care unit: a descriptive cohort study. J Parenter Enteral Nutr 2024. https://doi.org/10.1002/jpen.2672.
40. Singal A, Sahu MK, Trilok Kumar G, et al. Effect of energy- and/or protein-dense enteral feeding on postoperative outcomes of infant surgical patients with congenital cardiac disease: a systematic review and meta-analysis. Nutr Clin Pract 2022;37(3):555–66.
41. Winderlich J, Little B, Anderson A, et al. Feed modification for increased energy and protein density as nutrition therapy in critically ill children: a protocol for a scoping review. Clinical Nutrition Open Science 2022;46:13–9.
42. Marino LV, Eveleens RD, Morton K, et al. Peptide nutrient-energy dense enteral feeding in critically ill infants: an observational study. J Hum Nutr Diet : the official journal of the British Dietetic Association 2019;32(3):400–8.
43. Alten JA, Rhodes LA, Tabbutt S, et al. Perioperative feeding management of neonates with CHD: analysis of the pediatric cardiac critical care consortium (PC4) registry. Cardiol Young 2015;25(8):1593–601.
44. Tume LN, Balmaks R, da Cruz E, et al. Enteral feeding practices in infants with congenital heart disease across European PICUs: a european society of pediatric and neonatal intensive care survey. Pediatr Crit Care Med 2018;19(2):137–44.
45. Bell D, Suna J, Marathe SP, et al. Feeding neonates and infants prior to surgery for congenital heart defects: systematic review and meta-analysis. Children-Basel 2022;9(12).
46. Cognata A, Kataria-Hale J, Griffiths P, et al. Human milk use in the preoperative period is associated with a lower risk for necrotizing enterocolitis in neonates with complex congenital heart disease. J Pediatr 2019;215:11–6.
47. Fivez T, Kerklaan D, Mesotten D, et al. Early versus Late parenteral nutrition in critically ill children. New Engl J Med 2016;374(12):1111–22.
48. Vanhorebeek I, Verbruggen S, Casaer MP, et al. Effect of early supplemental parenteral nutrition in the paediatric ICU: a preplanned observational study of post-randomisation treatments in the PEPaNIC trial. Lancet Respir Med 2017;5(6):475–83.
49. Koletzko B, Goulet O, Jochum F, et al. Use of parenteral nutrition in the pediatric ICU. Curr Opin Clin Nutr Metab Care 2017;20(3):201–3.
50. Goulet O, Jochum F, Koletzko B. Early or late parenteral nutrition in critically ill children: practical implications of the PEPaNIC Trial. Ann Nutr Metab 2017;70:34–8. Switzerland.
51. Joosten K, Verbruggen S. PN administration in critically ill children in different phases of the stress response. Nutrients 2022;14(9):1819.
52. Mihatsch WA, Braegger C, Bronsky J, et al. ESPGHAN/ESPEN/ESPR/CSPEN guidelines on pediatric parenteral nutrition. Clin Nutr 2018;37(6 Pt B):2303–5.
53. Hunt MF, Pierre AS, Zhou X, et al. Nutritional support in postcardiotomy shock extracorporeal membrane oxygenation patients: a prospective, observational study. J Surg Res 2019;244:257–64.
54. Dennis JL, Jordan J, Rice M, et al. Enteral nutrition during extracorporeal membrane oxygenation in the neonatal and pediatric populations: a literature review. Pediatr Crit Care Med 2023;24(8).
55. Tatucu-Babet OA, Diehl A, Kratzing C, et al. Modified indirect calorimetry for patients on venoarterial extracorporeal membrane oxygenation: a pilot feasibility study. Eur J Clin Nutr 2023;77(9):888–94.

56. De Waele E, Jonckheer J, Pen JJ, et al. Energy expenditure of patients on ECMO: a prospective pilot study. Acta Anaesthesiol Scand 2019;63(3):360–4.

57. Ewing LJ, Domico MB, Ramirez R, et al. Measuring the resting energy expenditure in children on extracorporeal membrane oxygenation: a prospective pilot study. Am Soc Artif Intern Organs J 2023;69(1):122–6.

58. Li X, Yu X, Cheypesh A, et al. Non-invasive measurements of energy expenditure and respiratory quotient by respiratory mass spectrometry in children on extracorporeal membrane oxygenation-a pilot study. Artif Organs 2015;39(9):815–9.

59. Ohbe H, Jo T, Yamana H, et al. Early enteral nutrition for cardiogenic or obstructive shock requiring venoarterial extracorporeal membrane oxygenation: a nationwide inpatient database study. Intensive Care Med 2018;44(8):1258–65.

60. Li X, Fan L, Pan X, et al. Enteral nutrition in children and adolescents who receive extracorporeal membrane oxygenation and its impact on complications and mortality: a systematic review and meta-analysis. JPEN J Parenter Enteral Nutr 2024. https://doi.org/10.1002/jpen.2626.

61. Dresen E, Naidoo O, Hill A, et al. Medical nutrition therapy in patients receiving ECMO: evidence-based guidance for clinical practice. JPEN J Parenter Enteral Nutr 2023;47(2):220–35.

62. Kyle UG, Akcan-Arikan A, Orellana RA, et al. Nutrition support among critically ill children with AKI. Clin J Am Soc Nephrol 2013;8(4):568–74.

63. Jonckheer J, Demol J, Lanckmans K, et al. MECCIAS trial: metabolic consequences of continuous veno-venous hemofiltration on indirect calorimetry. Clin Nutr 2020;39(12):3797–803.

64. Vega MRW, Cerminara D, Desloovere A, et al. Nutritional management of children with acute kidney injury—clinical practice recommendations from the Pediatric Renal Nutrition Taskforce. Pediatr Nephrol 2023;38(11):3559–80.

65. Wong Vega M, Vuong KT, Chmielewski J, et al. Nutrition for critically ill children and neonates requiring dialysis: application of clinical practice recommendations. Nutr Clin Pract 2023;38(S2):S139–57.

66. Fomon SJ, Ziegler EE. Renal solute load and potential renal solute load in infancy. J Pediatr 1999;134(1):11–4.

67. Tume LN, Valla FV, Floh AA, et al. Priorities for nutrition research in pediatric critical care. JPEN J Parenter Enteral Nutr 2019;43(7):853–62.

68. Ong C, Lee JH, Leow MKS, et al. Skeletal muscle ultrasonography in nutrition and functional outcome assessment of critically ill children: experience and insights from pediatric disease and adult critical care studies. J Parenter Enteral Nutr 2017;41(7):1091–9.

69. Valverde Montoro D, Rosa Camacho V, Artacho González L, et al. Thigh ultrasound monitoring identifies muscle atrophy in mechanically ventilated pediatric patients. Eur J Pediatr 2023;182(12):5543–51.

70. Tume LN, Simons C, Latten L, et al. Association between protein intake and muscle wasting in critically ill children: a prospective cohort study. J Parenter Enteral Nutr 2024. https://doi.org/10.1002/jpen.2627. n/a(n/a).

71. McCarter DL, Morgan C, Bray L, et al. How is bioelectrical impedance used in neonatal intensive care? A scoping review. Eur J Pediatr 2024;183(7):3053–62.

72. Mehta N. PRotein optimization with eXercise to improve MUscle mass and functional outcomeS (PROXIMUS). 2024. Available at: https://classic.clinicaltrials.gov/ct2/show/NCT05296096. Accessed May 28, 2024.

73. Rogers MB, Firek B, Shi M, et al. Disruption of the microbiota across multiple body sites in critically ill children. Microbiome 2016;4(1):66.

74. Xu J, Kong X, Li J, et al. Pediatric intensive care unit treatment alters the diversity and composition of the gut microbiota and antimicrobial resistance gene expression in critically ill children. Front Microbiol 2023;14.

75. Fan L, Lee JH. Enteral feeding and the microbiome in critically ill children: a narrative review. Transl Pediatr 2021;10(10):2778–91.

76. Angurana SK, Mehta A. Probiotics in critically ill children: an updated review. J Pediatr Crit Care 2021;8(5):234–42.

77. O'Connor G, Sun Y, Gardiner B, et al. An open-label pilot single-subject study to monitor the impact of a Food-Based enteral formula on faecal short-chain fatty acid concentrations in children admitted to intensive care with sepsis. Clinical Nutrition Open Science 2024;53:1–10.

78. Maddux AB, Fink EL. The post-PICU growth curve. Pediatr Crit Care Med 2022;23(8).

79. Killien EY, Rivara FP, Dervan LA, et al. Components of health-related quality of life most affected following pediatric critical illness. Crit Care Med 2022;50(1): e20–30.

80. Winderlich J, Little B, Oberender F, et al. Nutrition support in children discharged from the pediatric intensive care unit: a bi-national prospective cohort study (ePICUre). J Pediatr Gastroenterol Nutr 2024;1–9. https://doi.org/10.1002/jpn3. 12387.

81. Jacobs A, Dulfer K, Eveleens RD, et al. Long-term developmental effect of withholding parenteral nutrition in paediatric intensive care units: a 4-year follow-up of the PEPaNIC randomised controlled trial. Lancet Child Adolesc Health 2020;4(7): 503–14.

82. Fink EL, Maddux AB, Pinto N, et al. A core outcome set for pediatric critical care. Crit Care Med 2020;48(12):1819–28.

83. Gadhvi KR, Valla FV, Tume LN. Review of outcomes used in nutrition trials in pediatric critical care. JPEN J Parenter Enteral Nutr 2020;44(7):1210–9. Epub 20200203.

84. Arias AV, Lintner-Rivera M, Shafi NI, et al. A research definition and framework for acute paediatric critical illness across resource-variable settings: a modified Delphi consensus. Lancet Glob Health 2024;12(2):e331–40. Epub 20240105.

Which Outcomes Should We be Using in Critical Care Nutrition Trials?

Naomi Watson, BMBCh, MA, PgDip, MRCP[a],*,
Saira Nazeer, Physiotherapy BSc(Hons)[b],
Zudin Puthucheary, MBBS, BMedSci, DUHM, PGCME, EDICM, FRCP, FHEA, FFICM, PhD[c]

KEYWORDS

- Core outcome sets • Exploratory outcomes • Surrogate markers

KEY POINTS

- Outcomes selected in critical care research should facilitate comparison between trials.
- Core outcome sets are valuable in improving the consistency of research, so that conclusive recommendations can be made.
- Exploratory outcomes are important in providing novel insights into disease pathophysiology and treatment response.

INTRODUCTION

Clinical trials are vital for the generation of high-quality evidence, to inform the development and delivery of patient-centred care. Selection of appropriate outcome measures is a key part of experimental trial design, ensuring relevance and feasibility. In well-established areas of research these may be relatively straightforward to define, based on previous research and the selection of outcomes, which facilitate comparison between the data. In rapidly expanding fields of research, standardized measures are less well-established, and there may be debate regarding the optimal time points, outcomes, and measurement instruments.[1]

[a] The William Harvey Research Institute, Barts and the London School of Medicine & Dentistry, Queen Mary University of London, London, UK; [b] Critical Care and Peri-Operative Medicine Research Group, The William Harvey Research Institute, Barts and the London School of Medicine & Dentistry, Queen Mary University of London, London, UK; [c] The William Harvey Research Institute, Barts and The London School of Medicine & Dentistry, Queen Mary University of London, Consultant in Intensive Care, Royal London Hospital, Barts Health NHS Trust, London, UK
* Corresponding author. The William Harvey Research Institute, Barts and the London School of Medicine & Dentistry, Queen Mary University of London, London, UK.
E-mail address: naomi.watson5@nhs.net

Crit Care Clin 41 (2025) 363–378
https://doi.org/10.1016/j.ccc.2024.09.005
criticalcare.theclinics.com
0749-0704/25/© 2024 Elsevier Inc. All rights reserved, including those for text and data mining, AI training, and similar technologies.

Research into nutrition and metabolism in critical illness are rapidly evolving and therefore require continuous appraisal of outcome measures as the evidence base expands. Developing standardized measures are critical to enable comparison between studies and facilitate systematic reviews and meta-analyses.[2] This improves the quality of evidence-based knowledge internationally, making research more valuable to decision makers and reducing avoidable research waste.[3] Alongside this approach, it is important to explore novel outcome measures, which may generate new insights and ultimately become standardized once the evidence base has been established.

There has been a shift in the past decade toward increasingly patient-focussed outcomes in critical care research, driven in part by improving mortality rates. Survivorship is characterized by physical, psychologic, and cognitive impairments, which have negative socioeconomic consequences and ultimately reduce patients' quality-of-life. Outcomes that address these limitations are therefore necessary and urgent, to facilitate a more patient-centric approach to critical care research.

Many of the physical functional limitations are associated with muscle wasting, which is a common and early feature of critical illness.[4] Critical illness has multiple etiologies; however, there is a significant overlap in physiologic characteristics and metabolic dysfunction. Glucose, amino acid, and fatty acid utilization is impaired, resulting in bioenergetic failure, organ dysfunction, and cell death.[4] This is associated with increased muscle breakdown, impaired protein synthesis, and intramuscular inflammation. Exercise rehabilitation and increased delivery of energy and protein have consistently failed to deliver improved outcomes.[5,6] Nutritional and metabolic strategies targeting muscle bioenergetics have shown some promise; however, the longer-term physical functional outcomes need careful evaluation.

Outcomes to assess muscle wasting and the associated functional impairment range from analysis of biochemical markers to muscle loss quantification and functional assessment. Longer term outcomes are increasingly important with increased survivorship, and some of the relevant assessment methods will be discussed.

CORE OUTCOME SETS

Defining relevant physical functional outcomes requires input from all relevant stakeholders. Input from patients and caregivers is increasingly being sought in defining research priorities, with a greater awareness and utilization of patient focus groups such as the Intensive Care Priority Setting Partnerships (PSP).[7] Another opportunity for meaningful patient input is in the development of Core Outcome Sets, which are the minimum outcomes that should be measured and reported in clinical trials undertaken in a specific area. The development of these involves 3 major stakeholders: healthcare professionals, clinical researchers, and patients and caregivers. The process utilizes the modified Delphi consensus methodology, using expert opinion to address questions where empirical data does not exist or is not in a useable format. Outcomes are selected from systematic reviews and participants undergo rounds of voting, conducted anonymously, on recommendations related to the study question. Each outcome is scored according to the Grading of Recommendations Assessment, Development and Evaluation (GRADE) scale ranging from 1 to 9; score 1 to 3 corresponds to 'Not Important', 4 to 6 is 'Important but Not Critical' and 7 to 9 is 'Critical'. Results of the voting rounds are discussed by a steering committee, who then decide whether outcomes should be deemed 'essential', 'recommended', or excluded from the process. Following identification of 'essential' outcomes, stakeholders then participate in a systematic process to identify the most appropriate measurement instruments. The use of these outcome sets improves the consistency of research, such that conclusive recommendations about the effectiveness of interventions can be made.

The Core Outcome Measures in Effectiveness Trials initiative provides a freely-available searchable database of all core outcome sets, including much relevance to critical illness. Three of these core outcome sets will be discussed, relating to nutritional and metabolic interventions, acute respiratory failure survivors, and post-intensive care syndrome. There is considerable overlap in outcomes between these outcomes sets (**Fig. 1**), partly due to common physiologic and metabolic changes characteristic of pro-longed critical illness resulting in muscle wasting, which is highly associated with a wide range of outcomes. An advantage of conducting studies to define core outcomes is that priorities of different stakeholders groups can be directly compared.

OUTCOMES FOR NUTRITIONAL AND METABOLIC INTERVENTIONS

A core outcome set for nutritional and metabolic interventions in critical illness (CONCISE) has defined the minimum set of outcomes relevant to this area of research, at 30-d and 90-d post-randomization.[1] Defining time points is challenging with metabolic and nutritional interventions, as the range is extremely broad. However, using fixed time points from randomization enables data alignment of future trials, increasing external validity. Stakeholders were recruited internationally from 24 countries, and included patients who have survived critical illness or their caregivers, clinicians who care for critically ill patients with an interest in metabolic and nutritional interventions, and clinical researchers who might apply the core outcome set. The 'essential' outcomes to include were survival, physical function, infection, activities of daily living (ADLs), nutritional status, and muscle/nerve function (**Table 1**). Additional 'recommended' outcomes included organ dysfunction, wound healing, and frailty and body composition.

Survival

Survival is a widely reported outcome and is fundamental to critical care medicine. There has been a substantial decline in mortality over the past few decades, which

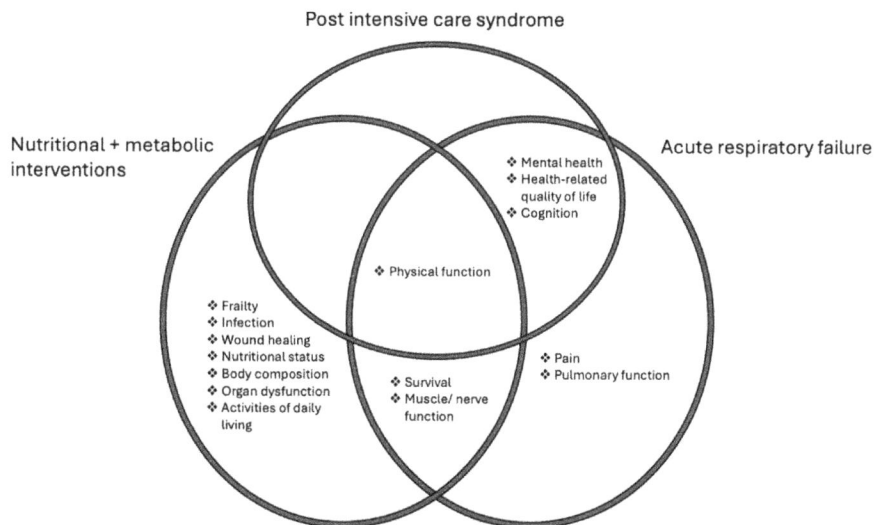

Fig. 1. Diagram demonstrating the overlapping important outcomes from relevant core outcome sets for critical illness.

Table 1
Common core outcome measures in critical care trials

	Outcome Measure	Instructor Burden	Patient Participation	Clinical Relevance
Muscle strength	Hand grip strength	• Objective measure providing quantifiable measurement • Requires a handheld dynamometer	• Requires patient volition • No need to have the ability to converse	• Association with mortality
Physical Function	CPAx	• Easy application • Requires a handheld dynamometer, but nil further additional equipment that would not otherwise be used during rehabilitation	• Does not rely on patient volition	• Association with place of residence at 90 d, critical care length of stay and duration of mechanical ventilation
	30 s STS	• Easy application, only requires a chair • Can be assessed remotely	• Does require the patient to be able to sit in a chair and follow instructions • No need to have the ability to converse	• Innately linked to function and ability to participate in activities of daily living
	SPPB	• Easy application • No specialist equipment required	• Requires patient volition • No need to have the ability to converse	• Highly reproducible • Functional tasks • Potential for incomplete results as asks for time taken to complete tasks (as opposed to number of repetitions in set time)
	PFS or PF domain of SF-36	• No equipment required • PFS: Once the patient has filled in the outcome measure, the instructor needs to produce the PFS using paid for software • PF domain: cumulative score of this domain	• Requires patient volition and ability to complete a questionnaire (either by speaking or writing)	• PCS widely used as a measure of physical function in the ICU population • PF has been shown to be more responsive than PCS when predicting persistent impairment trajectory

Quality of life	PICUPS + PICUPS-Community	• No equipment nor software required	• Reflects patient's needs • Used as a screening tool • Inform service provision.
		• Requires patient volition and ability to complete a questionnaire (either by speaking or writing)	
	WHODAS 2.0	• No equipment nor software required	• Reliable, valid and responsive measure of disability in ICU population • Correlates with physical function measures (ranks better than other self-reported outcome measures)
		• Requires patient volition and ability to complete a questionnaire (either by speaking or writing)	
	EQ5D	• No equipment nor software required	• Excellent psychometric properties • Better at providing an on-the-day health profile, rather than predictive value
		• Requires patient volition and ability to complete a questionnaire (either by speaking or writing)	
Socioeconomic position (SEP)	International Standard Classification of Occupations + International Standard Classification of Education and Income	• No specialist equipment required	• Lower SEP associated with worse survival outcomes and worse mental health outcomes • Lacking evidence for association with physical function
		• Residential area specific SEP data can be used when individual data are unattainable	
Nutritional status	GLIM	• Access to patient data required	• Association with critical care mortality and hospital length of stay • Subjectivity noted in scoring
		• Minimal participation required	

Abbreviations: CPAx, chelsea critical care physical assessment Tool; STS, sit-to-stand; SPPB, short physical performance battery; PFS, physical function score; PF, physical function; SF-36, short form-36 score; PICUPS, post intensive care presentation and screening; WHODAS, World Health Organization Disability Assessment Score; GLIM, global leadership initiative on malnutrition.

has implications for study design if using survival as a primary outcome. For interventions such as nutritional regimes, very large numbers of patients would be required to maintain sufficiently narrow confidence intervals.[8]

Physical Function

The inclusion of physical function as an 'essential' outcome at both timepoints reflects the increasing focus on patient-centred outcomes, and aligns with the Intensive Care PSP's top priorities for critical care research.[7] Four measurement instruments were deemed 'recommended': the Physical Component Score (PCS) Short Form-36 score (SF-36), 30 sec sit-to-stand (STS) test, 6-min walk test, and the short physical performance battery (SPPB). The lack of 'essential' measurement instruments may be indicative of a relative paucity of evidence in this emerging field of research, limiting confidence in decision-making regarding mandatory assessment tools.[1] Functional outcomes that require face-to-face measurement following hospital discharge can also be logistically challenging in critical care survivors.

Short Form-36 Score

The 36-Item Short Form survey is a self-reported outcome measure that is often used as a measure of a person or population's quality-of-life. This outcome measures comprise 36 questions covering 8 domains: physical functioning, role limitations due to physical health, role limitations due to emotional problems, energy/fatigue, emotional well-being, social functioning, pain, and general health. The total score can be used to indicate a range of low to high quality-of-life, as well as looking at 2 component scores: the PCS and the mental component score. The PCS has been widely used as a measure of physical function in the critical care population and was ranked 'essential' to include in the CONCISE outcome set; however, its ranking was down-graded due to the need to pay for this score, thereby reducing its accessibility.[9] An alternative option could be to use the physical function domain of the SF-36, which has been shown to be more responsive than the PCS when predicting persistent impairment trajectory in the sepsis population.[10]

Thirty Second Sit-To-Stand

The 30 second STS test is used as a measure of physical function. It is used extensively in a wide range of chronic diseases and in different settings, including remotely. The widespread use and acceptability of this test stems from the fact that the ability to stand from a seated position is so innately linked to function and ability to participate in ADLs. To perform this test, all that is needed is a chair with no arms, with the measurement being the number of times the participant is able to stand from the chair unaided in 30 sec. There is an adapted version where the participant is allowed to use their arms, the modified 30s STS, which is useful in the critical care population where it has been shown that roughly half will need to use their arms at point of discharge from intensive care unit (ICU) and hospital.[11] A floor effect has been noted when used on ICU; however, neither this was no longer observed nor was a ceiling effect at point of hospital discharge.[11] Due to this floor effect observed, the time-based sit to stand measurement is preferable in the critical care population where a reading of '0' can be scored as opposed to other STS measurements, which ask for the time taken to complete a set number of stands (such as in the SPPB).

Short Physical Performance Battery

SPPB is a group of measures used to assess physical function. It covers 3 test areas: chair stands (time taken to perform a single chair stand and 5 repeated chair stands), balance tests (unsupported stand for 10 sec in 3 positions: feet together, semi-tandem, and full-tandem) and gait speed (time taken to perform a 3 or 4 m walk). It is widely used due to its ease of application, lack of specialist equipment needed, and its reproducibility and discriminatory ability following ICU and hospital discharge.[12] However, this tool relies on patient volition and a patient unable to complete a task leads to an inability to score that element.

Infection

Infection features in the Intensive Care PSP top priorities, specifically identifying the best way to prevent, diagnose, and treat hospital-acquired infection.[7] Despite its inclusion as an 'essential' outcome, no measurement instruments were deemed 'essential' or 'recommended'. Infection-related core outcome measures have been included in other core outcome sets for critical illness, which may be relevant for consideration.[13]

Activities of Daily Living

Assessment of ADLs/instrumental ADLs was deemed 'essential', with the Barthel or Katz index voted 'essential' at 90 d post-randomization. These assess common ADLs such as feeding, washing, dressing, toileting and transfers on an ordinal scale, and do not require formal training to complete.

Nutritional Status

The Global Leadership Initiative on Malnutrition (GLIM) was 'recommended' to assess nutritional status at 90 d post-randomization. This is an outcome measure used to evaluate nutritional status, which covers 2 main domains: phenotypic criteria (non-voluntary weight loss, low body mass index, and reduced muscle mass) and etiological criteria (reduced food intake and inflammation). GLIM measured at admission to the critical care unit is predictive of critical care mortality and hospital length-of-stay; however, no such association has been noted for longer term outcomes. Subjectivity in scoring has been observed that may be a clinimetric limitation.[14,15]

Muscle/Nerve Function

Muscle/nerve function is an 'essential' outcome for many core outcome sets relating to critical illness, and hand-grip strength is the 'recommended' measurement instrument at 90 d post-randomization. This measures the force exerted by the forearm using a handheld dynamometer and is used as a screening tool for overall strength. Grip strength may also have use as a prognostic indicator for health outcomes, especially physical function in the aging population and more recently cognitive ability.[16–19] This less subjective measure can provide a more precise, quantifiable measurement of muscle strength, which can be compared to the opposite side, as well as normative values. It can be used as an alternative to the Medical Research Council Sum Score to identify ICU-associated weakness but retains the same requirement of patient volition, which limits the number of patients who are able to comply in a critical care setting.[20] It has demonstrated association with health outcomes in the critical care population, with one study finding an independent association with hospital mortality.[21,22]

OUTCOMES FOR STUDIES IN ACUTE RESPIRATORY FAILURE SURVIVORS

Acute respiratory failure is one of the most common reasons for admission to ICUs, and the core outcome set developed for these patients is relevant for a broader range of critical illness etiologies.[23] The pool of stakeholders for this Delphi panel was not restricted to acute respiratory failure, and comprised clinical researchers, clinicians and representatives of clinician professional associations, patients and caregivers, and representatives of United States' federal research funding organisations. The consensus criteria for inclusion were at least 70% of all respondents rating the measure as 'Critical' (a GRADE score of ≥ 7) and less than or equal to 15% rating the measure as 'Not Important'. The outcomes achieving these criteria were survival, physical function, mental health, pulmonary function, pain, muscle/nerve function, cognition, and satisfaction with life or personal enjoyment. Survival was deemed not to require a consensus-based process for selecting an appropriate measurement instrument. Of note, time points for the assessment of outcomes were not specified in this core outcome set, which may limit comparability particularly with physical function assessment, which has significant variability over time.

Satisfaction with Life and Personal Enjoyment

The recommended outcome measurement tools for satisfaction with life and personal enjoyment were the Short Form-36 and EuroQol-5-dimension (EQ-5D) questionnaires. The pain question of the EQ-5D was recommended for assessment of pain. The EQ-5D was developed by the EuroQol Group as a simple means of measuring health-related quality-of-life. This self-reported outcome measure captures an individual's evaluation of their health using a visual analogue scale and covers 5-dimensions of health: mobility, self-care, usual activities, pain, and anxiety/depression. The EQ-5D has been shown to have excellent psychometric properties, correlating well with more in-depth outcome measures such as in a study looking at pain in survivors of critical care.[24,25] The EQ-5D has not been shown to have good predictive validity, with its value in clinic trials being more associated in providing an on-the-day health profile of a patient or population.[26]

Mental Health and Cognition

The Hospital Anxiety and Depression Scale and Impact of Event Scale were recommended for assessment of mental health, and the Montreal Cognitive Assessment tool for cognition.

Physical Function, Muscle/Nerve Function, and Pulmonary Function

No consensus was achieved for outcome measures of physical function, muscle/nerve function, or pulmonary function in survivors of acute respiratory failure. Concerns were raised regarding the mandatory inclusion of performance-based measurement instruments, which tend to need face-to-face assessment with increased administrative skill, cost, and time requirements. This does not negate their value, as existing data demonstrate that performance-based tests measure distinct aspects of patient outcomes compared to patient-reported outcome measures.[27] The inclusion of several measurement instruments for physical function and muscle/nerve function in the CONCISE recommendations may reflect an expansion of the evidence base, as the nutritional and metabolic interventions core outcome set was published 5 y after the acute respiratory failure set.

OUTCOMES IN POST-INTENSIVE CARE SYNDROME RESEARCH

The core outcomes for post-intensive care syndrome (PICS) research include previously discussed outcomes such as health-related quality-of-life (EQ-5D-5 L and the 12-Item World Health Organization Disability Assessment Schedule [WHODAS 2.0]), mental health (Patient Health Questionnaire-4 and -8, Generalized Anxiety Disorder

Scale-7, and Impact of Event Scale-Revised), physical function (2-min walk test, hand-grip strength, and SPPB), and cognition (Repeatable Battery for the Assessment for Neuropsychological Status and Trail Making Test A and B).[28]

World Health Organization Disability Assessment Schedule 2.0

WHODAS 2.0 is an assessment tool covering 6 domains of function to assess health status and disability. These domains are cognition, mobility, self-care, getting along, life activities (household and work), and participation. A simple sum of the scores of the items across all the domains can be used to describe the degree of functional limitations. A more complex level of scoring can be adopted to enable comparison to the data on population norms. When tested in the critical care population, it was observed to be a reliable, valid, and responsive measure of disability.[29] It has been shown to correlate well with physical function measures in the critical care population, ranking better than other self-reported outcome measures such as the EQ-5D.[30]

ADDITIONAL OUTCOMES
Chelsea Critical Care Physical Assessment Tool

The Chelsea Critical Care Physical Assessment Tool (CPAx) was developed to assess physical and respiratory function in critically ill adults and has been validated as a tool to assist in the identification of patients at risk of developing ICU acquired weakness.[31] The CPAx can be used throughout a patients stay on critical care and after discharge from the unit to track their recovery. It assesses 10 domains: respiratory function, cough, moving within the bed, supine to sitting on the edge of the bed, dynamic sitting, standing balance, sit to stand, transferring bed to chair, stepping, and grip strength. It can be used to aid discussion as a multidisciplinary team (MDT) and with family about progression or regression in the critical care environment and can help focus rehabilitation plans, which have been shown to improve physical function.[32] It has demonstrated good validity when predicting place of residence at 90 d post-ICU discharge; however, this predictive validity was not demonstrated with regard to health-related quality-of-life.[33] It did, however, demonstrate good predictive validity for critical care length-of-stay and duration of mechanical ventilation when an assessment took place between 72 and 144 hr of mechanical ventilation.[33]

Post-intensive Care Presentation and Screening and Post-intensive Care Presentation and Screening-Community

The Post-intensive Care Presentation and Screening (PICUPS) Tool can be used to inform the rehabilitation needs after treatment in the critical care environment by identifying areas that are likely to require further assessment/treatment by members of the MDT. It can be used at an individual patient level to guide decision-making and inform rehabilitation plans, as well as at population level to enable understanding of shortfalls in service provision and aid future planning. It covers 5 main domains (with 3 additional in the PICUPS plus items): medical care, breathing/nutrition, physical movement, communication/cognition, and psychosocial (upper airway, physical and ADLs, and symptoms that interfere with daily activities). An adaptation of this tool is the PICUPS-Community, which works off the same foundations but is a self-reported measure to be used with the critical care population once they have been discharged into the community. It covers similar areas but groups questions into 4 domains: Breathing, upper airway and nutrition, Physical activities of everyday living, Symptoms and interferences with activities and Communication, cognition and psychosocial.

The PICUPS tool is for use in the hospital setting and is to be performed by healthcare professionals as a checklist. The PICUPS-Community is for use in the community and is a self-reported tool, which can subsequently be evaluated by a healthcare professional as a screening tool.

This tool is for use on the adult critical care population as a way of screening for post-intensive care syndrome It has been shown to have good utility amongst the MDT, reported as reflecting the patient's needs at that point in their journey.[34,35] Currently, we do not understand its predictive validity.

EXPLORATORY OUTCOMES

While standardized outcome measurements are important to ensure consistent reporting of essential outcomes and minimize bias from selective outcome reporting, they are not intended to be a limit. Additional outcomes are often appropriate and can provide novel insights into disease pathophysiology and treatment response. Surrogate outcomes developed through exploratory methods may enable intervention at an earlier stage in the development of functional disability, with the potential for prevention rather than management of the sequalae of muscle weakness (**Fig. 2**). Outcomes may also be highly informative but not feasible on a large scale, due to training or resources required for measurement.

Urea-creatinine Ratio

Survival is an essential outcome in most core outcome sets relating to critical illness. Biochemical markers associated with increased or reduced risk of mortality are therefore valuable outcome measures to explore. One such marker is the urea-creatinine ratio (UCR), which may be amenable to nutritional or metabolic interventions. Inability to utilize exogenous and endogenous amino acids results in decreased protein synthesis, and these amino acids may be oxidized, raising serum urea. Deamination of amino acids arising from protein breakdown may further contribute to hepatic urea synthesis. Muscle wasting and reduced muscle mass decreases serum creatinine,

PREVENTION AND TREATMENT OF ACQUIRED FUNCTIONAL DISABILITY

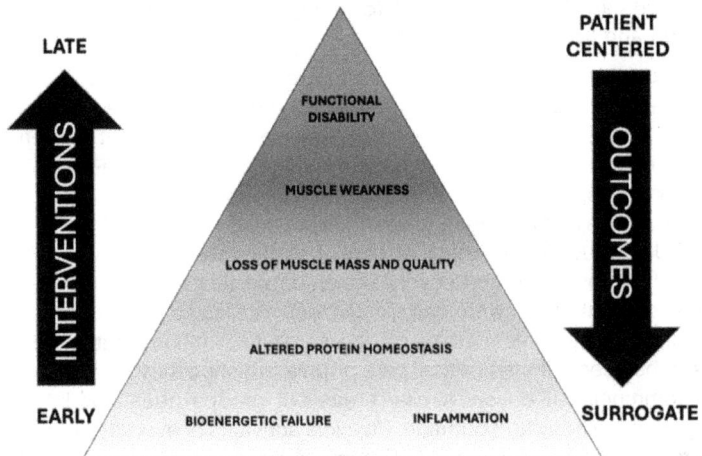

Fig. 2. Representation of the key features of critical illness, and the interventions and outcomes required to investigate these.

thereby altering the UCR. An elevated UCR is a biochemical signature of catabolism associated with prolonged critical illness.[36]

In a study of polytrauma patients admitted to ICU, UCR was found to be a more discriminative marker of persistent need for intensive care (defined as beyond 10 d) than premorbid characteristics or other biologic characteristics such as persistent inflammation or relative immunosuppression.[36–38] This finding was replicated in further data sets (MIMIC-III), in which UCR discriminated both persistent critical illness and differing ICU length-of-stay.[39] A rising UCR was found to correlate with lower muscle mass on serial imaging, supporting the biologic relevance of the UCR. Re-analysis of a trial investigating glutamine supplementation in critical illness (REDOXS) found that a higher UCR trajectory was associated with greater mortality risk, which remained after adjustment for development of organ failure over the time course of critical illness.[40,41]

Metabolomic Data

Metabolomics refers to the study of the products of metabolism at a cellular, tissue, or circulating level, and provides a functional view of an individual's metabolic state.[42] Many factors influence the metabolome, including environmental factors such as nutrient and drug delivery, cellular function, and disease state. It is, therefore, of potential value in assisting diagnosis of disease, prediction of response to an intervention, and monitoring of a response. Many disease states common to critical care, such as sepsis and acute respiratory disease syndrome, have been resistant to novel interventions and management remains largely supportive, alongside treatment of any underlying infection.[43] Re-analyses of negative trials have found subgroups of patients that appear to respond to interventions, highlighting the need to better identify markers indicative of treatment responsiveness.[44,45] The metabolome offers a potential tool for this identification, in addition to defining biologic biomarkers of disease and enhancing mechanistic understanding of pathophysiologic processes. Lactate is a metabolic product, which has historically been used in critical care trials to monitor response to treatment or to aid prognostication.[43,46,47] Outcomes which include more detailed analyses of the metabolome are interesting to explore as the evidence base expands.

The development of high-resolution accurate mass spectrometry, alongside expanding big data analytical tools, is crucial in the expansion of personalized and precision nutritional support.[48] In the Alternative Substrates in the Critically Ill Subject (ASICS) study, investigating a novel ketogenic feed, plasma metabolomic analyses were used to identify differential metabolite abundance in the ketogenic feeding arm compared to controls.[49] This is beneficial firstly in identifying a clear separation of treatment arms at the end of the intervention, and secondly in identifying metabolic profiles that are potentially associated with better outcomes, giving insight into the metabolic processes induced by ketogenic enteral feeding.

Intermittent versus continuous feeding in critically-ill patients has gained increased interest in nutritional research, with intermittent feeding potentially benefitting circadian rhythm and sleep, and influencing ghrelin secretion, insulin resistance, and autophagy.[50] In contrast to the clear trial arm separation in the ASICS trial, investigation of the metabolite features of intermittent, and continuously found that there was no difference in metabolite patterns over time between the 2 groups.[50] This suggests that the metabolism of critically unwell patients is not significantly affected by the feeding regime; however, there may be other clinical benefits of intermittent feeding not examined in this study.

Metabolic signatures of septic patients have been studied to investigate their potential for prognostication. In a retrospective analysis of the Community Acquired

Pneumonia and Sepsis Outcome Diagnostics study, levels of proteins involved in fatty acid transport and β-oxidation, gluconeogenesis, and the citric acid cycle were significantly higher in patients who died.[51] The predictive value of these metabolic features was then validated in an independent cohort. Identifying reliable predictors of morbidity and mortality would be hugely beneficial in critical to aid treatment planning and prognostication.

Assessment of Muscle Wasting

Given the association of muscle wasting with many important outcomes including ICU length-of-stay, ICU and hospital mortality, acquired weakness and numerous functional outcomes, quantification of muscle wasting, and the rate of muscle mass loss is highly valuable. Ultrasound and computed tomography (CT) at different time points have been used in conjunction with ratio of protein to DNA, histopathologic analyses, bioelectrical impedance analysis, and UCR.[52] The commonly assessed muscles are the rectus femoris, quadriceps and biceps brachii, measuring cross-sectional area, or thickness. Of note, studies measuring both rectus femoris and bicep brachii cross-sectional area and thickness found that the thickness measurement can significantly underestimate muscle loss compared with cross-sectional area.[53–55]

Ultrasound is more commonly used than CT, likely reflective of the risks of transferring critically-ill patients to the scanner compared to the relative ease of bedside ultrasound scanning. Interobserver correlation for quantitative analysis of muscle parameters shows ultrasound to be a reliable method (intraclass correlation coefficient >0.75); however, methodologic variability may limit comparisons between studies.[56] Inconsistency in measurement methods and time points for measurement limits meta-analyses of studies investigating the rate of muscle loss and quantification of muscle wasting, which should be addressed as the evidence base expands in line with the CONCISE Delphi consensus.

SUMMARY

Outcomes in critical care need to encompass comparable outcomes as defined in the Core Outcome Sets, while enabling research groups to explore new associations and develop techniques for capturing novel outcomes. The primary core outcome relevant to all stakeholders in critical illness is physical function, and outcomes directly measuring this or acting as surrogate measures should continue to inform the development of critical illness research trials.

CLINICS CARE POINTS

- Physical function a key outcome measure recognised by all stakeholders in critical illness.
- Important outcomes relevant to physical function range from clinical measures of functional disability and muscle weakness, to surrogate markers of altered protein homeostasis, inflammation and bioenergetic failure.
- Exploratory outcomes such as urea-to-creatinine ratio and metabolomic data provide novel insights into critical illness pathophysiology.

DISCLOSURE

Z. Puthucheary has received honoraria for consultancy from Nestle, Nutriticia, BioAge, Faraday Pharmaceuticals and Fresenius-Kabi, and speaker fees from Baxter,

Fresenius-Kabi, Nutriticia, Sedana and Nestle. Z. Puthucheary is a named inventor for a ketogenic feed with a patent submission.

REFERENCES

1. Davies TW, van Gassel RJJ, van de Poll M, et al. Core outcome measures for clinical effectiveness trials of nutritional and metabolic interventions in critical illness: an international modified Delphi consensus study evaluation (CONCISE). Crit Care 2022;26(1):240.
2. Kirkham JJ, Williamson P. Core outcome sets in medical research. BMJ Med 2022;1(1):e000284.
3. Chan AW, Song F, Vickers A, et al. Increasing value and reducing waste: addressing inaccessible research. Lancet 2014;383(9913):257–66.
4. Puthucheary ZA, Astin R, McPhail MJW, et al. Metabolic phenotype of skeletal muscle in early critical illness. Thorax 2018;73(10):926–35.
5. Bear DE, Parry SM, Puthucheary ZA. Can the critically ill patient generate sufficient energy to facilitate exercise in the ICU? Curr Opin Clin Nutr Metab Care 2018;21(2):110–5.
6. Heyland DK, Patel J, Compher C, et al. The effect of higher protein dosing in critically ill patients with high nutritional risk (EFFORT Protein): an international, multicentre, pragmatic, registry-based randomised trial. Lancet 2023;401(10376):568–76.
7. Partnerships JLAPS. Available at: https://www.jla.nihr.ac.uk/priority-setting-partnerships/intensive-care/top-10-priorities/. Accessed May 20, 2024.
8. Bear DE, Puthucheary ZA. Designing nutrition-based interventional trials for the future: addressing the known knowns. Crit Care 2019;1:53.
9. Wright SE, Thomas K, Watson G, et al. Intensive versus standard physical rehabilitation therapy in the critically ill (EPICC): a multicentre, parallel-group, randomised controlled trial. Thorax 2018;73(3):213–21.
10. Puthucheary ZA, Gensichen JS, Cakiroglu AS, et al. Implications for post critical illness trial design: sub-phenotyping trajectories of functional recovery among sepsis survivors. Crit Care 2020;24(1):577.
11. O'Grady HK, Edbrooke L, Farley C, et al. The sit-to-stand test as a patient-centered functional outcome for critical care research: a pooled analysis of five international rehabilitation studies. Crit Care 2022;26(1):175.
12. Files D, Morris P, Shrestha S, et al. Randomized, controlled pilot study of early rehabilitation strategies in acute respiratory failure. Crit Care 2013;Suppl 2(P540). Copyright © 2013 Files et al.; licensee BioMed Central Ltd.
13. Dinglas VD, Cherukuri SPS, Needham DM. Core outcomes sets for studies evaluating critical illness and patient recovery. Curr Opin Crit Care 2020;26(5):489–99.
14. Levy D, Giannini M, Oulehri W, et al. Long term follow-up of sarcopenia and malnutrition after hospitalization for COVID-19 in conventional or intensive care units. Nutrients 2022;14(4).
15. Shahbazi S, Hajimohammadebrahim-Ketabforoush M, Vahdat Shariatpanahi M, et al. The validity of the global leadership initiative on malnutrition criteria for diagnosing malnutrition in critically ill patients with COVID-19: a prospective cohort study. Clin Nutr ESPEN 2021;43:377–82.
16. Cui M, Zhang S, Liu Y, et al. Grip strength and the risk of cognitive decline and dementia: a systematic review and meta-analysis of longitudinal cohort studies. Front Aging Neurosci 2021;13:625551.

17. Wiśniowska-Szurlej A, Ćwirlej-Sozańska A, Wołoszyn N, et al. Association between handgrip strength, mobility, leg strength, flexibility, and postural balance in older adults under long-term care facilities. BioMed Res Int 2019;2019: 1042834.
18. Miljkovic N, Lim JY, Miljkovic I, et al. Aging of skeletal muscle fibers. Ann Rehabil Med 2015;39(2):155–62.
19. Porto JM, Nakaishi APM, Cangussu-Oliveira LM, et al. Relationship between grip strength and global muscle strength in community-dwelling older people. Arch Gerontol Geriatr 2019;82:273–8.
20. Leong DP, Teo KK, Rangarajan S, et al. Prognostic value of grip strength: findings from the Prospective Urban Rural Epidemiology (PURE) study. Lancet 2015; 386(9990):266–73.
21. Ali NA, O'Brien JM, Hoffmann SP, et al. Acquired weakness, handgrip strength, and mortality in critically ill patients. Am J Respir Crit Care Med 2008;178(3): 261–8.
22. Bragança RD, Ravetti CG, Barreto L, et al. Use of handgrip dynamometry for diagnosis and prognosis assessment of intensive care unit acquired weakness: a prospective study. Heart Lung 2019;48(6):532–7.
23. Needham DM, Sepulveda KA, Dinglas VD, et al. Core outcome measures for clinical research in acute respiratory failure survivors. an international modified delphi consensus study. Am J Respir Crit Care Med 2017;196(9):1122–30.
24. Docherty C, Shaw M, Henderson P, et al. Evaluating pain in survivors of critical illness: the correlation between the EQ-5D-5L and the Brief Pain Inventory. BMJ Open Respir Res 2023;10(1). https://doi.org/10.1136/bmjresp-2022-001426.
25. Feng YS, Kohlmann T, Janssen MF, et al. Psychometric properties of the EQ-5D-5L: a systematic review of the literature. Qual Life Res 2021;30(3):647–73.
26. Granja C, Teixeira-Pinto A, Costa-Pereira A. Quality of life after intensive care–evaluation with EQ-5D questionnaire. Intensive Care Med 2002;28(7):898–907.
27. Needham DM. Understanding and improving clinical trial outcome measures in acute respiratory failure. Am J Respir Crit Care Med 2014;189(8):875–7.
28. Spies CD, Krampe H, Paul N, et al. Instruments to measure outcomes of post-intensive care syndrome in outpatient care settings - results of an expert consensus and feasibility field test. J Intensive Care Soc 2021;22(2):159–74.
29. Higgins AM, Neto AS, Bailey M, et al. The psychometric properties and minimal clinically important difference for disability assessment using WHODAS 2.0 in critically ill patients. Crit Care Resusc 2021;23(1):103–12.
30. Paton M, Lane R, Paul E, et al. Correlation of patient-reported outcome measures to performance-based function in critical care survivors: predictable. Aust Crit Care 2023;36(4):485–91.
31. Corner EJ, Wood H, Englebretsen C, et al. The Chelsea critical care physical assessment tool (CPAx): validation of an innovative new tool to measure physical morbidity in the general adult critical care population; an observational proof-of-concept pilot study. Physiotherapy 2013;99(1):33–41.
32. Whelan M, van Aswegen H, Corner E. Impact of the Chelsea critical care physical assessment (CPAx) tool on clinical outcomes of surgical and trauma patients in an intensive care unit: an experimental study. S Afr J Physiother 2018;74(1):450.
33. Eggmann S, Verra ML, Stefanicki V, et al. Predictive validity of the chelsea critical care physical assessment tool (CPAx) in critically ill, mechanically ventilated adults: a prospective clinimetric study. Disabil Rehabil 2023;45(1):111–6.
34. Turner-Stokes L, Corner EJ, Siegert RJ, et al. The post-ICU presentation screen (PICUPS) and rehabilitation prescription (RP) for intensive care survivors part I:

development and preliminary clinimetric evaluation. J Intensive Care Soc 2022; 23(3):253–63.

35. Puthucheary Z, Brown C, Corner E, et al. The Post-ICU presentation screen (PI-CUPS) and rehabilitation prescription (RP) for intensive care survivors part II: clinical engagement and future directions for the national Post-Intensive care Rehabilitation Collaborative. J Intensive Care Soc 2022;23(3):264–72.

36. Haines RW, Zolfaghari P, Wan Y, et al. Elevated urea-to-creatinine ratio provides a biochemical signature of muscle catabolism and persistent critical illness after major trauma. Intensive Care Med 2019;45(12):1718–31.

37. Pradhan S, Ghimire A, Bhattarai B, et al. The role of C-reactive protein as a diagnostic predictor of sepsis in a multidisciplinary intensive care unit of a tertiary care center in Nepal. Indian J Crit Care Med 2016;20(7):417–20.

38. Boomer JS, To K, Chang KC, et al. Immunosuppression in patients who die of sepsis and multiple organ failure. JAMA 2011;306(23):2594–605.

39. Johnson AE, Pollard TJ, Shen L, et al. MIMIC-III, a freely accessible critical care database. Sci Data 2016;3:160035.

40. Heyland D, Muscedere J, Wischmeyer PE, et al. A randomized trial of glutamine and antioxidants in critically ill patients. N Engl J Med 2013;368(16):1489–97.

41. Haines RW, Fowler AJ, Wan YI, et al. Catabolism in critical illness: a reanalysis of the reducing deaths due to oxidative stress (REDOXS) trial. Crit Care Med 2022; 50(7):1072–82.

42. Christopher KB. Nutritional metabolomics in critical illness. Curr Opin Clin Nutr Metab Care 2018;21(2):121–5.

43. Pacheco-Navarro AE, Rogers AJ. The metabolomics of critical illness. Handb Exp Pharmacol 2023;277:367–84.

44. Calfee CS, Delucchi K, Parsons PE, et al. Subphenotypes in acute respiratory distress syndrome: latent class analysis of data from two randomised controlled trials. Lancet Respir Med 2014;2(8):611–20.

45. Puskarich MA, Jennaro TS, Gillies CE, et al. Pharmacometabolomics identifies candidate predictor metabolites of an L-carnitine treatment mortality benefit in septic shock. Clin Transl Sci 2021;14(6):2288–99.

46. Jansen TC, van Bommel J, Schoonderbeek FJ, et al. Early lactate-guided therapy in intensive care unit patients: a multicenter, open-label, randomized controlled trial. Am J Respir Crit Care Med 2010;182(6):752–61.

47. Mikkelsen ME, Miltiades AN, Gaieski DF, et al. Serum lactate is associated with mortality in severe sepsis independent of organ failure and shock. Crit Care Med 2009;37(5):1670–7.

48. Li K, Tong HHY, Chen Y, et al. The emerging roles of next-generation metabolomics in critical care nutrition. Crit Rev Food Sci Nutr 2024;64(5):1213–24.

49. McNelly A, Langan A, Bear DE, et al. A pilot study of alternative substrates in the critically Ill subject using a ketogenic feed. Nat Commun 2023;14(1):8345.

50. Wilkinson D, Gallagher IJ, McNelly A, et al. The metabolic effects of intermittent versus continuous feeding in critically ill patients. Sci Rep 2023;13(1):19508.

51. Langley RJ, Tipper JL, Bruse S, et al. Integrative "omic" analysis of experimental bacteremia identifies a metabolic signature that distinguishes human sepsis from systemic inflammatory response syndromes. Am J Respir Crit Care Med 2014; 190(4):445–55.

52. Fazzini B, Märkl T, Costas C, et al. The rate and assessment of muscle wasting during critical illness: a systematic review and meta-analysis. Crit Care 2023; 27(1):2.

53. Puthucheary ZA, McNelly AS, Rawal J, et al. Rectus femoris cross-sectional area and muscle layer thickness: comparative markers of muscle wasting and weakness. Am J Respir Crit Care Med 2017;195(1):136–8.
54. Nakanishi N, Oto J, Tsutsumi R, et al. Upper and lower limb muscle atrophy in critically ill patients: an observational ultrasonography study. Intensive Care Med 2018;2:263–4.
55. Parry SM, El-Ansary D, Cartwright MS, et al. Ultrasonography in the intensive care setting can be used to detect changes in the quality and quantity of muscle and is related to muscle strength and function. J Crit Care 2015;30(5). 1151.e9-e14.
56. Sarwal A, Parry SM, Berry MJ, et al. Interobserver reliability of quantitative muscle sonographic analysis in the critically ill population. J Ultrasound Med 2015;34(7): 1191–200.

Recent Insights into the Evolving Role of the Gut Microbiome in Critical Care

Seoho Lee, BA[a], Paul E. Wischmeyer, MD[b],
Cyrus D. Mintz, MD, PhD[a], Mara A. Serbanescu, MD[b],*

KEYWORDS

- Microbiome • Critical care • Nutrition • Gut hyperpermeability
- Bacterial extracellular vesicles

KEY POINTS

- *Impact of ICU Environment on Gut Microbiota*: Acute illness and ICU exposures, such as inflammation, nutrient deprivation, and antibiotics, disrupt the gut microbiota, leading to a loss of beneficial microbes and an increase in pathogenic species, which are linked to higher mortality and infections.
- *Need for Tailored Treatments*: The lack of efficacy in current microbiome interventions may stem from their non-specific application across diverse ICU patients. Understanding microbial dynamics and unique dysbiotic states during ICU stays is crucial for developing effective, tailored therapies.
- *Microbiota Impact on Gut Barrier and Immune Activation*: Inflammation and ICU-induced microbiota changes weaken gut barrier defenses, contributing to the translocation of immune-activating microbial components and secondary infections.
- *Research Focus Areas*: Future studies should clarify how gut microbiota influence critical illness, identify the impact of patient-specific factors and the ICU environment, and develop therapies that address or account for the disturbances in gut microbial communities and barrier integrity unique to ICU patients.

INTRODUCTION

Over the past decade, there has been an exponential increase in our understanding of crucial roles played by the human microbiota (ie, complex community of bacteria, fungi, and other microbes residing throughout the human body), and their collective

[a] Department of Anesthesiology and Critical Care, Johns Hopkins University School of Medicine, Phipps 455 1800 Orleans Street, Baltimore, MD 21212, USA; [b] Department of Anesthesiology, Duke University School of Medicine, 5692 HAFS Box 3094, 2301 Erwin Road, Durham, NC 27710, USA
* Corresponding author. Duke University Hospital, 5692 HAFS Box 3094, 2301 Erwin Road, Durham, NC 27710.
E-mail address: Mara.serbanescu@duke.edu

Crit Care Clin 41 (2025) 379–396
https://doi.org/10.1016/j.ccc.2024.11.002
0749-0704/25/Published by Elsevier Inc.

criticalcare.theclinics.com

genomes (ie, microbiome). With increasing accessibility of tools to study microbiota structures and functions, explorations of how the microbiota regulate host responses to impact disease susceptibility, severity, and response to therapy have permeated nearly all disciplines of health. For example, changes in the microbiota are responsible for conditions such as Crohn's Disease, *Clostridium Difficile* Infection (CDI), periodontitis, and bacterial vaginosis, and microbiota-targeted therapies that ameliorate microbial derangements are already in use in clinical practice.[1] However, while most critically-ill patients demonstrate pathologic disruption of gut microbial communities (a state referred to as dysbiosis), developing microbiota-targeted interventions for use in the intensive care unit (ICU) remains an unmet challenge and a possible opportunity to improve care for vulnerable patients. Despite clinical benefits observed in various conditions in non-critically ill patients, the currently extant therapeutic trials of prebiotics and pro/synbiotics have had inconsistent effects on mortality and most other outcomes in the ICU. As case in point, the largest randomized controlled trial (RCT) to date assessing the impact of probiotics on ventilator-associated pneumonia failed to show a clinical benefit.[2] Subsequently, a comprehensive meta-analysis of RCTs with trial sequential analysis concluded that there is little value in conducting additional studies of pro/synbiotics in critically-ill patients due to little anticipated gain.[3] Accompanying concern for lack of benefit, reports of extra-intestinal seeding after live microbial therapeutics have understandably lessened excitement for these interventions as potential therapeutic options.[4] However, rather than being viewed as evidence of treatment failure, these findings simply underscore the complexity of host-microbe interactions in the context of critical illness, and our currently incomplete understanding of these processes. It is challenging to delineate relevant mechanisms of microbiome-related pathology (and therapeutic targets) in the ICU when a plethora of factors contribute to dynamic changes in the microbiome, which often happen simultaneously with changes in clinical condition.

Geared to clinicians and scientists alike, this review aims to highlight our evolving understanding of microbiota-mediated responses that may impact clinical trajectory in critical illness, while underscoring gaps in knowledge and their implications. We begin with a background discussion of the gut microbiota in states of health and critical illness. Then, we continue with an examination of dynamic factors in critical illness that account for characteristic changes within the ICU gut microbiota, highlighting the crucial role of ecological interactions within the gut microbial community and disturbances rendered by ICU exposures. Lastly, we discuss the downstream consequences of these disturbances, examining several mechanisms by which changes in the ICU gut microbiota may cause injury and impact clinical trajectory. Ultimately, we aim to provide readers with a more nuanced understanding of the clinical relevance of the gut microbiota in ICU patients, which both accounts for current challenges faced in clinical trials of microbiota therapeutics, and suggest a path forward for this potentially valuable treatment approach.

The Healthy Human Gut Microbiome and Dysbiosis in the Intensive Care Unit

In states of health, the human gut microbiome (HGM) is comprised of roughly 100 trillion bacteria that occupy the gastrointestinal (GI) tract. Of these, over 99% are obligate anaerobes and require specific growth conditions provided by the intestinal microenvironment.[5] As a result, only a fraction of gut microbes (estimated 20%–30%) can be grown using routinely used in clinical microbiology laboratories.[6] With the development of culture-independent techniques in the past 2 decades, and increasingly advanced bioinformatics pipelines, researchers are now able to characterize these microbes and begin to understand how they interact with their host and environment to regulate health and disease. In clinical microbiome studies, the most widely used characterization approaches are amplicon techniques, which provide information on the relative abundance of a microbe (generally to the genus or species level) based on recognition of a marker gene and its surrounding sequences. Commonly used examples include 16S ribosomal RNA (rRNA) sequencing, which leverages identification of the 16 rRNA gene sequence universally expressed by bacteria and some archeobacteria, and internal transcribed spacer sequencing for identification of the fungal species.[7] "Shotgun sequencing" or whole genome metagenomic approaches provide additional resolution into functional gene expression, including those of antimicrobial resistance (ie, "the resistome"), while other -omics techniques can identify products derived from the microbiota (ie, microbiota-derived metabolites by metabolomics).[8]

Though every individual's HGM is unique, there are universal trends characterized by a tendency toward homeostasis.[9] For example, in states of good health, over 90% of these microbes belong to the phyla Bacillota (formerly Firmicutes), and Bacteroidota (formerly Bacteroidetes), while the remaining 10% are classified as Actinomycetota (Actinobacteria), Pseudomonadota (Proteobacteria), Verrucomicrobiota (Verrucomicrobia), and Fusobacteriota (Fusobacteria).[10] Despite high inter-individual variation, at the genus-level, a set of 15 to 20 genera—again, primarily represented by Bacillota and Bacteroidota—are noted to be highly prevalent across healthy populations, and are major regulators of key homeostatic functions like the modulation of immune responses, maintenance of gut barrier, and regulation of metabolic processes.[1] Gut microbes regulate these functions through direct actions on intestinal epithelial and immune cells, and via secreted components including small molecule metabolites, immunomodulatory compounds, extra-cellular vesicles, and neurotransmitters and hormones that enter the lymph and circulation and signal to peripheral immune cells.[11] Importantly, many species within the HGM have overlapping functional repertoires, often working synergistically to maintain these key homeostatic processes.[12] Thus, both the loss of certain microbes, and widespread disruption of the gut microbial community (ie, following antibiotic depletion), have been shown to have profound implications on derangements in host responses relevant to the critically-ill patient. For example, Lachnospiraceae and Ruminococcaceae spp. metabolize undigested fibers to produce short-chain fatty acids (SCFAs), like butyrate, acetate, and propionate, which serve as energy sources for intestinal epithelial cells (IECs) and modulate systemic immune cell activation and differentiation through inhibition of histone deacetylases and signaling to G-protein coupled receptors.[13] Additionally, leukocyte differentiation, activation, and cytokine responses can be mediated by tryptophan derivatives, secondary bile acids, and other microbiota-derived metabolites, as well as by polyamines and molecules produced de-novo by certain commensals.[11]

In contrast to the healthy HGM, it is now well-established that critically ill patients exhibit profound and deleterious changes in gut microbial composition, which have negative consequences on host responses (ie, dysbiosis).[14–18] Dysbiosis is observed within 48 h of admission and progress over the first weeks of ICU stay, with further remodeling throughout the course of treatment and recovery. Characteristic features of ICU-associated dysbiosis include a loss of the total number of species, and depletion of prevalent health-promoting commensals including Bifidobacterium and species from the Lachnospiraceae and Ruminococcaceae family, including Faecalibacterium, Ruminococcus, Roseburia, among others that all perform key immunoregulatory roles[19] (Fig. 1). Indeed, studies measuring functional profiles demonstrate corresponding reductions in fecal SCFAs and changes in serum microbiota-derived metabolites.[16,20,21] The loss of these beneficial microbes almost always co-occurs with expansion of gut microbes with high pathogenic potential (pathobionts) like members

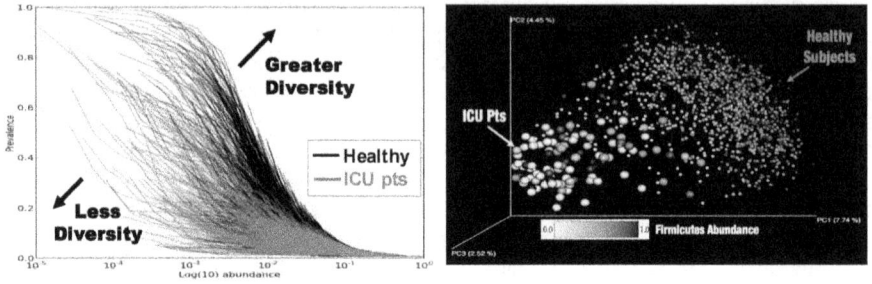

Fig. 1. The intensive care unit (ICU) gut microbiota features a reduction in biodiversity and loss of Firmicutes (ie, Bacillota by current nomenclature). Panels depict unpublished work from landmark study by McDonald *et al.* that used 16S rRNA sequencing of fecal samples from 162 ICU patients and 199 healthy controls from the American Gut Project (AGP) to identify significant changes in the gut microbiota throughout ICU stay. Left panel demonstrates differences in diversity. Right panel demonstrates Principal-coordinate (PC) plot of distributions of Firmicutes representation (vast majority belonging to the Clostridiales order) among ICU patients (n = 135 samples) and healthy patients (n = 2640 samples) with sphere color denoting relative abundance within each sample. (*Data used with permission from* Dr McDonald and Dr Knight; see reference #15 for full article.)

of the *Enterobacteriaceae* family (*Escherichia Coli [E. coli], Klebsiella Pneumonia*), *Enterococcus* species, *Clostridium Difficile*, and *Candida* spp., many of which express genes associated with antimicrobial resistance.[22–24] In fact, expansion of 1 or multiple pathobionts is often reported to be a feature of over half of included patients.[25,26] For example, *Enterobacteriaceae* and/or *Enterococcus* spp., which ordinarily represent less than 1% of the HGM in healthy patients,[9,27] are frequently reported to occupy 10% to 80% of the gut microbial community in ICU patients.

The potential negative consequences of ICU-associated dysbiosis have been elucidated by studies demonstrating that several of these features—either present on admission or emerging during ICU stay—are uniquely associated with clinical outcomes. In particular, increased mortality and risk of secondary infection has been repeatedly observed in patients with a high intestinal burden of *Enterococcus* (genus) or colonization with vancomycin-resistant *Enterococcus*,[17,19,22,28] as well as those with progressive enrichment of *Enterobacteriaceae* (family).[17,26,28,29] Though less frequently reproduced, reduced abundances of SCFA-producers (*Faecalibacterium prausnitzii, Blautia* spp, and *Bifidobacterium*), reduced concentrations of fecal SCFAs, and alterations in the composition of *Candida* spp. (mycobiome) have also been implicated in morbidity and mortality.[18,30,31] This body of work has been foundational to our understanding of harmful versus protective gut microbial features, and while many are mentioned herein, comprehensive assessments of ICU-associated dysbiosis and clinical outcomes have been the focus of several excellent recent reviews.[32–34] What remains less well-understood are the specific mechanisms by which different elements of disease progression and corresponding medical care, which change over time during a patient's course in the ICU in ways that are unique for each patient but do fall into some predictable patterns, contribute to these dysbiotic changes.

DYNAMIC FACTORS CONTRIBUTING TO CHANGES IN MICROBIAL COMPOSITION IN THE INTENSIVE CARE UNIT

Intensive care is highly dynamic and involves numerous elements of both disease and medical care that alter the gut microbiota composition such that its role in maintaining homeostatic healthy physiology across multiple organ systems is compromised. What follows forthcoming is primarily a discussion of the effects of inflammation, nutrient deprivation, and antimicrobial therapy as they pertain to intensive care. These topics are by no means a comprehensive list of factors in the ICU that are relevant to microbiome health, but they represent critical elements for which we have some direct evidence and some extrapolated data that define them as productive areas of further research.

Inflammation

Hyperinflammatory states are nearly universal in intensive care patients, and although they vary widely in the specifics, all are predicted to have profound effects on the gut microbiota. Several studies of the ICU microbiome have demonstrated evidence of dysbiosis—namely, *Enterobacteriaceae* expansion and loss of SCFA-producers—even prior to administration of antimicrobials, suggesting that intrinsic changes in the microbiota may accompany critical illness.[19,26,35] Though pinpointing a definitive cause is challenging in patients, abundant data from preclinical models demonstrate that inflammation itself may be responsible for these early derangements. Gut inflammation from various etiologies (eg, infection, chemically-induced colitis, and immunosuppression) has been shown to alter the intestinal microenvironment in several ways, all of which provide a more favorable environment for pathobionts.[36] For example, inflammation induces hypoxia in the intestinal mucosa but increases luminal oxygen concentration, which in turn favors growth of facultative anaerobes including *Enterobacteriaceae*, *Enterococcus,* and other pathobionts.[37] Further, signaling by proinflammatory cytokines promotes the release of reactive oxygen and nitrogen species by IECs and migrating neutrophils; the nitrate-rich environment can be leveraged by *Enterobacteriaceae,* which are capable of nitrate respiration, but not by commensal Bacteroidiales and Clostridiales spp. (which lack expression of nitrate reduction).[38,39] Inflammation additionally alters nutrient availability in the GI microenvironment, and iron, zinc, and lipid byproducts (released from dying epithelial cells) can all be preferentially used by commensal and opportunistic *Enterobacteriaceae* for growth.[37,40] However, expansion of *Enterobacteriaceae* under these conditions is not always harmful. In fact, the ability of commensal *E. coli* to perform aerobic respiration is crucial to mediating protection against colonizing *Salmonella enteritica* serovars, a subset of pathogenic *Enterobacteriaceae*.[41,42] Importantly, this protective effect was further traced to the ability of commensal *E. Coli* to outcompete *Salmonella* not only for oxygen, but also for access to substrates liberated by co-occurring Clostridiales species in a study using assembled HGM communities.[43] Taken together, these studies suggest that inflammation may account for changes in the microbiota observed early in ICU course and serve to "prime" the intestinal microenvironment to favor the expansion of certain species (namely, pathobionts). However, they also underscore the importance of community membership and interactions like cross-feeding, and the distinction between commensal and opportunistic *Enterobacteriaceae*—recurring themes throughout this review.

Nutrient Availability and Implications of Enteral Nutrient Deprivation

Changes in diet significantly alter the gut microbiota, and absence of nutrition, and micro/macronutrients provided are additional environmental factors, which likely shape the ICU gut microbiota dynamically over the course of illness and care. Prolonged periods of enteral nutrient deprivation are common in ICU patients, and have previously been shown to impact gut barrier defenses and reduce abundances of beneficial microbes like *Bifidobacterium* and *Ruminococcaceae*.[44–46] In the past years, alterations in microbial responses to dietary interventions, and the processes responsible for these changes, have been the focus of a growing body of literature. Increasingly, studies have demonstrated that abundances of beneficial gut microbes are shaped by the combined influences of 3 factors: (1) the carbohydrates available in the environment; (2) the metabolic capabilities of the specific microbe; and (3) metabolic interactions between the microbe and community members occupying the same ecologic niche.[47] For example, *Bacteroidaceae* are capable of efficiently metabolizing a wide range of diet- and host-derived carbohydrates (including mucins). This metabolic capacity not only assures resilience of *Bacteroidaceae* in environmental stress, but also provides growth substrates for other community members.[48] In contrast, beneficial Bacillota (*Lactobacillus, Lachnospiraceae and Ruminococcaceae* spp) and Actinomycetota (*Bifidobacterium*) have restrictive carbohydrate metabolizing capabilities, and thus rely on simple carbohydrates provided through diet or liberated by *Bacteroidaceae*.[49]

In settings of homeostasis, microbial composition is largely driven by a habitat-filtering process, and diets that provide a surplus of nutrients preferred by a subset of the community will increase the abundance of those species.[50] However, nutrient scarcity alters these dynamics, and instead favors survival and expansion of resilient and fast-growing species.[51] In a sequence of experiments using HGM communities, investigators demonstrated that while community architecture was maintained when simple carbohydrates were provided in excess, in environments where these resources were limited, *Bacteroidaceae* and *Enterobacteriaceae* spp. preferentially expanded, due to their abilities to outcompete *Lachnospiraceae* and *Ruminococcaceae*.[51] The investigators further showed that expansion of *Bacteroides* and *Enterobacteriaceae* was able to thrive in this nutrient-limited environment by forming a unique, mutually beneficial alliance based on metabolic cross-feeding. A similar context-dependent synergism between these microbes was also demonstrated in undernourished children who were subsequently provided a diet rich in carbohydrates but deficient in protein, with animal models further demonstrating that this gut microbial signature promoted intestinal inflammation.[52] These rules of community assembly likely have profound implications on gut microbial dynamics in the ICU—where both absent nutrition and undernutrition are nearly universal[46]—and may explain the loss of Bacillota observed in settings of nutrient deprivation, as well as other features observed in the ICU gut microbiota, including the coordinate expansion of *Bacteroides* and *Enterobacteriaceae* that has been demonstrated to be a feature of septic patients.[14] Metabolic preferences and community dynamics may also have implications on microbial responses to nutritional interventions. These ecological interactions, in the context of selection pressures faced in the ICU, may account for lack of consistent improvement in abundances of Bacillota and *Bifidobacterium* observed after fiber administration in the ICU[53] and mouse models of antibiotic-induced dysbiosis,[54] despite success in other settings. Indeed, in our own preliminary work,[55] we have observed that providing prebiotic supplementation with short-chain fructooligosaccharides in the setting of severe dysbiosis may provide a context-dependent advantage to *Bacteroides spp.*, further benefiting *Enterobacteriaceae* at the expense of less resilient commensals.

Antimicrobials

Treatment with antimicrobials, particularly periods of broad-spectrum coverage are an exceedingly common feature of ICU care and few patients pass through an ICU without some course of antibiotic treatment. While effects of host factors on the gut microbiota are largely based on conclusions from animal models, abundant studies in patients have demonstrated the pervasive effects of antimicrobials on the HGM. Indeed, antibiotics, even in healthy patients, have been shown to induce changes in the gut microbiota that mirror those observed in the ICU, namely: (1) a rapid decline in microbial diversity; (2) loss of key beneficial commensals; (3) increased representation of pathobionts; and (4) increased expression of virulence genes and emergence of antimicrobial-resistant organisms (AROs).[56] Patients receiving antibiotics repeatedly demonstrate a reduction in *Lachnospiraceae* and *Ruminococcaceae* species, as well as reductions in *Bacteroides* and *Bifidobacterium*, with concurrent increases in *Enterobacteriaceae* and other Proteobacteria, as well as *Enterococcus*.[56–59] Although the mechanisms of colonization resistance in humans are less well-defined, preclinical studies have demonstrated how disturbances in commensals contribute to expansion of pathobionts. For example, similar to selection pressures observed in inflammation, antibiotic depletion of butyrate-producing species increases the concentration of oxygen and contributes to expansion of *Enterobacteriaceae;* a finding that has been traced to the importance of butyrate in maintaining luminal hypoxia through its effects on colonocyte metabolism.[60] Inverse correlations between *Lachnospiraceae* (common butyrate producers) and *Enterobacteriaceae* have also been observed in critically-ill patients,[26] suggesting that at least some protective mechanisms are likely conserved across various host species.

Studies further incorporating metagenomic techniques demonstrate that selective pressures induced by antibiotics further promote emergence of AROs. Pathobionts often intrinsically express antimicrobial resistance genes (ARGs), and *Enterobacteriaceae* and *Enterococcus* have been shown to readily engage in horizontal gene transfer to assimilate ARGs from other community members.[37,61] As exposure to any antibiotic preferentially selects for the survival of bacteria resistant to its effect, pathobionts with ARGs are at an advantage and will out-survive other species. A major focus of ongoing research is identifying mechanisms of colonization resistance that can combat AROs. For instance, a recent study on carbapenem-resistant *Enterobacteriaceae* (CRE) found that the depletion of beneficial commensals induced by anti-anaerobic agents (eg, Piperacillin/Tazobactam, carbapenems, ciprofloxacin, and cephalosporins) allowed the preferential expansion of CRE. This expansion was linked to a loss of inhibitory microbiota-mediated metabolites and changes in nutrient availability.[62] Separately, a longitudinal study of multidrug-resistant *Enterobacteriaceae* (MDR-E) involving over 800 samples from 100 patients with acute leukemia identified specific cooperative interactions between *Lactobacillus rhamnosus* and Clostridiales spp. that prevented the expansion of MDR-E by creating a hostile environment for resistant strains through increased butyrate levels and reduced nutrient sources.[63]

Other Exposures

We cannot summarize all potential factors in the ICU that can cause dysbiosis, given the sheer number of possibilities and the lack of direct or extrapolated data; however, there is evidence that many other common features of ICU care would be expected to impact the gut microbiota. Some examples include the use of supplemental oxygen, opioid analgesics, proton-pump inhibitors, and anesthetics/sedatives, all of which have been shown to cause dysbiosis in different contexts.[60,64,65] Colonization and transmission of AROs is endemic in ICUs and may have a substantial effect on gut microbial communities. For example, a recent study exploring potential ARO sources throughout ICU surfaces and built environments demonstrated that sink drains within ICU rooms had the highest density of AROs. The investigators further demonstrated that several *P. aeruginosa* strains within these reservoirs could be detected in a subset of patient blood samples, suggesting movement of this clone between the environment and patients.[66] There are likely dozens, if not hundreds, of other elements of ICU care that can and do contribute to dysbiosis. This leads to the question of what the impact of poor microbiome health is on outcomes for patients undergoing intensive care.

MECHANISMS OF INJURY MEDIATED BY ICU-ASSOCIATED DYSBIOSIS

Growing evidence indicates that the derangements in the gut microbiota in the ICU (sustained by inflammation and/or effects of environmental exposures) modulate host responses in acute critical illness and phases of recovery. While there are numerous potential mechanisms, here we primarily focus on recent advances in understanding that impact the conceptualization of ICU-associated dysbiosis specifically as it pertains to gut barrier hyperpermeability, translocation of microbial components into circulation, and secondary infections. This is not a comprehensive list of key factors, and in particular we do not discuss the numerous potential effects of microbial-derived metabolites, an important topic that is well-studied outside the ICU setting and remains poorly understood in this context.[11,67]

Gut Barrier Hyperpermeability

Hyperpermeability of the gut barrier induced by inflammation is thought to play a central role in immune dysregulation and organ dysfunction in many infectious and non-infectious conditions encountered in the ICU (e,g, sepsis, acute respiratory distress syndrome, trauma, and pancreatitis).[68] Comprehensive reviews of intestinal barrier defenses have been published in greater details elsewhere,[69–71] and here we have focused on alterations in the physical barrier given accumulating recent research exploring the role of host-microbe interactions on gut barrier hyperpermeability. Specifically, independent of its effects on the gut microbiota, inflammation directly impairs both the physical and functional barriers in the GI tract, which ordinarily prevent entry of luminal factors (host- and microbe-derived molecules) into mesenteric lymph and circulation.[69] Gut hyperpermeability is a result of inflammation-induced insults to several physical barriers in the gut including mucin degradation, increased tight-junction mediated paracellular permeability, and IEC death.[69,71] IEC death, in particular, is induced in the presence of tumor necrosis factor (TNF)[72] and IL-13,[73] as well as programmed cell death networks, the last of which features prominently in the pathobiology of sepsis.[74] While the mechanisms of gut barrier hyperpermeability have only been clarified recently, the ramifications of impaired intestinal defenses on the potentiation of systemic inflammation date back to over 2 decades ago. Then, foundational studies demonstrated that gut-derived Microbial- or Pathogen-Associated Molecular Patterns (PAMPs) can signal to TLRs and other pattern recognition receptors on endothelial and immune cells within and outside the gut, inducing release of pro-inflammatory cytokines. The most well-known of these PAMPS is lipopolysaccharide (LPS), a glycoconjugate expressed by gram-negative bacteria consisting of a hydrophobic domain known as lipid A (or endotoxin), a non-repeating "core" oligosaccharide, and a distal polysaccharide (or O-antigen).[75] Landmark experiments using LPS derived from E. Coli have shown that in the setting of sepsis and other conditions of gut barrier hyperpermeability, LPS induces MyD88 and MyD88-independent pathways following binding of toll-like receptor 4 (TLR4) on systemic endothelial and immune cells, thus promoting release of pro-inflammatory cytokines and potentiating end-organ dysfunction.[76,77] Indeed, indirect evidence of gut barrier permeability has been demonstrated by elevations in serum markers of enterocyte damage (zonulin and intestinal fatty acid binding protein) in patients with both chronic inflammation and acute critical illness.[78] Patients with surgical and non-surgical sepsis, trauma, and cirrhosis, the extent of gut permeability on or within 7 days of admission has also been shown to correlate with clinical outcomes like end-organ dysfunction and mortality,[79–81] supporting the relationship between gut barrier hyper-permeability and sustained inflammation.

Compositional changes in the gut microbiota in the ICU may further modulate intestinal inflammatory responses and directly impact permeability, with recent data highlighting the complexity and nuances of microbial features in regulating these responses. For example, recent data suggests that inflammatory signals generated by LPS derived from gut microbes are not uniformly pro-inflammatory, but rather, are variable and dependent upon the LPS isoform.[82] Moreover, using computational and experimental approaches to characterize effects of gut microbiota LPS, investigators additionally found that the majority of LPS in human gut communities is derived from Bacteroidales spp. and, in fact, antagonizes the immunostimulatory effect of Proteobacteria-derived LPS TLR4-mediated signaling.[83] However, Proteobacteria and other pathobionts additionally employ other mechanisms beyond LPS to weaken barrier defenses. For example, preclinical models demonstrate that colonization by Enterobacteriaceae and Enterococcus can directly disrupt intestinal endothelial integrity, including commensal and pathogenic E. Coli (via upregulation of zonulin)[84]; K. Pneumoniae (via increasing pore formation)[85]; and, E. faecalis (via promoting secretion of matrix metalloproteinase).[86]

Though these studies underscore the potential negative consequences of pathobiont Enterobacteriaceae, it is important to note that the LPS isoform and designated genus are not always enough to inform the effect of a microbe. For example, despite the immunogenicity of its LPS, the probiotic Escherichia coli Nissle 1917, exerts protective effects on gut barrier defenses, down-regulating the expression of matrix metalloproteinase-2 and TNF, and promoting the expression of tight junction proteins in IECs.[87] It has been used as a probiotic for treatment of IBD and demonstrated success in a mouse model of sepsis,[88] further showing promise as a platform for engineered E. Coli with additional therapeutic capabilities.[89]

Translocation of Gut-derived Microbial Components

In the context of intestinal hyperpermeability, the composition of the ICU gut microbiota may additionally impact the translocation of microbial components and subsequent host responses. Importantly, the permeability that occurs from IEC death does not have a size or charge restriction,[69] and thus potentially allows larger DNA components, including live microorganisms or bacterial extracellular vesicles (BEVs), to enter systemic circulation. BEVs are nanometer-sized membrane particles secreted by gram-negative and gram-positive microbes, used to transport nucleic acids (including the 16s rRNA gene), as well as metabolites, proteins, and toxins (including LPS in the case of gram-negative EVs).[90] Although there are no current studies directly assessing BEVs in the context of critical illness, in patients with chronic inflammatory conditions associated with gut hyperpermeability, investigators reported that EV-associated LPS, rather than lower-density soluble LPS products, was the primary source of systemic TLR4 activation.[91]

Both live microorganisms and BEVs of gut-origin that enter the circulation have the potential to elicit a variety of immunologic and metabolic responses that may be crucial to acute host responses in critical illness, and have the potential to serve as therapeutic targets.[92] Thus, characterizing these microbial DNA components using culture-independent techniques is a growing area of interest with the potential for highly fruitful advances in understanding. Nonetheless, there are methodologic considerations to using 16S sequencing in blood and other low biomass samples, including a high potential for contamination, particularly in healthy patients (ie, with low suspicion for translocation).[93,94] Moreover, 16S sequencing cannot determine viability, and the source of blood microbial DNA identified may vary based on processing techniques. This microbial DNA may represent (1) live gut microbes (de-facto translocation); (2) DNA associated with BEVs; (3) free-floating DNA fragments (ie, from lysed bacteria); or (4) DNA fragments that were phagocytosed by leukocytes.[94] Given these complexities, we use the term "blood microbial DNA signatures" to describe these findings until definitive validation through culture is achieved.

Despite the limitations of sequencing techniques, there are growing direct and indirect evidences that the amount and composition of these microbial DNA signatures may contribute to shaping host responses in critical illness. For example, in a study using 16S rRNA sequencing to analyze blood collected from healthy volunteers (n = 23) and patients with sepsis (n = 62), the investigators found a significant difference in community composition between groups (beta-diversity), as well as relative increase of Proteobacteria-derived DNA in septic patients.[95] A separate investigation focusing on translocation in the setting of ST-segment elevation myocardial ischemia (MI) further the potential importance of microbial DNA signatures recovered from blood leukocytes. Specifically, investigators found that compared to healthy controls (n = 49) and those with stable coronary heart disease (n = 50), those with ST-elevation MI had a greater proportion of gut-derived microbial DNA components in blood (Lactobacillus, Bacteroides, and Streptococcus), and that markers indicative of gut bacterial translocation (LPS and D-lactate) correlated with systemic inflammation (CD14^{++} CD16^{+} monocytes, C-reactive protein).[96]

Moreover, microbial DNA signatures and live micro-organisms have also been recovered from distal tissues and implicated in local inflammation at these sites. For example, a study of post-mortem brain tissue samples from patients who died from sepsis or non-infectious causes found discrete gut-derived microbial signatures specific to the sepsis group. These findings were corroborated in a murine sepsis model, where cultivatable live gut bacteria were found in brain tissue.[97] In ICU patients with Acute Respiratory Distress Syndrome (ARDS), landmark studies profiling microbial communities in bronchoalveolar lavage samples demonstrated that gut-associated microbes, including Enterobacteriaceae and Lachnospiraceae, correlated with greater disease severity and mortality.[98,99] A comprehensive study by Montassier and colleagues further validated the role of gut microbial translocation in ARDS pathobiology. Using 16S rRNA sequencing data pooled from 17 studies involving 1029 critically-ill patients (21.7% with ARDS and 26.3% with hospital-acquired pneumonia [HAP]) and 327 healthy controls, the investigators found that endotracheal aspirates from ARDS patients were enriched with pathobionts (Staphylococcus, Ralstonia, and Enterococcus), whereas those from HAP patients had reduced lung commensals.[100] Together, these studies underscore the importance of understanding microbial DNA signatures and the species-specific responses they may trigger upon immune cell stimulation, highlighting a promising area for future research with significant therapeutic implications. Establishing consistent protocols and nomenclature will be crucial for accurately defining the impact of microbial DNA, and the actual biologic material they represent, from various sources.

Dysbiosis in the Intensive Care Unit and Secondary Infection

In addition to the potential modulation of acute processes by microbial components (of unclear source), an association between expansion of pathobionts and development of nosocomial infections has repeatedly been demonstrated in critically-ill and immunocompromised patients. Two potential mechanisms have been identified that may be responsible for these associations. The first is elucidated from countless studies demonstrating a direct association between pathobiont expansion and/or colonization by AROs and the subsequent development of infection by the same organism. Indeed, translocation of live pathobionts from the gut with seeding at distal sites has been implicated in the development of bacteremia, nosocomial pneumonia, and biofilm-related infections.[101–104] In some instances, rather than translocating as live microorganisms, these pathogens may be carried by neutrophils to distant sites, potentially facilitating secondary infections.[105] Although the processes determining which pathobionts cause disease are not fully understood, some data suggest that pathobionts may become virulent only in the context of a disrupted microbiota. For instance, a model of pathobiont-induced intestinal inflammation revealed that *Helicobacter bilis* only causes disease in the presence of a disturbed microbiota and that the disease was driven by the intestinal Th17 response against other gut microbes rather than the pathobiont itself.[106] Nonetheless, translocation alone cannot explain results from other groups showing an association between *Enterobacteriaceae* expansion and the subsequent development of nosocomial infection by any organism.[22,26] Insights into these mechanisms were provided by Schectle and colleagues, who investigated approximately 50 mixed ICU patients using longitudinal gut microbiota sampling (rectal swabs), extensive immunophenotyping, and single-cell sequencing. They found that patients with "progressive *Enterobacteriaceae* enrichment" (ie, doubling of Enterobacteriaceae on sequential samples) exhibited a unique immunosuppressed phenotype characterized by hypofunctional neutrophils. This study integrates systems biology approaches to explore microbiota-immune cross-talk, suggesting that alterations in the gut microbiota may impair the host's ability to defend against secondary infections, including those potentially translocating from the gut. Thus, derangements in gut microbiota may compromise the host's immune defenses against secondary infections by other microbes.[26]

SUMMARY

The data we have summarized all lead to the conclusion that disturbances in the gut microbiota sustained throughout critical illness—some of which are potentially modifiable—may contribute to injury that is independent of the primary cause of the patient's need for ICU care. However, clinical studies of microbiome-targeted interventions including the administration of prebiotic fiber and pro/synbiotics have failed to show consistent benefit in large RCTs or systematic meta-analyses, even despite strong signals indicating clinical benefit in individual studies. While these findings are at odds with numerous conditions faced in the outpatient setting where prebiotic/probiotic therapy have had readily demonstrable positive impacts (eg, autoimmune mediated diseases, cancer therapy, GI disorders, and COVID-19 pneumonia)[107,108] and it implies a knowledge gap that will require substantial future research both in the clinical and translational settings. We hypothesize that the absence of benefit observed in the current literature is due to a lack of specificity of treatment—all ICU patients at all times in their treatment course do not benefit from the currently available therapies, which may be poorly targeted to the type of dysbiosis seen in this setting. We propose that focus should be centered in several areas that are likely to be highly productive: 1. Understanding how to parse different types of ICU patients and different phases of their care as it relates to putatively harmful states of dysbiosis through both clinical and translational approaches; 2. Clarifying mechanisms under control of the HGM in the context of the ICU environment and identifying in which patients these mechanisms are clinically relevant; and 3. Designing therapies for the microbiome that are reflective of what is known about ICU-induced dysbiosis, taking into account the implications of disturbances in gut microbial ecological interactions, as well as gut barrier integrity. The types of microbiome-targeted interventions are rapidly increasing, and a better understanding of which therapies should be provided, and at what point in disease course, and to what population of patients has the potential for high impact in intensive care medicine.

CLINICS CARE POINTS

- Characteristic disturbances in the gut microbiota—including loss of beneficial microbes and increased abundance of potentially pathogenic bacterial and fungal species (pathobionts)—are present to varying degrees in nearly all ICU patients. Certain features, namely high intestinal burden of pathobionts *Enterococcus* and *Enterobacteriaceae*, have repeatedly been associated with increased in-hospital mortality and development of nosocomial infection.

- Inflammation and exposure to ICU care (ie, alterations in diet, antibiotics) alter the intestinal microenvironment and ecological interactions within the gut microbial community, thus impairing various mechanisms of colonization resistance and providing an environment that preferentially favors expansion of pathobionts like *Enterobacteriaceae* and *Enterococcus* and development of AROs.

- Inflammation in acute critical illness leads to gut barrier hyperpermeability, which further promotes innate immune cell activation. Disruptions in the gut microbiota and increased burden of *Enterobacteriaceae* and *Enterococcus* provoked in the ICU setting may potentially further impact these responses by 1) weakening physical barriers via effects on intestinal endothelial cells and 2) regulating systemic immune cell activation via signals from gut-derived microbial components, with variations in blood microbial composition potentially impacting clinical phenotypes.

- Development of nosocomial infections in ICU patients may be the result of translocation of live pathobionts. Disruptions in the gut microbiota in the ICU may further contribute to this risk by enhancing virulence and impairing innate immune defenses.

- Improved stratification of ICU patients and the development of tailored microbiome interventions could enhance treatment outcomes. Ongoing advancements in microbiome science offer potential for significant impact but therapies must be better matched to the unique disturbances in the gut microbiota and GI microenvironment encountered in the ICU.

ACKNOWLEDGMENTS

We extend our sincere gratitude to Dr Daniel McDonald and Dr Robert Knight for their collaboration and for graciously allowing us to incorporate their data for the presentation of **Fig. 1**.

DISCLOSURES

The authors have no disclosures to report.

FUNDING

This publication was made possible by the NIH-funded post-doctoral Integrated Training in Anesthesiology Research fellowship at Duke University School of Medicine

(5T32-GM008600-27) and the International Anesthesiology Mentored Research Award for M.S.

REFERENCES

1. Wang B, Yao M, Lv L, et al. The human microbiota in health and disease. Engineering 2017;3(1):71–82.
2. Johnstone J, Meade M, Lauzier F, et al. Effect of probiotics on incident ventilator-associated pneumonia in critically ill patients: a randomized clinical trial. JAMA 2021;326(11):1024.
3. Lee Z-Y, Lew CCH, Ortiz-Reyes A, et al. Benefits and harm of probiotics and synbiotics in adult critically ill patients. A systematic review and meta-analysis of randomized controlled trials with trial sequential analysis. Clin Nutr 2023; 42(4):519–31.
4. Yelin I, Flett KB, Merakou C, et al. Genomic and epidemiological evidence of bacterial transmission from probiotic capsule to blood in ICU patients. Nat Med 2019;25(11):1728–32.
5. Bellali S, Lagier JC, Raoult D, et al. Among live and dead bacteria, the optimization of sample collection and processing remains essential in recovering gut microbiota components. Front Microbiol 2019;10:1606.
6. Almeida A, Nayfach S, Boland M, et al. A unified catalog of 204,938 reference genomes from the human gut microbiome. Nat Biotechnol 2021;39(1):105–14.
7. Gao B, Chi L, Zhu Y, et al. An introduction to next generation sequencing bioinformatic analysis in gut microbiome studies. Biomolecules 2021;11(4):530.
8. Wang WL, Xu SY, Ren ZG, et al. Application of metagenomics in the human gut microbiome. World J Gastroenterol 2015;21(3):803–14.
9. Human Microbiome Project Consortium. Structure, function and diversity of the healthy human microbiome. Nature 2012;486(7402):207–14.
10. Vliex LMM, Penders J, Nauta A, et al. The individual response to antibiotics and diet — insights into gut microbial resilience and host metabolism. Nat Rev Endocrinol 2024;20(7):387–98.
11. Schlechte J, Skalosky I, Geuking MB, et al. Long-distance relationships - regulation of systemic host defense against infections by the gut microbiota. Mucosal Immunol 2022;15(5):809–18.
12. Horrocks V, King OG, Yip AYG, et al. Role of the gut microbiota in nutrient competition and protection against intestinal pathogen colonization. Microbiology (Reading) 2023;169(8). https://doi.org/10.1099/mic.0.001377.
13. Martin-Gallausiaux C, Marinelli L, Blottière HM, et al. SCFA: mechanisms and functional importance in the gut. Proc Nutr Soc 2021;80(1):37–49.
14. Liu W, Cheng M, Li J, et al. Classification of the gut microbiota of patients in intensive care units during development of sepsis and septic shock. Dev Reprod Biol 2020;18(6):696–707.
15. McDonald D, Ackermann G, Khailova L, et al. Extreme dysbiosis of the microbiome in critical illness. mSphere 2016;1(4). https://doi.org/10.1128/mSphere.00199-16.
16. Ojima M, Shimizu K, Motooka D, et al. Gut dysbiosis associated with antibiotics and disease severity and its relation to mortality in critically ill patients. Dig Dis Sci 2022;67(6):2420–32.
17. Salameh TJ, Roth K, Schultz L, et al. Gut microbiome dynamics and associations with mortality in critically ill patients. Gut Pathog 2023;15(1):66.

18. Wei R, Chen X, Hu L, et al. Dysbiosis of intestinal microbiota in critically ill patients and risk of in-hospital mortality. Am J Transl Res 2021;13(3):1548–57.
19. Evans T, Ali U, Anderton R, et al. Lower gut dysbiosis and mortality in acute critical illness: a systematic review and meta-analysis. Intensive Care Med Exp 2023;11(1):6.
20. Shimizu K, Ogura H, Goto M, et al. Altered gut flora and environment in patients with severe SIRS. J Trauma Inj Infect Crit Care 2006;60(1):126–33.
21. Shimizu K, Yamada T, Ogura H, et al. Synbiotics modulate gut microbiota and reduce enteritis and ventilator-associated pneumonia in patients with sepsis: a randomized controlled trial. Crit Care 2018;22(1):239.
22. Freedberg DE, Zhou MJ, Cohen ME, et al. Pathogen colonization of the gastrointestinal microbiome at intensive care unit admission and risk for subsequent death or infection. Intensive Care Med 2018;44(8):1203–11.
23. Ivanova V, Chernevskaya E, Vasiluev P, et al. Hi-C metagenomics in the ICU: exploring clinically relevant features of gut microbiome in chronically critically ill patients. Front Microbiol 2021;12:770323.
24. Shen Y, Qu W, Yu F, et al. Dynamic associations between the respiratory tract and gut antibiotic resistome of patients with COVID-19 and its prediction power for disease severity. Gut Microb 2023;15(1):2223340.
25. Ravi A, Halstead FD, Bamford A, et al. Loss of microbial diversity and pathogen domination of the gut microbiota in critically ill patients. Microb Genom 2019; 5(9). https://doi.org/10.1099/mgen.0.000293.
26. Schlechte J, Zucoloto AZ, Yu I-L, et al. Dysbiosis of a microbiota–immune metasystem in critical illness is associated with nosocomial infections. Nat Med 2023; 29(4):1017–27.
27. Martinson JNV, Pinkham NV, Peters GW, et al. Rethinking gut microbiome residency and the Enterobacteriaceae in healthy human adults. ISME J 2019; 13(9):2306–18.
28. Agudelo-Ochoa GM, Valdes-Duque BE, Giraldo-Giraldo NA, et al. Gut microbiota profiles in critically ill patients, potential biomarkers and risk variables for sepsis. Gut Microb 2020;12(1):1707610.
29. Chanderraj R, Baker JM, Kay SG, et al. In critically ill patients, anti-anaerobic antibiotics increase risk of adverse clinical outcomes. Eur Respir J 2023;61(2). https://doi.org/10.1183/13993003.00910-2022.
30. Prevel R, Enaud R, Orieux A, et al. Gut bacteriobiota and mycobiota are both associated with Day-28 mortality among critically ill patients. Crit Care 2022; 26(1):105.
31. Zhou P, Zou Z, Wu W, et al. The gut-lung axis in critical illness: microbiome composition as a predictor of mortality at day 28 in mechanically ventilated patients. BMC Microbiol 2023;23(1):399.
32. Adelman MW, Woodworth MH, Langelier C, et al. The gut microbiome's role in the development, maintenance, and outcomes of sepsis. Crit Care 2020; 24(1):278.
33. Serbanescu MA, Da Silva M, Zaky A. Impact of intensive care unit nutrition on the microbiome and patient outcomes. Anesthesiol Clin 2023;41(1):263–81.
34. Cho NA, Strayer K, Dobson B, et al. Pathogenesis and therapeutic opportunities of gut microbiome dysbiosis in critical illness. Gut Microb 2024;16(1):2351478.
35. Gamage H, Venturini C, Tetu SG, et al. Third generation cephalosporins and piperacillin/tazobactam have distinct impacts on the microbiota of critically ill patients. Sci Rep 2021;11(1):7252.

36. Stecher B. The roles of inflammation, nutrient availability and the commensal microbiota in enteric pathogen infection. Microbiol Spectr 2015;3(3). https://doi.org/10.1128/microbiolspec.MBP-0008-2014.
37. Zeng MY, Inohara N, Nunez G. Mechanisms of inflammation-driven bacterial dysbiosis in the gut. Mucosal Immunol 2017;10(1):18–26.
38. Winter SE, Thiennimitr P, Winter MG, et al. Gut inflammation provides a respiratory electron acceptor for Salmonella. Nature 2010;467(7314):426–9.
39. Winter SE, Winter MG, Xavier MN, et al. Host-derived nitrate boosts growth of E. coli in the inflamed gut. Science 2013;339(6120):708–11.
40. Garsin DA. Ethanolamine utilization in bacterial pathogens: roles and regulation. Nat Rev Microbiol 2010;8(4):290–5.
41. Litvak Y, Mon KKZ, Nguyen H, et al. Commensal Enterobacteriaceae protect against Salmonella colonization through oxygen competition. Cell Host Microbe 2019;25(1):128–139 e5.
42. Wallace N, Zani A, Abrams E, et al. The impact of oxygen on bacterial enteric pathogens. Adv Appl Microbiol 2016;95:179–204.
43. Eberl C, Weiss AS, Jochum LM, et al. E. coli enhance colonization resistance against Salmonella Typhimurium by competing for galactitol, a context-dependent limiting carbon source. Cell Host Microbe 2021;29(11):1680–1692 e7.
44. McClave SA, Taylor BE, Martindale RG, et al. Guidelines for the provision and assessment of nutrition support therapy in the adult critically ill patient: society of critical care medicine (SCCM) and American society for parenteral and enteral nutrition (A.S.P.E.N.). JPEN J Parenter Enteral Nutr 2016;40(2):159–211.
45. Moron R, Galvez J, Colmenero M, et al. The importance of the microbiome in critically ill patients: role of nutrition. Nutrients 2019;11(12). https://doi.org/10.3390/nu11123002.
46. Wischmeyer PE. Overcoming challenges to enteral nutrition delivery in critical care. Curr Opin Crit Care 2021;27(2):169–76.
47. Langlands SJ, Hopkins MJ, Coleman N, et al. Prebiotic carbohydrates modify the mucosa associated microflora of the human large bowel. Gut 2004;53(11):1610–6.
48. Tramontano M, Andrejev S, Pruteanu M, et al. Nutritional preferences of human gut bacteria reveal their metabolic idiosyncrasies. Nat Microbiol 2018;3(4):514–22.
49. Kircher B, Woltemate S, Gutzki F, et al. Predicting butyrate- and propionate-forming bacteria of gut microbiota from sequencing data. Gut Microb 2022;14(1):2149019.
50. Levy R, Borenstein E. Metagenomic systems biology and metabolic modeling of the human microbiome: from species composition to community assembly rules. Gut Microb 2014;5(2):265–70.
51. Aranda-Diaz A, Willis L, Nguyen TH, et al. Assembly of gut-derived bacterial communities follows "early-bird" resource utilization dynamics. bioRxiv 2023. https://doi.org/10.1101/2023.01.13.523996.
52. Huus KE, Hoang TT, Creus-Cuadros A, et al. Cross-feeding between intestinal pathobionts promotes their overgrowth during undernutrition. Nat Commun 2021;12(1):6860.
53. Majid HA, Cole J, Emery PW, et al. Additional oligofructose/inulin does not increase faecal bifidobacteria in critically ill patients receiving enteral nutrition: a randomised controlled trial. Clin Nutr 2014;33(6):966–72.

54. Tao C, Zeng W, Zhang Q, et al. Effects of the prebiotic inulin-type fructans on post-antibiotic reconstitution of the gut microbiome. J Appl Microbiol 2021; 130(3):634–49.

55. Serbanescu MA, Wright MC, Arnold J, et al. Impact of fiber-containing enteral nutrition on microbial community dynamics in critically ill trauma patients: a pilot-randomized trial. Preprint 2024. https://doi.org/10.21203/rs.3.rs-4583745/v1.

56. Lange K, Buerger M, Stallmach A, et al. Effects of antibiotics on gut microbiota. Dig Dis 2016;34(3):260–8.

57. Marfil-Sanchez A, Zhang L, Alonso-Pernas P, et al. An integrative understanding of the large metabolic shifts induced by antibiotics in critical illness. Gut Microb 2021;13(1):1993598.

58. Palleja A, Mikkelsen KH, Forslund SK, et al. Recovery of gut microbiota of healthy adults following antibiotic exposure. Nat Microbiol 2018;3(11):1255–65.

59. Reijnders D, Goossens GH, Hermes GD, et al. Effects of gut microbiota manipulation by antibiotics on host metabolism in obese humans: a randomized double-blind placebo-controlled trial. Cell Metabol 2016;24(2):341.

60. Rivera-Chavez F, Zhang LF, Faber F, et al. Depletion of butyrate-producing clostridia from the gut microbiota drives an aerobic luminal expansion of Salmonella. Cell Host Microbe 2016;19(4):443–54.

61. Bäumler AJ, Sperandio V. Interactions between the microbiota and pathogenic bacteria in the gut. Nature 2016;535(7610):85–93.

62. Yip AYG, King OG, Omelchenko O, et al. Antibiotics promote intestinal growth of carbapenem-resistant Enterobacteriaceae by enriching nutrients and depleting microbial metabolites. Nat Commun 2023;14(1):5094.

63. Djukovic A, Garzon MJ, Canlet C, et al. Lactobacillus supports Clostridiales to restrict gut colonization by multidrug-resistant Enterobacteriaceae. Nat Commun 2022;13(1):5617.

64. Serbanescu MA, Mathena RP, Xu J, et al. General anesthesia alters the diversity and composition of the intestinal microbiota in mice. Anesth Analg 2019;129(4): e126–9.

65. Lukovic E, Moitra VK, Freedberg DE. The microbiome: implications for perioperative and critical care. Curr Opin Anaesthesiol 2019;32(3):412–20.

66. Sukhum KV, Newcomer EP, Cass C, et al. Antibiotic-resistant organisms establish reservoirs in new hospital built environments and are related to patient blood infection isolates. Commun Med (Lond) 2022;2:62.

67. Ghosh S, Whitley CS, Haribabu B, et al. Regulation of intestinal barrier function by microbial metabolites. Cell Mol Gastroenterol Hepatol 2021;11(5):1463–82.

68. Klingensmith NJ, Coopersmith CM. The gut as the motor of multiple organ dysfunction in critical illness. Crit Care Clin 2016;32(2):203–12.

69. Ghosh SS, Wang J, Yannie PJ, et al. Intestinal barrier dysfunction, LPS translocation, and disease development. J Endocr Soc 2020;4(2):bvz039.

70. Yoseph BP, Klingensmith NJ, Liang Z, et al. Mechanisms of intestinal barrier dysfunction in sepsis. Shock 2016;46(1):52–9.

71. Zuo L, Kuo WT, Turner JR. Tight junctions as targets and effectors of mucosal immune homeostasis. Cell Mol Gastroenterol Hepatol 2020;10(2):327–40.

72. Gitter AH, Bendfeldt K, Schulzke JD, et al. Leaks in the epithelial barrier caused by spontaneous and TNF-alpha-induced single-cell apoptosis. Faseb J 2000; 14(12):1749–53.

73. Heller F, Fromm A, Gitter AH, et al. Epithelial apoptosis is a prominent feature of the epithelial barrier disturbance in intestinal inflammation: effect of pro-inflammatory

interleukin-13 on epithelial cell function. Mucosal Immunol 2008;1(Suppl 1): S58–61.

74. Yang CS, Coopersmith CM, Lyons JD. Cell death proteins in sepsis: key players and modern therapeutic approaches. Front Immunol 2023;14:1347401.

75. Raetz CR, Whitfield C. Lipopolysaccharide endotoxins. Annu Rev Biochem 2002;71:635–700.

76. Joffre J, Hellman J, Ince C, et al. Endothelial responses in sepsis. Am J Respir Crit Care Med 2020;202(3):361–70.

77. Hoshino K, Takeuchi O, Kawai T, et al. Cutting edge: toll-like receptor 4 (TLR4)-deficient mice are hyporesponsive to lipopolysaccharide: evidence for TLR4 as the Lps gene product. J Immunol 1999;162(7):3749–52.

78. Camilleri M, Vella A. What to do about the leaky gut. Gut 2022;71(2):424–35.

79. Ardehali SH, Eslamian G, Malek S. Associations between systemic inflammation and intestinal permeability with Onodera's prognostic nutritional index in critically ill patients. Acute Crit Care 2021;36(4):361–8.

80. Klaus DA, Motal MC, Burger-Klepp U, et al. Increased plasma zonulin in patients with sepsis. Biochem Med (Zagreb) 2013;23(1):107–11.

81. Vermette D, Hu P, Canarie MF, et al. Tight junction structure, function, and assessment in the critically ill: a systematic review. Intensive Care Med Exp 2018;6(1):37.

82. Stephens M, von der Weid PY. Lipopolysaccharides modulate intestinal epithelial permeability and inflammation in a species-specific manner. Gut Microb 2020;11(3):421–32.

83. d'Hennezel E, Abubucker S, Murphy LO, et al. Total lipopolysaccharide from the human gut microbiome silences toll-like receptor signaling. mSystems 2017; 2(6). https://doi.org/10.1128/mSystems.00046-17.

84. El Asmar R, Panigrahi P, Bamford P, et al. Host-dependent zonulin secretion causes the impairment of the small intestine barrier function after bacterial exposure. Gastroenterology 2002;123(5):1607–15.

85. Nakamoto N, Sasaki N, Aoki R, et al. Gut pathobionts underlie intestinal barrier dysfunction and liver T helper 17 cell immune response in primary sclerosing cholangitis. Nat Microbiol 2019;4(3):492–503.

86. Steck N, Hoffmann M, Sava IG, et al. Enterococcus faecalis metalloprotease compromises epithelial barrier and contributes to intestinal inflammation. Gastroenterology 2011;141(3):959–71.

87. Behrouzi A, Mazaheri H, Falsafi S, et al. Intestinal effect of the probiotic Escherichia coli strain Nissle 1917 and its OMV. J Diabetes Metab Disord 2020;19(1): 597–604.

88. Guo S, Chen S, Ma J, et al. Escherichia coli Nissle 1917 protects intestinal barrier function by inhibiting NF-κB-mediated activation of the MLCK-P-MLC signaling pathway. Mediat Inflamm 2019;2019:1–13.

89. Lynch JP, Gonzalez-Prieto C, Reeves AZ, et al. Engineered Escherichia coli for the in situ secretion of therapeutic nanobodies in the gut. Cell Host Microbe 2023;31(4):634–649 e8.

90. Ellis TN, Kuehn MJ. Virulence and immunomodulatory roles of bacterial outer membrane vesicles. Microbiol Mol Biol Rev 2010;74(1):81–94.

91. Tulkens J, Vergauwen G, Van Deun J, et al. Increased levels of systemic LPS-positive bacterial extracellular vesicles in patients with intestinal barrier dysfunction. Gut 2020;69(1):191–3.

92. Schorey JS, Harding CV. Extracellular vesicles and infectious diseases: new complexity to an old story. J Clin Invest 2016;126(4):1181–9.

93. Tan CCS, Ko KKK, Chen H, et al. No evidence for a common blood microbiome based on a population study of 9,770 healthy humans. Nat Microbiol 2023;8(5): 973–85.

94. Castillo DJ, Rifkin RF, Cowan DA, et al. The healthy human blood microbiome: fact or fiction? Front Cell Infect Microbiol 2019;9:148.

95. Gosiewski T, Ludwig-Galezowska AH, Huminska K, et al. Comprehensive detection and identification of bacterial DNA in the blood of patients with sepsis and healthy volunteers using next-generation sequencing method - the observation of DNAemia. Eur J Clin Microbiol Infect Dis 2017;36(2):329–36.

96. Zhou X, Li J, Guo J, et al. Gut-dependent microbial translocation induces inflammation and cardiovascular events after ST-elevation myocardial infarction. Microbiome 2018;6(1):66.

97. Singer BH, Dickson RP, Denstaedt SJ, et al. Bacterial dissemination to the brain in sepsis. Am J Respir Crit Care Med 2018;197(6):747–56.

98. Dickson RP, Schultz MJ, van der Poll T, et al. Lung microbiota predict clinical outcomes in critically ill patients. Am J Respir Crit Care Med 2020;201(5): 555–63.

99. Dickson RP, Singer BH, Newstead MW, et al. Enrichment of the lung microbiome with gut bacteria in sepsis and the acute respiratory distress syndrome. Nat Microbiol 2016;1(10):16113.

100. Montassier E, Kitsios GD, Radder JE, et al. Robust airway microbiome signatures in acute respiratory failure and hospital-acquired pneumonia. Nat Med 2023;29(11):2793–804.

101. Serbanescu MA, Apple CG, Fernandez-Moure JS. Role of resident microbial communities in biofilm-related implant infections: recent insights and implications. Surg Infect (Larchmt) 2023;24(3):258–64.

102. McMahon S, Sahasrabhojane P, Kim J, et al. Contribution of the oral and gastrointestinal microbiomes to bloodstream infections in leukemia patients. Microbiol Spectr 2023;11(3):e0041523.

103. Tamburini FB, Andermann TM, Tkachenko E, et al. Precision identification of diverse bloodstream pathogens in the gut microbiome. Nat Med 2018;24(12): 1809–14.

104. Taur Y, Xavier JB, Lipuma L, et al. Intestinal domination and the risk of bacteremia in patients undergoing allogeneic hematopoietic stem cell transplantation. Clin Infect Dis 2012;55(7):905–14.

105. Krezalek MA, Hyoju S, Zaborin A, et al. Can methicillin-resistant Staphylococcus aureus silently travel from the gut to the wound and cause postoperative infection? Modeling the "trojan horse hypothesis". Ann Surg 2018;267(4):749–58.

106. Gomes-Neto JC, Kittana H, Mantz S, et al. A gut pathobiont synergizes with the microbiota to instigate inflammatory disease marked by immunoreactivity against other symbionts but not itself. Sci Rep 2017;7(1):17707.

107. Gulliver EL, Young RB, Chonwerawong M, et al. Review article: the future of microbiome-based therapeutics. Aliment Pharmacol Ther 2022;56(2):192–208.

108. Wischmeyer PE, Tang H, Ren Y, et al. Efficacy of probiotic treatment as post-exposure prophylaxis for COVID-19: a double-blind, Placebo-Controlled Randomized trial. Clin Nutr 2024;43(1):259–67.

www.ingramcontent.com/pod-product-compliance
Lightning Source LLC
Chambersburg PA
CBHW050458190326
41458CB00005B/1334